Conduct Disorders
of
Childhood and Adolescence

A Social Learning Perspective

2nd Edition

Martin Herbert

University of Leicester

JOHN WILEY & SONS

Chichester . New York . Brisbane . Toronto . Singapore

Library of Congress Cataloging in Publication Data:

Herbert, Martin.
    Conduct disorders of childhood and adolescence.

    Bibliography: p.
    Includes index.
    1. Problem children. 2. Juvenile delinquency.
3. Behavior therapy for children 4. Behavioral
assessment of children. I. Title. [DNLM:1. Behavior
Therapy. 2. Child Behavior Disorders. 3. Juvenile
Delinquency. 4. Social Behavior Disorders—in infancy
& childhood. WS 350.2 H537c]
RJ506.P63H47 1987 618.92′858 86–18915

ISBN 0 471 91230 1
ISBN 0 471 91231 X (pbk.)

British Library Cataloguing in Publication Data:

Herbert, Martin
    Conduct disorders of childhood and
adolescence: a social learning perspective.
— 2nd ed.
1. Problem children
I. Title
618.9′289142   RJ506.P63

ISBN 0 471 91230 1
ISBN 0 471 91231 X Pbk

Printed and bound in Great Britain

For Gaynor

Acknowledgements

It is impossible to acknowledge by name all those to whom I am indebted for ideas and research findings which appear in this book. However, I would like to express my appreciation for the stimulating influence of my friends and colleagues at the Centre for Behavioural Work with Families (formerly the Child Treatment Research Unit).

Contents

PART I THE NATURE AND DEVELOPMENT OF THE CONDUCT DISORDERS

PART II THE ASSESSMENT AND TREATMENT OF CONDUCT DISORDERS

APPENDIXES

Preface

This revised and updated book is a theoretical and practical guide to the behavioural assessment and treatment of conduct and delinquent disorders of childhood and adolescence. It is therefore written with various professional groups in mind: psychologists, psychiatrists, probation officers, social workers, teachers, and school counsellors. The book is also intended for care and teaching staff in residential establishments such as community homes, assessment centres, and schools for the maladjusted. Given readers from such different professional and training backgrounds, I have attempted to provide a brief account of the basic theories and techniques that make up behaviour modification (and therapy). The emphasis is very much on the 'nuts and bolts' of designing and implementing treatment programmes, with illustrations of the practical difficulties that always arise when working with people. These are illustrated in detailed case analyses.

A view expressed in this book is that antisocial (abnormal) behaviour in children and adolescents is not very different from prosocial (normal) behaviour in its development, in its persistence, and in the ways in which it can be changed. Many problem behaviours can be viewed as a consequence of a failure to learn successful ways of dealing with the environment or as the result of acquiring inappropriate and deviant strategies for coping with life. The conduct and delinquent disorders — ranging from hyperactivity and violence to truancy and theft — are dealt with in a developmental framework, an approach which is thought to be crucial given the fraught task of assessing the complex and often obscure events of childhood.

Because many of the problems dealt with in the book tend to be less transitory and more intractable than the more common range of 'emotional' problems of childhood, I have included a chapter on parent training for this second edition. Parents and/or other caregivers are an important part of the therapeutic alliance which is essential if conduct and delinquent disorders are to be prevented, managed, or remedied successfully.

Martin Herbert
September, 1986.

Part I

The Nature and Development of the conduct Disorders

Two things fill the mind with ever-increasing wonder and awe, the more often and the more intensely the mind of thought is drawn to them: the starry heavens above me and the moral law within me.

IMMANUEL KANT
(Critique of Practical Reason)

Introduction

This book has a great deal to do with the 'moral law' within us and, thus, a complex and controversial area of human values. The reason is that 'conduct disorders' generally refer to a variety of disruptive behaviours of childhood and adolescence which give rise to social disapproval because of their antisocial qualities. They are antisocial in the sense that they are explicitly harmful or disturbing to others, or, in some other way, an adverse influence upon the environment. It is plain to see that there is a large element of subjective judgement in such criteria. The problems, after all, range from legally defined delinquent acts, such as violence, stealing, vandalism, truancy, and arson, to a variety of non-delinquent behaviours, such as fighting, bullying, lying, destructiveness, and defiance. The conduct problems also include the more or less troublesome and involuntary behaviours commonly associated with childhood: temper-tantrums, bouts of screaming and crying, surliness, and episodes of commanding or pestering behaviour.

The children manifesting these problems in severe form should be of serious concern to society; they cause themselves and those who are close to them the utmost misery. Antisocial activities tend to disrupt and hinder the acquisition of crucial adaptive skills. Their presence in childhood is predictive of problems of adjustment in later adolescence and adulthood. The empirical results of several investigations suggest that children with more extreme forms do not 'outgrow' their problem behaviours (Robins, 1966; West and Farrington, 1973). The case histories of delinquents repeatedly indicate the onset of serious antisocial behaviour when they were very young (Glueck and Glueck, 1960).

There is a pressing need, therefore, to identify, at an early age, those children who are at risk of developing conduct and delinquent problems, and to find and develop methods for their modification. Glueck (1966) believes that it

3

is not only possible to discriminate between potential delinquents and non-delinquents at the age of five or six, when they first enter school and have to fulfil behavioural standards set by adults (other than their parents) in authority over them, but that it might be possible to identify vulnerable children even earlier in life. We shall be looking at the issue in more detail in Chapter 2.

It needs to be emphasized that a child who has broken the law does not necessarily have a conduct disorder. As we shall see, many young people — most of them free of behavioural disorder — technically transgress the law. On the other hand, a child who *is* thought to have a conduct disorder may never have appeared in court nor committed a delinquent act. His activities may, or may not, be restricted to his home. The point is that his behaviours (be they aggression, dishonesty, disruptiveness, or non-compliance) have reached a level which is considered 'deviant' or 'abnormal' in his social and cultural setting. Essentially, a social (and therefore, non-objective) judgement is made that the child's conduct constitutes a 'social impairment'.

These behaviours are often referred to as subdelinquent or predelinquent because of the continuity (mentioned earlier) between many of the conduct disorders of childhood and the generally more serious delinquent acts which society proscribes by legal means.

Approximately one-third of the referrals for professional help made by parents and teachers involve conduct problems (Patterson, 1982). Reports by Robins (1966, 1972) and O'Neal and Robins (1958) on the follow-up of child guidance clinic attenders reveal the paradox that children with neurotic problems* who are more likely to reach adult life without psychiatric problems, whether or not they receive systematic psychotherapy (Levitt, 1971), are the ones who are most likely to receive psychological or psychiatric help as children. This situation is beginning to change as we become more knowledgeable about the conduct disorders.

Fortunately, most neurotic children become reasonably well-adjusted adults; they are almost as likely to grow up 'normal' as children drawn at random from the general population. By comparison, the outcome for seriously antisocial aggressive children is generally poor. The majority of children in the O'Neal and Robins sample who grew up to be psychopathic displayed clear antisocial behaviour between the ages of seven and ten. The most striking finding concerning the antisocial children is the very broad spectrum of disturbances they showed when grown up. This group was most likely to be dealt with by the courts rather than by the psychological professions.

Not only is the prognosis for the 'natural history' of the more severe conduct disorders a grave one (West and Farrington, 1973), but they tend to be resistant to traditional therapeutic interventions whether carried out in residential institutions (Clarke and Cornish, 1978) or in clinic settings (Wolff, 1977).

Among the more optimistic developments in recent years has been the application of behavioural treatments to conduct disorders, an application

* Also referred to as children with 'emotional' or 'personality' problems.

linked fruitfully — given the psychosocial definition and evolution of these problems — to social learning theory. Several authors (e.g. Herbert and Iwaniec, 1981; Jones and Kazdin, 1981; and Patterson, 1982) report the successful treatment of serious conduct disorders by means of behavioural methods mediated by parents and teachers who have been specially trained or guided in their use. We shall be reviewing the evidence for this approach (the so-called triadic model) in Chapter 6.

A consistent theoretical framework (see Figure 3, page 45) is necessary in order to make reasonable predictions concerning a child's future behaviour and to alter current maladaptive patterns of behaviour. Such consistency demands a clear conceptualization of what constitutes a psychological problem. This is no easy task. In this book, dealing with the treatment of conduct problems, we shall be concerned with the particular strategies developed by individual children to meet the specific needs and problems of *their* life situations. This means finding out what advantages there are to the child (seen from *his* perspective) in hitting, screaming, pestering, truanting, or stealing at particular times, or in particular situations.

A view put forward (Achenbach, 1982; Herbert, 1974) is that abnormal behaviour in children does not differ, by and large, from normal behaviour in its development, its persistence, and the way in which it can be modified. It is hypothesized that much of a child's behaviour is learned, maintained, and regulated by its effects upon the natural environment and the feedback it receives with regard to these consequences. Behaviour does not occur in a vacuum. It is a resultant of a complex transaction between the individual, with his inborn strengths and weaknesses, acting and reacting within an environment which sometimes encourages and sometimes discourages his behaviour. The theoretical position adopted in this book, while not underestimating the contribution of biological determining factors, is summarized in the proposition that many behaviour problems are the result of failures or distortions of learning. The laws of learning which apply to the acquisition and changing of normal socially approved behaviour are assumed to be relevant to the understanding and managing of socially disapproved (problem) behaviour.

Basically a *social learning* approach is adopted here (see Bandura, 1977). Learning occurs within a social nexus: rewards, punishments, and other events are mediated by human agents and within attachment systems, and are not simply the impersonal consequences of behaviour. Unfortunately — and it is the case with all forms of learning — the very processes which help the child adjust to life can, under certain circumstances, contribute to his maladjustment. An immature child who learns by imitating an adult is not necessarily to know when it is deviant behaviour that is being modelled. The young person who learns (adaptively) on the basis of classical and instrumental conditioning processes to avoid dangerous situations can also learn in the same way (maladaptively) to avoid school. Parents may reinforce overdependent behaviour by endlessly, and solicitously, responding to it.

If deviant behaviours of childhood are acquired as a function of faulty learning processes, then there is a case for arguing that problems can most effectively be modified where they occur, by changing the 'social lessons' the child receives and the reinforcing contingencies supplied by the social agents. This concept of problem behaviour as a learned response has led to the evolution of behavioural methods of treatment based on the assumption that behaviour that has been learned can be unlearned or modified directly and often in brief periods of treatment; the behavioural approach has crucial implications not only for the way in which therapists work but also where they work. It affects the manner in which they listen to the parent's complaints about their child's behaviour and the methods by which they later explore the specific details of the problem. Among the identifying features of the behavioural approach is a concern with present difficulties, a focus (whenever possible) on observable behaviour, and the specificity of the assessment process and intervention procedures which flow from it.

Behavioural work starts from a clear objective of producing change. The assessment (in which the client is closely involved) attempts to identify precisely what are the behaviours to be changed. What can be said about them is that they bring disadvantage and disablement to a multitude of troubled and troublesome children. Behaviour modification, however, is *not only* about changing the undesirable behaviour of 'problem children'. It is also about altering the behaviour of the persons — parents, teachers, and others — who form a significant part of the child's social world. The underlying assumptions about behaviour change lead inexorably to the proposition that maladaptive behaviour can most effectively be changed by the therapeutic application of principles of learning to the natural environment in which it has developed. There is, indeed, growing evidence — the subject of Chapter 6 — that effective assessment and treatment of certain childhood disorders requires observation and intervention in the young person's home or classroom.

This development has broadened the concept and scope of the therapeutic endeavour. It still requires rigorous training and safeguards, but it need not remain so elitist or esoteric in the sense of requiring an expensive training analysis on the part of a member of only one or two privileged professions. The practitioners of behaviour modification increasingly include members of professional groups other than psychologists and psychiatrists. Social workers, general medical practitioners, nurses, teachers, and residential child-care staff have been trained to carry out effective programmes. There is more flexibility in what is increasingly becoming a community-based therapeutic approach. Depending upon the requirements of the particular case, a behaviour modification programme may involve work in the consulting room, office, classroom or institution, the parental home, or even in the street, and the use of specific techniques by a professional, the parents, or the child himself.

To summarize the main premises of this book: the diagnostic task is to assess, within a developmental and learning framework, the implications and consequences of a child's general life-style and the stratagems he has adopted in order to cope with the demands of growing towards maturity. Our experience at the Centre for Behavioural Work with Families (formerly the Child Treatment Research Unit), based at the University of Leicester, in treating large numbers of conduct problems, has led us to adopt an approach to children's problems (Herbert, 1980a and b; Herbert and Iwaniec, 1981; Iwaniec, Herbert and McNeish, 1985; Iwaniec, 1983) which might more aptly be called behavioural psychotherapy or behavioural casework. This is an elaboration of the usual behavioural orientation insofar as the framework for therapeutic change is provided by the available literature on normal development and this, to a large extent, involves us in adolescent and parent 'counselling'.

This aspect of our approach is informative in the sense of disseminating the knowledge we have of child development (e.g. what is normal or appropriate to the child's age, sex, and level of ability) and of suggesting to parents what are reasonable expectations for their child. This transmission of information about normal child development is often as important as suggestions about ways of dealing with difficult behaviour. In the approach it is assumed that a primary aim of our work is essentially educative for parents, and it is hypothesized that the upbringing of children is itself a skill. Another aim is less didactic and involves exploring ideas, attributions, notions about self-efficacy and attitudes which undermine treatment. Not infrequently, those difficulties between parent and child (relationships and interactions) which have contributed to the child's behaviour problems get in the way of the parents' practical efforts to implement a programme. They may have special sensitivities or anxieties with regard to *this* child which make it impossible for them to be firm or consistent when he behaves in a certain manner. Or they may have fixed ideas about rearing children which represent the standard of *their* parents or reactions against them. These matters may require discussion and a sympathetic hearing before the parents can sustain the modification of their own behaviour that is being required of them.

This is only to put the negative or preventive side of the approach. There is also the aspect which facilitates a shared therapeutic endeavour. The behavioural approach is only too susceptible to the accusation of being impersonal, unfeeling, or mechanistic. The philosophy of home-based therapy and counselling as practised at the Centre is to present a form of behaviourism which has a human face. Parents (and children) are asked to share in the decisions (e.g., negotiating treatment goals with the therapist) and to participate in the treatment process. This gives back to parents who often feel demoralized, the dignity of caring for their own child. Such a philosophy requires personal contact in the home, detailed discussion and debate with clients, as the therapy is explained as fully as possible at all times. This is an exacting requirement for all concerned, but one (and it is the purpose of this book to argue the case) which has great advantages.

1

The Conduct Disorders

The concept of a conduct disorder is imprecise, but then the taxonomies applied to childhood behaviour are imprecise. There have been many classificatory systems in the field of childhood psychopathology — none of which are fully satisfactory (see Achenbach, 1982). The phrase 'conduct disorders', in particular, has an archaic ring to it, redolent of the comments about 'good' or 'bad' conduct which children used to get (perhaps still get) in their school reports. And, sadly, the technical term is not too far removed from the value judgements which informed those schoolmasterly remarks. It has moralistic overtones. But then we are dealing, *inter alia*, with moral problems. Not surprisingly, therefore, the category is overinclusive and untidy, but hopefully it *is* meaningful enough to justify its use as a shorthand term for the problems which are the concern of this book. To answer this we need to know how the problems listed earlier come together under the rubric 'conduct disorders'.

A TAXONOMY OF CHILDHOOD BEHAVIOUR PROBLEMS

The traditional approach to the classification of childhood psychopathology was that of providing a conceptual framework built upon a multitude of assumptions and constructs regarding the nature and development of personality and behaviour problems (see Anthony, 1970). More recently, attempts have been made to arrive at meaningful and uniform dimensions of behaviour disorder (as opposed to types or disease entities) along which all children range. What is advocated is an empirical approach which involves a minimum of assumptions and constructs regarding the causation of behavioural disorders. It endeavours to tease out, from masses of data culled from clinic records and epidemiological surveys, dimensions of disturbed behaviour which are explicit and operational.

Many instruments have been constructed to describe and classify the behaviour of children. More than 50 measures have appeared since the nineteen seventies. Alongside this development of methods for measuring behaviour as many as 30 dimensions of child behaviour have been identified. Despite the range of instruments that are available and the number of dimensions measured by these instruments, two dimensions emerge from most analyses: those of emotional and conduct disorders (Achenbach and Edelbrock, 1978).

The various researchers find, despite further diversity in subjects, settings, nationalities, raters, and statistical analyses, that empirical investigations consistently elicit problems of the undercontrolled type (conduct disorder, aggressive, externalizing, acting out) and the overcontrolled type (emotional disturbance, personality disorder, inhibited, internalizing, anxious). There is a convergence between clinical and factor analytic studies with regard to these dimensions, and they tend to uphold the early work of researchers like Peterson (1961) who demonstrated that conduct disorder was a cluster (or constellation) of problems characterized by non-compliance, restlessness, irresponsibility, boisterousness, and aggression. It was often associated with hyperactivity and might include, especially in older children, delinquent activities (see Table 1).

The common theme running through this rather heterogeneous collection of problems is antisocial disruptiveness, and the social disapproval they earn because they flout society's sensibilities and rules and because their consequences are so disturbing or explicitly harmful to others. This represents one extreme of what is essentially a directional and dichotomous concept of maladaptive responses — those directed towards the child's environment ('externalizers') or, in the case of emotional problems away from the environment towards oneself ('internalizers'). In practice, a sizeable proportion of children have behaviour problems which, to an important extent, share characteristics of both *emotional* and *conduct* disorders.

In other words, there is a category of 'mixed disorders' which, in many respects, have most in common with the conduct disorders, but in other respects occupy an intermediate position.

Wolff's (1971) study of the behaviour of 100 problematic English primary school children produced four dimensions of behaviour on the basis of a principal component analysis of the intercorrelations. The first of these had high loadings on non-delinquent conduct problems, namely, tantrums, fighting, quarrelling, disobedience, overactivity, poor concentration and attention, overdominating, overtalkative, high-strung, and discontented. This factor accounted for 14.8 per cent. of the variance and describes an aggressive, acting out, but non-delinquent pattern of behaviour. Clearly, a social criterion is being applied here to certain categories of behaviour; any definition of conduct problems must involve a consideration of the social judgements that lead to their being labelled as such.

Table 1 Factor loadings on conduct disorder variables in kindergarten children (Peterson, 1961, p.207)

Factor Conduct problem	Rotated factor loadings Conduct Disorder	Personality disorder
Disobedience	74	03
Disruptiveness	73	−04
Boisterousness	68	−16
Fighting	54	−09
Attention-seeking	54	−12
Restlesness	64	04
Negativism	56	12
Impertinence	57	02
Destructiveness	59	−05
Irritability	53	01
Temper-tantrums	54	08
Hyperactivity	51	−06
Profanity	30	−07
Jealousy	23	06
Uncooperativeness	67	09
Distractibility	56	29
Irresponsibility	60	22
Inattentiveness	54	39
Laziness in school	44	29
Shortness of attention span	48	37
Dislike of school	38	06
Nervousness	22	40
Thumb sucking	29	09
Skin allergy	−16	01

ANTISOCIAL BEHAVIOUR

To summarize the evidence: it would appear that there are important links between the various specific conduct problems, particularly the disregard of society's rules. However, children with conduct disorders are far from constituting a homogeneous group. This is scarcely surprising given the many points in the socialization of the child at which distortions or failures may occur. This chapter can touch upon only a few of the complex issues involved, the subject being large enough for several monographs.

The distribution by sex of the behaviour problems is one such issue. Whereas the emotional problems are displayed marginally more often by girls than boys, the conduct disorders are three times more common in boys than in girls (Rutter, Tizard, and Whitmore, 1970). Such a male predominance is further underlined in the case of delinquency (West, 1967), where male delinquents outnumber female delinquents in a ratio of up to ten to one. In the United States the ratio is smaller with a higher increase, of late, in female as compared with male cases.

Three main conduct problem areas can be isolated: serious antisocial behaviour, overactivity, and aggression. We analyse the first of these in this chapter, as childhood and adolescent antisocial problems constitute such a central and broadly coherent developmental and clinical theme. Young people with conduct and delinquent disorders demonstrate a fundamental inability or unwillingness to adhere to the rules and codes of conduct prescribed by society at its various levels. Such failures may be related to the temporary lapse of poorly established learned controls, to the failure to learn these controls in the first place, or to the fact that the behavioural standards a child has absorbed do not coincide with the norms of that section of society which enacts and enforces the rules. For whatever reason this failure has occurred, the serious implications of persistent and intense non-compliant, and therefore antisocial, behaviour in children are not in doubt.

Several retrospective and longitudinal studies have investigated the intercorrelations among behavioural and personality ratings over the years — an exercise fraught with methodological and interpretive problems. However, it is evident that despite variation in the patterns and strength of the continuities according to the type of behaviour or disorder under consideration, there are significant links between childhood and adolescence and between adolescence and adulthood. For example, there is general agreement — in the area of psychopathology — that it is those disorders involving disruptive, aggressive, or antisocial behaviour that are most likely to persist into adolescence (Robins, 1966; Rutter, 1977a). There are also links between childhood and adult life in the area of antisocial personality (Farrington, 1978; Wadsworth, 1979).

In the Rutter studies (e.g., Rutter, Tizard, and Whitmore, 1970), Isle of Wight children who were diagnosed initially at 10 years were followed up at 14 or 15. Three-fourths of those diagnosed earlier as having a conduct disorder still manifested a handicapping disorder at adolescence. More specifically, aggression — of problematic proportions — has been shown to persist (from as early as 8 years to the middle and late teens) in British and American studies (Farrington, 1978; Leftkowitz et al., 1977). Overactivity is another specific behaviour with grave prognostic implications, especially when it shows the sort of generality that is rated high by both parents and teachers.

General population surveys show that just under half of adolescent disorders have an onset before adolescence, whereas clinic-based studies suggest that the majority of adolescent psychiatric disorders have been manifesting themselves from early or middle childhood (Rutter, 1977a). There is a degree of continuity between early conduct disorder and juvenile delinquency. West and Farrington's (1973) study of London boys indicates the marked relationship between troublesome, difficult, and aggressive behaviour in boys ages 8 to 10 (combined ratings by teachers and social workers on a measure of 'combined conduct disorder', also combined ratings by peers and teachers on a measure of 'troublesomeness') and later juvenile delinquency. These measures powerfully predicted severe and persistent delinquency continuing into adult life.

Robins (1966), in her longitudinal studies of American males, demonstrates that most adult antisocial behaviour is antedated by similar behaviour in childhood. The behaviour of childhood, and in particular the *extremeness* and *variety* of antisocial actions, provided better predictors of adult functioning — and, in particular, antisocial adult life style — than the family background, social class of rearing, or particular type of childhood behaviour.

Of interest is the finding, with regard to the former, that many of these antisocial children in the Robins (1966) study had parents who were lax in providing discipline and supervision. Many of these children opposed requirements set by their parents, their schools, and their communities in general. Their parents were unable or unwilling to cope with the problem. Robins attests to the importance of such disciplinary problems by describing instances in which strict or adequate discipline decreased the probability for some of the children of developing adult sociopathic disorders. Similar findings are reported by Kallarackal and Herbert (1976), although not with regard to a long-term follow-up. Indian children, carefully supervised and strictly disciplined in loving homes, showed remarkably low rates of maladjustment compared with an English contrast group, despite the cultural and educational difficulties of being immigrants to Britain and the stresses of living in the twilight areas of an industrial city.

The evidence suggests that the earlier children started to commit offences, the graver is the outlook. Gibbens (1963) demonstrated that Borstal boys in the United Kingdom who were convicted before the age of 11 had a 65 per cent. relapse rate while the figure was 46 per cent. for those who had their first conviction between the ages of 16 and 21. Glueck and Glueck (1960) concluded, from their American findings, that those who offend at a young age are likely to continue in this way and go on to commit the more serious crimes.

The difficulties of treating antisocial adolescents are legendary and yet it is usually at the stage at which a conduct disorder has been labelled as delinquency that a probation officer, social worker, psychologist or psychiatrist is most likely to be asked to provide a therapeutic solution to an intractible personal and social problem. The importance of discovering the effective treatment (or, better still, preventive) techniques for antisocial children is certainly illustrated by all these studies. Let us examine some of these problems as they present themselves at an early stage of life.

The most common complaints from parents and teachers about the children who present as conduct problems tend to be as follows: 'He acts first and thinks (if he ever thinks) afterwards', 'He doesn't seem to know right from wrong', 'He never listens', 'He is *so* selfish; he never thinks of anyone but himself'. The theme that underlies these complaints about lack of self-control, dishonesty, disobedience, and self-centredness is, first of all, uncompromisingly non-compliant behaviour, and beyond that a defiance (or lack of appreciation) of rules. These children, in the short and/or long term do not obey adult requests, commands, and prohibitions. This is what makes conduct-disordered children so disturbing to parents and teachers and others who have to care for them. Obedience of rules — whether they are prescribed by convention, codified in laws, or internalized in what we call our consciences — is a prerequisite for

Factor Analysis
— non compliant ken
extreme disobedience in
conduct disorders.

social living. Non-compliant behaviour has consistently been identified by factor analytic studies as a significant factor in several forms of child psychopathology, but notably it is in the conduct disorders that extreme disobedience has been of prime importance (Jenkins, 1966; Lapouse and Monk, 1958; Quay, Morse, and Cutler, 1966; Rutter, 1965).

The problem for the therapist carrying out an assessment is that all children are disobedient some of the time — a fact of life all parents have to contend with. At what point is non-compliance maladaptive? This is a sensitive issue given the lip service paid by society to individualism; a precarious balance is required by society between 'reasonable' conformity and 'unreasonable' or slavish conformity. There are also other types of behaviour which come under the heading of the conduct disorders. They include, as we saw, disruptiveness, boisterousness, fighting, attention seeking, restlessness, negativism, impertinence, destructiveness, irritability, temper-tantrums, hyperactivity, profanity, jealousy, and uncooperativeness. Again, most children manifest these 'problems' to some extent. The diagnostic problem lies in the fact that there is no clear-cut distinction between the characteristics of 'abnormal' children and other children; the differences are relative — a matter of degree. Like it or not, we are in an area of social value judgements rather than objective scientific criteria. Behaviour problems, signs of psychological abnormality, are, by and large, exaggerations, deficits, or handicapping combinations of behaviour patterns common to all children.

Take 'delinquent acts' as an example. A 6-year study was conducted by the Survey Research Centre of the London School of Economics (Belson, 1975) on a random sample of 1,425 London youths between the ages of 13 and 16 from all social levels. They were encouraged to reveal their antisocial secrets during the intensive interviewing. Belson wished to find out whether they had ever been guilty of any of 44 different types of theft, ranging from keeping something found to stealing a car or lorry. Belson's study is unusual because it used a population which included non-delinquents and undetected delinquents, as well as boys already known to police and courts. So much research in the delinquency area is rendered useless because it is based on young people who have come before the courts or are inmates of penal institutions. The detected offender is almost certainly a biased sample of the delinquent population in general. And such bias makes it impossible to draw valid inferences about the characteristics of offenders in general or about the motives for their offences. Nearly all the London boys of all backgrounds and classes admitted to some stealing — mainly petty — at some time or other. Ninety-eight per cent. admitted having kept something that they had found (but in only 40 per cent. of these cases was the article in question worth more than £1.00). 70 per cent. had stolen from a shop, 35 per cent. from family or friends; 25 per cent. from work, and from a car, lorry or van; 18 per cent. from a telephone box, while 5 per cent. admitted having stolen a car or lorry. Seventeen per cent. had 'got in a place and stolen'. Apparently boys from all classes are given to thieving but *what* they steal differs somewhat. Public school boys specialize in travelling without paying their fare and in thefts from their relatives or from changing rooms, while their state school contemporaries are more disposed to stealing cigarettes or sweets from shops and also find great temptation in motor vehicles. Clearly, a majority of the boys in this study had indulged in at least one offence which, if detected and prosecuted, would have swollen the official statistics bearing on 'delinquency' rates.

DIAGNOSTIC DECISION-MAKING

This finding highlights the difficulty of deciding when problem behaviour is sufficiently serious to merit further investigation and therapeutic intervention. The remarkable thing about this by no means untypical survey (see Elmhorn, 1965; Malewska and Muszynski, 1970) is that these were ordinary boys of school age, most of whom had never been suspected of being juvenile delinquents. It cannot be assumed that youths who have been found guilty of an offence are the only ones committing antisocial or delinquent acts.

This begs the question: what is antisocial? In a sense young children are all antisocial and, judged by adult criteria, 'delinquent'. Even 'innocent' toddlers lash out at each other, inflicting pain; they 'steal' each other's possessions and appear to show no remorse after transgressing the rules. In a sense they do not need to learn 'delinquent' behaviours or attitudes. These tendencies occur quite spontaneously and to the child they have an internal logic which is dazzling in its simplicity (see page 23). What happens, as the child matures, is that he has to learn to avoid certain behaviours; that is to say, he must be trained to check certain impulses and to regulate his behaviour in terms of certain informal and formal rules of conduct (including the law). This socialization process is a slow continuing process, involving countless 'lessons' from parents, siblings, peers, and adults in authority over the child. To a significant degree the rules continue to be flouted by a wide range of young people, some in a minor and relatively painless manner. Others give vent to their impulses in a blatant and highly aversive fashion. As this kind of child gets older and ranges more widely outside the confines of his home, the implications of his conduct become more serious. His misdemeanours are quite likely to take him and his parents into the juvenile courts. In other words, his acts are legally defined as delinquent and, in the manner society has of categorizing and labelling people, he becomes a juvenile delinquent.

This process of labelling is highly selective. Certain children are more likely than others to avoid detection. Children who attend a school which is conscious of its good name are, if caught stealing, likely to have the incident dealt with privately between headmaster and parents. A boy who is caught shoplifting is more likely to be dealt with leniently if he is known to come from a 'respectable' middle-class home. Issues like these make it impossible to draw the unambiguous line of demarcation between delinquents and non-delinquents.

Delinquent behaviour is often no more than an transitory incident in the pattern of a youth's normal development. We know that although a large number of young people commit isolated crimes, few develop into offenders. Among delinquent youths brought to court, half are never reconvicted. Many of these youngsters are essentially normal and do not have a conduct disorder in the sense used in this book. Given the poor prognosis for an early established conduct disorder, there is an onus on the clinician to know the developmental evidence (and particularly data from longitudinal studies) before making a diagnosis. We know that *isolated* antisocial or delinquent acts are common and therefore of relatively little diagnostic significance.

What is apparent from facts like these is that early identification of conduct disorders may be a crucial matter, but that diagnostic decisions rest on somewhat vague criteria and conflicting reports. For example, the findings of several studies (e.g., Rutter, Tizard, and Whitmore, 1970) suggest that maternal and teacher accounts of child behaviour are only modestly correlated. This is possibly due to the effects of situational factors; it has been suggested that since mothers and teachers see children in different contexts governed by different rules, there is no strong reason to expect that their ratings of behaviour will be similar.

While maternal and teacher ratings of particular children are only modestly correlated, there is quite marked stability in their ratings over time; in other words their individual judgements tend to be consistent, even if they do differ somewhat. Rater-specific factors (e.g. maternal depression) as well as situation-specific factors may influence behaviour ratings (Iwaniec, 1983).

At the same time, it seems possible that there may be a minority of children whose behavioural characteristics persist over both time and situation and these are the children who turn out to be those with persistent and marked conduct disorder (or those with a complete absence of such tendencies). The presence of such children would account for the fact that parent and teacher ratings do show some modest positive correlation.

In any event, these considerations suggest that the interpretation of parent and teacher reports of child behaviour is a complex matter and that probably relatively little information can be gained about a child's behavioural tendencies from a *single* measure taken at one particular time using a solitary source of information. Clearly a crucial (if inconvenient) clinical implication of these findings is that the evaluation of children referred for an alleged conduct disorder should include consideration not only of the child's behaviour but of the situation in which this behaviour occurs and the characteristics of the individual describing the conduct disorder.

There is an intensity/frequency dimension which can be taken into account in assessment. Ryall (1974) examined in depth the characteristics of some 150 consecutive entrants to a fairly typical Approved School which admitted boys aged 13 and 14 years, mainly from small- to medium-sized connurbations. These boys admitted committing offences over a period of at least 4 years (on average) prior to their committal. At the time of commital they were routinely offending at least once a fortnight. The level of delinquent activity was so high that it was impossible to determine accurately the average total number of offences which had been committed by the boys; a minimum estimate would be about 100 for each boy, but the true figure was probably several times higher. The great majority of the offences were acts of theft and many were relatively minor offences of shoplifting. However, it was easier to estimate more accurately the quantity of breaking and entering offences which had been committed and the average number of these far more serious offences was well over 20 per boy. The population also contained a minority of boys whose offending was of a rather different nature (e.g., taking and driving specialists), but for these boys the frequency and intensity of offending was just as great as for the majority who indulged in more generalized forms of antisocial behaviour.

Ryall notes that the peculiar feature of approved school children was the *quantity* of their law breaking. He emphasizes that the *intensity* of the offending of the persistent delinquent is at the centre of the treatment problem. For these boys delinquent behaviour had become a habit or, more precisely, a self-reinforcing learned behaviour pattern. Each delinquent act was producing excitement, peer-group status, and possible material rewards, thus generating the motivation for further offences.

CRITERIA FOR DEFINING PROBLEMS

The point of this discussion is that there *are* criteria for making diagnostic judgements, albeit less precise ones than we might choose in an ideal world. Diagnostic decisions about treatment are too important to shirk simply because there is a dangerous element of subjectivity involved. Granted, we are not carrying out a diagnosis in the medical sense. Delinquency, after all, is an administrative term and subject to all the foibles of bureaucratic processes. The range of delinquent acts is enormous. Even with the more 'psychological' term 'conduct disorder' there are *no* absolute signs or symptoms of psychological abnormality. We are not in fact dealing with disease equivalents, but with social and psychological phenomena. This is not to deny the contribution of biological influences (e.g., genetics, brain damage, etc.) to the evolution of some conduct or delinquent disorders. What is rejected is the claim that the medical model provides a satisfactory framework for describing, explaining, or changing such problems (see Bandura, 1969).

The term 'problem' as used in this context is closely bound up with the concept of a deviation from some *social* norm. Terms like normal and abnormal, delinquent and non-delinquent, are commonly applied in a global manner to characterize certain children and adolescents. They are used as if they are mutually exclusive concepts like good and bad. Thus the label 'conduct disorder' attached to a particular youth seems to suggest that he is deviant in some generalized and absolute sense. This is misleading; the most that can be said of any child is that certain of his actions or attributes are more or less abnormal (in the sense of deviating from a social standard) and maladaptive (in the developmental sense of hindering the child's adaptation to the demands of growing up to live in society).

In the pages that follow, conduct is called disordered or problematic if it has unfavourable consequences, particularly in terms of its frequency, intensity, duration, and developmental appropriateness. The unfavourable consequences may be for the child himself — his behaviour affecting his ability to learn, to enjoy life in general, or, indeed, to remain at liberty. The consequences may be painful to others in the sense of, say, bullying affecting the victim or persistent screaming forcing the parent 'to give in' on important child-rearing issues, and so on. The problem behaviours also tend (although not in every case) to deviate widely from accepted social standards. It is tempting to add 'reasonable' standards. Of course, the problem behaviours may represent appropriate reactions to highly pathological home influences. It is at this point that ethical and political issues become particularly poignant (see page 291). They are still viewed as problematic because, although wholly understandable and proportionate to their cause (in other words, normal reactions to abnormal conditions), they have disabling consequences for the child in the broader context of life and society (e.g., school and work).*

This statement begs several questions. Johnson et al. (1973) point to the example of 'attention-to-task' behaviour in the classroom. Obviously poor attention of a gross kind in a classroom in handicapping to a child, and it is laudable when the therapists (e.g., Walker, Mattson, and Buckley, 1971) can report an increase of concentration following a behavioural programme. But what is the norm? Does a rise from a pre-intervention average of 39 per cent. to a follow-up average of 66 per cent. represent not only an 'improvement' relative to a problem group's baseline but, indeed, the attainment of a performance level which is needed, as Johnson and his colleagues (1973) put it, 'to survive in this environment'? The provision by Walker, Mattson, and Buckley (1971) of normative data for the peers of the problem group is a happy but rare event in the behaviour modification literature. The clinician has to hope for guidance from the developmental literature and the data he wants may often not be found there either.

Behaviour problems in general, and conduct disorders in particular, when they do not represent deficit problems (a failure to learn adaptive responses), are conceptualized in this book as strategies of adjustment which the child has learned to his own disadvantage (*and* to the disadvantage of others) in the attempt to cope with the demands of life. These maladaptive strategies are by-products of the stresses and strains of growth and development for an imperfect organism functioning in an imperfect world. The development of inappropriate strategies (or the failure to acquire appropriate strategies) for coping with life-tasks may be due to faulty training and example or other environmental deficiencies. They may be a result of neurological defects or other inherited or acquired impairments. Senn (1959) makes the perceptive comment that the problem child is invariably trying to solve a problem rather than be one; sadly his methods are often crude and his conception of his problem faulty. Until the therapist has patiently sought, and in a sympathetic

---

* See the case of Freddie, page 216.

fashion found, what the child is trying to achieve he is in no position to offer advice.

It is not only a matter of trying to see things from the child's point of view; it is also essential to look at his behavioural strategies in terms of their consequences, in the short and long term. In the short term they may bring rewards which are reinforcing; in the long term they may be self-defeating and destructive.

2

The Development of Social and Moral Behaviour

PSYCHOLOGICAL FACTORS: RULES OF CONDUCT

A major component of the conduct disorder 'syndrome' is serious non-compliance which is also referred to as 'negativism' or 'oppositional' behaviour. It takes many forms. In the classroom, the child may defy the teacher, may refuse to work, getting out of his seat at will, leaving the classroom, talking loudly to his neighbour, or molesting him. The net effect is the disruption of all order and concentration. In the home, the mother may be driven to distraction because she is unable to cope with her child. He refuses to obey her slightest command, or prevaricates, or, indeed, does the opposite of what she asks (negativism). In several studies, such negativism has been isolated as an important class of behaviour pathology in early childhood (Ausubel, 1950).

The development of compliance in young children is an important aspect of socialization. Piaget (1932) defines the essential core of morality as the tendency to accept and follow a system of rules which regulate interpersonal behaviour. The human species is unique in having as its main mechanism of social regulation a system of conceptually formulated rules, values, and conventions. These norms of conduct, of course, vary widely from culture to culture.

INFANCY

The earliest signs of obedience begin to appear in the last quarter of the baby's first year of life. They consist in complying with the mother's simple commands and prohibitions, such as 'Come here!' and 'No, don't do that!' With this achievement, the child has embarked on a long journey of rule learning. On the

19

one hand, there are the conventional rules of good manners and of correct behaviour with regard to particular persons or situations. On the other, there exist rules concerning sympathy and respect for others, keeping faith, honesty, and so on. These are moral issues. A willingness (in broad terms) not only to heed but to see the necessity for moral rules is essential to the maintenance of social life. The induction of the child into the social system (socialization) involves the transmission to him of social and moral codes by the family and other agents of society. For the child it involves incredibly subtle and complex processes of learning. The hoped-for end-result of socialization is the transformation of an apparently asocial, amoral infant into a mature adult, who accepts the norms of his society and who will act upon them without continual supervision. He, in turn, will transmit these norms to his own children. We have seen that many of the conduct problems involve the flouting of moral rules, and it is when children break these rules that parents get most perturbed. Youngsters are forbidden to lie, steal, cheat, and hurt others; parents strive to make their offspring check their impulses — irrational, sexual, aggressive, and acquisitive.

THE TODDLER AND PRE-SCHOOL CHILD

It does not take long for problems of disobedience to appear as the child grows up.* These are quite likely to be wilful acts of rebellion — a deliberate countering of the mother's will. Negativism is an exaggerated form of resistance, occurring when a child becomes stubborn and 'contrary', often doing quite the opposite of what the parents wish. Levy (1955) points out that in the course of normal development there is a period, usually during the second year, when the child refuses to do what he is told; he wants to do things for himself, and his most frequent word is 'No'. In the younger child, extreme negativism takes the form of refusal to take food, to move his bowels, to go to the toilet, and refusal to talk. Levy considers that it represents the child's initial efforts to establish himself as an independently functioning organism. He notes that the stage at which it usually occurs coincides approximately with the time when the mother would ordinarily be having her next child. It may represent, in his view, a built-in behaviour pattern which has had selective value in man's evolutionary history in the sense of enabling the child to achieve some independence at about the time that he will be supplanted by a newborn sibling.

Loevinger (1966), too, believes that the child is confirming his separate existence from parents by the exercise of his own will. She refers to this period as the 'impulsive' stage of ego-development. The child's interpersonal rela-

* Many factors (including early individual differences) are known to be of importance in the development of the conduct disorders. What we do know is that temperamentally many of the children are unusual from the outset in being impulsive, unpredictable, and unmalleable.

tionships are interpreted as being predominantly exploitive and dependent. People are seen as sources of supply.

Parents, however, are prepared to nurture and indulge the child with a massive commitment only for as long as he is palpably helpless and vulnerable. The age deemed appropriate for terminating what Ausubel and Sullivan (1970) call 'the stage of volitional independence and executive dependence' (viz. infancy) varies between 2 and 4 years in age in different cultures — nearer to 2 years in Western society. During this so-called transitional phase* they withdraw much of the attentive and uncritical deference they previously allowed the child because of his helpless status as a baby; furthermore, they begin to make fairly exacting demands of the child's self-control. During the toddler stage parents became somewhat less tolerant, attentive and deferential towards the child. As Ausubel and Sullivan (1970, p.260) put it:

> They comfort the child less and demand more conformity to their own desires and to cultural norms. During this period the child is frequently weaned, is expected to acquire sphincter control, approved habits of eating and cleanliness, and to do more things for himself. Parents are less disposed to gratify his demands for immediate gratification, expect more frustration tolerance and responsible behaviour, and may even require performance of some household chores. They also become less tolerant towards displays of childish aggression. In short, all of these radical changes in parent behaviour tend to undermine environmental supports for infantile self-perceptions of volitional independence and omnipotence . . . As a consequence of ego devaluation, the situation is precisely reversed: increased *executive* independence is required along with greater volitional dependence.

Not surprisingly, this transitional phase is marked by 'problematic' behaviour in the child — a period sometimes referred to as the 'terrible two's' or 'three's'. He often displays oppositional and aggressive behaviour together; the negativistic child, if coerced by parent or teacher, may react with rage and aggression. Oppositional behaviour in the very young child does not always have this hostile aspect, but as others in his environment, especially the main caregivers (and therefore usually the mother), begin to oppose his negative behaviour, hostility becomes directed towards them. Such problems are common among pre-school children, and the age of 3 years sees the peak for the incidence of temper-tantrums, particularly among boys (MacFarlane, Allen, and Honzik, 1954). In a statistical and developmental respect this behaviour is 'normal', and as such represents one of the many transitory crisis periods that children pass through as they grow up. In the setting of a reasonably robust family, such outbursts are managed by most parents without seeking professional advice.

*These transitional phases are often conceptualized as 'crises of development'.

It is obviously essential to be familiar with these norms when making a behavioural assessment (see Herbert, 1974, 1980a; MacFarlane, Allen, and Honzik, 1954; Rutter, Tizard, and Whitmore, 1970; Shepherd, Oppenheim, and Mitchell, 1971). When dealing with a case on an advice basis, these norms can be reassuring to the parents; they indicate that during the development of normal children most have problems which last a short time, then disappear. The child's problems — provided they are not severely disruptive or inappropriate to his chronological or mental age and circumstances — are by no means unique and will be outgrown given time *and* sensible parental management.

At another level, there is small comfort for the mother who still has to cope with the irksome problem. Problem behaviour tends to be very annoying behaviour; this does not mean, of course, that all behaviours which irritate and create problems for parents are to be thought of as maladaptive and requiring a therapeutic intervention. However, yet again the diagnostic judgement is a vexed one. Johnson et al. (1973) made a study of 33 American children (ages 4 to 6 years) with no history of treatment for behaviour problems, living in unbroken homes with psychiatrically healthy parents. They demonstrated that the average child emitted responses which parents considered deviant at the rate of one every 3·17 minutes. In addition, the probability was one in four that the child would not obey any command which his parents gave him. Doubtless, cultural thresholds for this kind of non-compliance vary; it is difficult to see Indian families (Kallarackal and Herbert, 1976) tolerating this level of disobedience.

Certainly the 'annoyance threshold' as Kanner (1953) calls it, with regard to children, differs from individual to individual, which is to say that parents vary in what they can tolerate in the way of 'bad' behaviour. It has been found (Shepherd, Oppenheim, and Mitchell, 1971) that the reason behind the referral of a child to a clinic is as closely related to the tolerance threshold of his parents (i.e., whether they are anxious, easily upset, and lacking in ability to cope with children) as to whether he actually has an independently assessed psychological problem. This is an important consideration in evaluating the resourcefulness of the family for initiating a treatment programme or the implications (perhaps dangerous ones like child abuse) if nothing is done. Oppositional behaviour in a child can provoke intense anger, frustration, resentment, helplessness, and indignation in the person against whom it is directed. Some parents feel exasperated, hurt, and puzzled when their young offspring, once so dependent, begins to reject their solicitude and care and to assert his independence of them. When his self-assertion takes extreme forms, they sometimes react with counter-aggression or they may seek to prolong the child's dependence on them by becoming overattentive and overindulgent.

Within the broad developmental theme described above there are marked and early individual differences in behavioural attributes. Some of these characteristics cluster together to make for a particularly defiant, hostile, and demanding kind of child as opposed to the type who is generally calm, cooperative and compliant. There is nothing absolute about these distinctions. They represent the child's position relative to several behavioural dimensions or continua (Becker and Krug, 1964).

Kohn (1969) found that children who were high on apathy/withdrawal in pre-school scored high on Peterson's personality problem factor, while children who scored high on anger/defiance scored high on Peterson's conduct problem factor.

These children continued to display behaviours in first grade that were similar to those exhibited earlier in their pre-school period (day-care centres), despite changes in school and teachers. It would thus appear that aggression and withdrawal are behavioural characteristics that provide, quite early in life, a reliable classification for the behaviour of young children whether they are found in special treatment clinics or in the general population.

THE SCHOOL-GOING CHILD AND ADOLESCENT

Towards the end of the pre-school age-range children enter what Loevinger (1966) calls a 'conformist' stage. Rules are partially internalized. They are obeyed just because they are the rules. The chief sanction for transgression is shame. Piaget (1932) demonstrates how the logic of the child's moral reasoning changes radically from the age of 4 until adolescence. During the early stages of moral development the rules are felt to be absolute, unquestionable, and sacred. Morality is a unilateral system based, essentially, upon authority and, as such, external to the child. The rules have behind them the mystical authority of parents, older children, other powerful adults, or God; therefore they are not subject to change. From the age of about 7 years onwards, the child increasingly experiences relationships which involve mutual respect — relationships between people of equal status. Thus he meets children who do not always share his views.

By the age of 10 years the system of morality has undergone considerable change so that the child now perceives rules to be manmade. He understands that they can be changed if agreement can be obtained. Piaget believes that the mature understanding of rules goes with an ability to keep them. On this point Kohlberg (1970) is particularly critical of both learning and psychoanalytic approaches to moral development. In his view behaviour psychology and psychoanalysis have always upheld the Philistine view that fine moral words are one thing and moral deeds another. Kohlberg suggests that morally mature reasoning is quite a different matter and does not really depend on 'fine words'. The man who understands justice *is more likely to practise it*.

For the child of 10 morality is still very much a matter of obedience, but to an increasing extent he sees it as a matter of cooperation and agreement. With the onset of adolescence the youth enters the final phase of moral development when morality is seen as a matter of individual principles. The adolescent begins to appreciate that without certain basic principles there would be no morality at all. He usually understands that although there may be endless debates and arguments over how these principles should be applied in particular circumstances, the principles themselves are constant. He is often very idealistic, a state of mind that tends to give way to bouts of cynicism. For his parents, the stage of adolescence often represents a flare-up of rebellious, resentful behaviour — a time when their principles and values (or lack of them) are challenged.

After all, it is during adolescence (roughly the years from 11 or 12 to 15) that the child begins to free his thinking from its roots in his own *particular* experience. He becomes capable of *general* propositional thinking, i.e., he can propose hypotheses and deduce consequences. His language is now fast, versatile, and extensive in its use. It is public, so that the child not only gains from his own thoughts but also from the articulated thoughts of others. His world has become larger and richer intellectually and conceptually. Both opportunity and training are essential to the development of logical and rational thinking and problem solving. It is not an innate characteristic; it depends upon the right sort of environmental stimulation and encouragement (particularly in the pre-school period), and it also depends on natural growth processes. Logical thinking or rationality is an important requirement for adjusting to life's demands; it is also a vital criterion of mental health. It can constitute a 'trial' for parents as teenagers flex their intellectual 'muscles' by asking 'why?' or 'why not?', and questioning parental social and moral values (see Herbert, 1987b)

In urban environments, pre-adolescent, as well as adolescent, children tend to acquire their values more and more from outside the family; to some extent, their peers replace the parents as interpreters and enforcers of the moral code. This tendency is accelerated in an era of swift social change and easy communication. Changes in attitudes and values are so quick to occur and so radical in nature that we get a hiatus between one generation and the next — the so-called generation gap. Such alienation between parent and child generations adds to the role of the peer group in the socialization process.

It has been found that the climate or atmosphere of his group can have an important influence on a child's personality (Campbell, 1964). One type of group (e.g., a delinquent gang) can foster hostile, disobedient, uncreative individuals; another can develop confused, purposeless drifters; and still another produces cooperative, flexible, purposeful, altruistic children. In turn, the atmosphere of the group is determined by the qualities of its leaders and those of the other group members. When the peer group takes over some of the functions of parents (see Bronfenbrenner, 1970), the child's attachment to it tends to be pathological (Wright, 1971).

SOCIAL BEHAVIOUR

Many children and adolescents, for reasons we do not fully understand, lack the essential social repertoire required to cope with social life in a satisfactory manner. Consequently, they behave maladaptively in response to a variety of stresses, frustrations, and challenges. If such youngsters could be helped to become more flexible and competent, then they might have less recourse to problem behaviour. Deficiences in social skills are implicated in a wide range of problems (marital discord, depression, problem drinking, drug abuse, sexual dysfunction, dependency, antisocial aggressive problems) in later life (see Herbert, 1986). Thus the possibility of pre-empting such disorders by the successful treatment or training of children is very attractive to the practitioner with a concern for preventive as well as remedial work.

Socially skilled individuals, it is postulated, are better able to deal with provocative situations by compromise actions, persuasion, relaxation, humour and other appropriate verbal responses, which not only reduce the provocation but also preserve self-esteem without resort to extremes. By contrast, persons who lack social and verbal skills have few choices when it comes to dealing with aggravations and are likely to become (say) aggressive, more readily. Socially successful children have at their command more potential techniques for solving difficult (and everyday) person-to-person dilemmas. The processes involved here are sensitivity to when problems occur, ability to imagine alternative courses of action and sensitivity to the consequences of an action. Children (and adults) who are good at these skills are less likely to have to rely on ways of behaving which are negative – they usually have alternatives available to them.

Most older children are able to take for granted these social skills simply because — for much of the time — they operate at a natural, spontaneous and barely conscious level. It is a very different matter for those who lack these skills; the anguish and apprehension they suffer in daily social intercourse can easily be overlooked or played down by parents and teachers. That we are dealing with a serious issue is borne out by the empirically established correlation between children's social dysfunctioning (notably their inability to get on with peers) and a wide range of indices of more general maladaptation. Academic performance (Asher et al., 1976), mental health and emotional wellbeing (Cowen et al., 1973), school adjustment (Gronlund and Anderson, 1963), proneness to delinquency (Henderson and Hollin, 1983), peer relationships (Hartup, 1979), adult adjustment (Robins, 1966), are some of the areas adversely affected by extreme and continuing deficits in social functioning.

This is not to say that social skills deficits cause later difficulties in and of themselves. This would be too simple. We know that linear causality seldom holds in child development and psychopathology (Herbert, 1980a). As they grow up children have to master many different social skills, and the confidence they develop and the attitude they have towards their *competence* — their general ability to cope with social situations — are generalized to other areas of adaptation. 'Success breeds success' may be a cliché, but it has a respectable empirical basis (see McCandless, 1969). For those children who fail to exhibit the requisite skills for gaining peer acceptance, failure breeds failure. Take the example of a vicious spiral in a case of poor peer relationships. Children with peer problems tend to become aggressive or antagonistic towards other children, or they withdraw from them. Not surprisingly, they are rejected by their peer group. If children fail to develop social confidence they tend to feel generally inadequate; the more inadequate they feel, the more likely they are to fail. Because the ability to get on with peers, to make friends, is so crucial to a child's wellbeing, this aspect of friendship-formation requires special attention in clinical work.

MORAL BEHAVIOUR

When a child has developed a conscience it is generally thought that he is able to restrain himself from doing wrong much of the time, even when no one else will ever know about his misdemeanour. If he does give way to temptation he feels guilty afterwards. However, contrary to what one might expect, the ability to resist temptation does not correlate highly with proneness to guilt. A sense of guilt, although crucial in the development of the child as a social and moral being, is only a second line of defence in his compliance with the rules. There are several components to moral behaviour: the braking mechanism against misbehaviour even when unobserved (resistance to temptation); the acute emotional discomfort that follows transgression of the rules and leads to confession, reparation, or blaming oneself (guilt); acts of kindness, generosity, sympathy, and service to others (altruism); and all the things which people think and say about morality (moral insight and belief).

Those who resist temptation well are not always those who experience the most intense guilt when they err. The imperfect correlation between the various aspects of moral behaviour is reflected in the finding that although there are those older children and adults who are highly moral in all four components, there are others who are 'moral' in some but not others, and yet another group which is scarcely, if at all, moral in any of them.

According to Wright (1971), the evidence suggests that moral self-restraint is one aspect of a more general control factor — a generalized capacity to check or suppress one's impulses in situations which *do not* raise moral issues. This is the factor called 'ego control' (or ego strength). This concept — the 'will' of earlier times — involves non-moral capacities like the ability to maintain attention, the capacity to delay a response, and intelligent task performance.

SOCIAL LEARNING AND MORAL DEVELOPMENT

Learning theorists (e.g. Hoffman, 1970; Mowrer, 1960) base their investigations of conscience development upon the assumption that there is nothing about moral learning to distinguish it qualitatively from other forms of learning. A child acquires, through learning and identification, both the *content* of his parents' moral code and a *willingness* to act in accordance with the rules. Stayton, Hogan and Ainsworth (1971) point out that usually no distinction is made between the process of learning the rules of society and that first (and most important) step in the socialization of the child, which occurs when he develops a willingness to do as he is told. What he learns will depend on the nature of the parents' demands, but the development of an initial disposition towards compliance may be critical for the effectiveness of all further attempts at training the child. If the child lacks this tendency he will remain, in many ways, a stranger to his society, unidentified with it, regarding its rules and values from an external point of view. The family, like other socializing agents of society (such as his school) makes use of various techniques other than physical and psychological rewards and punishments to teach and control the child in its care. Among those used are direct instruction, setting an example, and providing explanations of rules.

Social learning theorists view the family as being particularly significant in the child's social and moral development because it is the first and most potent agent, deciding which social stimuli he is exposed to and what he is taught. It determines the categories of behaviour which are defined as 'good', and therefore rewarded and encouraged, and those which are labelled 'bad', and therefore punished and suppressed. Positive experiences, in particular, gradually give shape and substance to the prosocial patterns of behaviour with which they are associated, and the more often these experiences are repeated the more enduring the responses become. When the family fails in providing appropriate and consistent socialization experiences, the child is particularly vulnerable.

FAMILY INFLUENCES

When one considers the intimate, protracted and highly influential nature of parents' relationships with their children, it seems self-evident that the quality of such relationships must have a vital bearing on the development of the child's personality and general adaptation. The scientific inquiry into human parental behaviour arises, in part, from a conviction about the power and reach of the early experiences they provide for their offspring (see Sluckin and Herbert, 1986).

This quest has produced disappointingly meagre results. The reasons are not difficult to find: the sheer complexity of the subject, a daunting number of methodological problems, and some quirky biases in scientists' approach to this area of research. Leaving aside the complexity issue which is self-evident, there are particular doubts about many of the studies of human parenting due largely to flawed research designs, biases in sampling, and a tendency for social-class and ethnocentric values to determine the questions asked and the assumptions made, in various investigations (Herbert, 1974, 1980a).

Of more immediate concern is a theoretical issue. Ever since the publication of Mischel's critique of trait psychology (Mischel, 1968) there has been a controversy as to whether or not social behaviours demonstrate stability across situations and across time. One result of this debate has been the emergence of the 'interactionist perspective' (Bell and Harper, 1977) which has had relatively little impact on research into parental behaviour, the emphasis still being on intrinsic dispositions (motives, traits, attitudes, etc.) in the individual parent. The finding that children *initiate* approximately 50 per cent. of interactions with their parents (see Bell, 1971), helps explain the paucity of generalizations about parent–child transactions: the traditionally unidirectional (parent-to-child) account of what occurs. Interpretations of socialization in terms of social reinforcement have shared a common model of the child as a 'tabula rasa' — an essentially passive organism under the control of a socializing agent (e.g., parent) who dispenses rewards and punishments. This preconception has resulted in the neglect of those factors which are not under the control of external agents: e.g., maturational processes, as well as hereditary and congenital conditions. Among the latter are the temperamental attributes found in certain 'difficult' children, which make them highly resistant to socialization. Even the simplest training requirements may involve an uphill struggle (Thomas, Chess, and Birch, 1968). In many ways a child's behaviour can have as much effect on his parents' actions as their behaviour has on his (Bell and Harper, 1977).

Whatever the deficiencies of research methodology (an excessive reliance on interviews of parents rather than direct observations or information from children; on field studies rather than experimental work), studies consistently produce evidence of a reasonably predictable structure underlying parental and other interpersonal transactions (Schaefer, 1959). A wide range of behaviours reduce to two major dimensions, with orthogonal axes described as warm–hostile and control–autonomy (see Figure 1 below). It is possible to summarize the major factors which foster prosocial behaviour (Staub, 1975):

(a) parental affection and nurturance;
(b) parental control;
(c) induction — the use of reasoning in disciplinary encounters;
(d) modelling; and
(e) assigning responsibility.

The balancing of these components is perhaps best illustrated in the philosophy of what (on the basis of her investigations) Baumrind (1971) calls the 'authoritative' parent. This kind of mother (for example) attempts to direct her child's activities in a rational manner determined by the issues involved in particular disciplinary situations. She encourages verbal give-and-take and shares with the child the reasoning behind her policy. She values both the child's self-expression and his so-called 'instrumental attributes' (respect for authority, work, and the like); she appreciates both independent self-will and disciplined conformity. Therefore, she exerts firm control at points where she and the child diverge in viewpoint, but does not hem in the child with restrictions. She recognizes her own special rights as an adult, but also the child's individual interests and special ways.

Disruption of socialization

Although it is not usually made explicit, substantial deviations from this ideal, as represented by authoritarian parenting at one extreme and permissive (laissez-faire) parenting at the other, are regarded, if not as pathological, at least as undesirable.

Certain parental attitudes and actions facilitate such developments; others, such as rejection, produce adverse outcomes.

An empirical approach to the issue of rejection and its 'effects' and, indeed, outcomes of other parental practices, has provided the findings (Caldwell, 1964; Yarrow, Campbell, and Burton, 1968) summarized in Figure 1. Schaefer's dimensions in Figure 1 have been combined with evidence (summarized by Becker, 1964) of the sort of behaviour problems associated with different combinations of parental attitudes and behaviours. The outcomes of these combinations — trends, of course — appear below the figure.

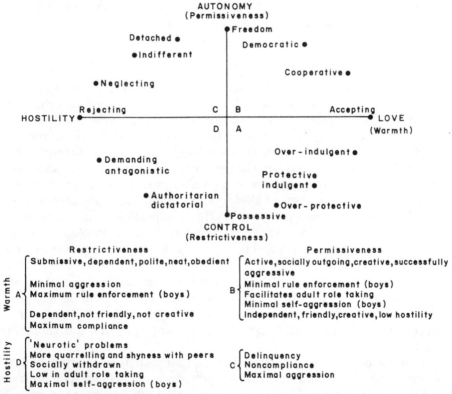

Figure 1 The range of parental behaviour-types within two major dimensions: autonomy-control/hostility-warmth; below are the outcomes (trends) in child/adolescent behaviour patterns.
Sources: Schaefer (1959) and Becker (1964) respectively.

Parental hostility

The most serious consequences (see Herbert, 1985b) result from punitive methods persistently used against a background of rejecting, hostile parental attitudes. These methods are often referred to as power-assertive; the adult asserts dominant and authoritarian control through physical punishment, harsh verbal abuse, angry threats and deprivation of privileges. There is a positive relationship between the extensive use of physical punishment in the home by parents and high levels of aggression in their offspring outside the home (see Becker, 1964). It would seem that physical violence is the least effective form of discipline or training when it comes to moulding a child's behaviour. All the evidence to date (Johnson and Medinnus, 1965) shows that physical methods of punishment (the deliberate infliction of pain on the child) may for the time being suppress the behaviour that they are meant to inhibit, but the long-term effects are less impressive. Violence begets violence. What the child appears to learn is that might is right. Delinquents have more commonly been the victims of adult assaults — often of a vicious, persistent, and even calculated nature — than non-delinquents.

Parental permissiveness

According to Baumrind (1971) the technical meaning of the designation 'permissive parent' is that the mother (or father) attempts to behave in a non-punitive, accepting, and affirmative manner towards the child's impulses, desires, and actions; consults with him about policy decisions and gives explanations for family rules; makes few demands for household responsibility and orderly behaviour; presents herself or himself to the child as someone to call upon for help and company as he wishes, not simply as an active agent responsible only for shaping or altering his ongoing or future behaviour; allows the child to regulate his own activities as much as possible; avoids the excessive exercise of control, does not encourage him to obey absolute, externally defined standards; and attempts to use reason but not overt power to accomplish her or his ends.

This empirical analysis is very different from the popular usage of the word 'permissiveness', which tends to be restricted to the extreme end of the dimension with its connotations of 'laissez-faire' parenting. The emotional background to this pattern of 'lax discipline' is only too often outright indifference.

It would appear that, notwithstanding variations in family pattern and style of parenting, all societies seem to be broadly successful in the task of transforming helpless, self-centred infants into more or less self-supporting, responsible members of their particular form of community. Indeed, there is a basic 'preparedness' on the part of most infants to be trained — an inbuilt bias towards all things social. The baby *responds* to the mother's characteristic infant-orientated overtures (see Stern, 1977) in a sociable manner that produces in her (in her turn) a happy and sociable reaction. He also initiates social encounters with vocalizations or smiles directed to the mother which cause her in turn to smile back and to talk, tickle or touch him. In this way she elicits further responses from the baby. A chain of mutually rewarding interactions is thus initiated on many occasions. Parents and child learn about each other in the course of these interactions (Sluckin, Herbert, and Sluckin, 1983).

Temperamental individuality

Some babies get off to a bad start, as we saw earlier. Not all infants are as rewarding or as cooperative as expected in this process of socializing and socialization. Parents are sometimes taken by surprise by the 'difficult' temperament of their newborn baby, and by his resistance to changes of routine and other demands of the socializing process.

Although it might seen far-fetched to propose that the stimulus characteristics of the child can constitute a sufficient or necessary provocation to maltreatment, factor analytic studies do indicate that abnormal attributes in the child are at least as substantial a factor in explaining incidents of abuse as deviance in the parents (Gil, 1970).

There is evidence (reviewed by Rutter, 1977b) that temperamental characteristics have a significant association with the later development of behaviour disorders of various kinds. Children who are hostile, restless, impulsive, and manifest poor concentration and who, in addition, display insensitivity to the feelings of others are predisposed to delinquent tendencies. It is not, of course, a simple matter of some children having 'adverse temperamental attributes' — e.g., poor adaptability — which make them difficult to rear. Children's characteristics interact with parental attributes; a mismatch of temperament can make for an extended series of mutually unrewarding interactions. They can also lead to faulty or incomplete socialization (Herbert, 1980a).

Predisposing factors

Of all the factors listed by Staub (1975) the establishment of an affectional bond between parent and child is perhaps the most critical — the foundation on which all social training is based (Hoffman, 1970). The factors which make for a rejecting parent are likely to be multiple and additive in their influence. They may be, in part, situational. A baby might be born at a particularly bad time for the parents — a time of emotional vulnerability and/or financial hardship. Parents identified as abusers of children are disproportionately represented among the under-20s at the birth of their first child, have produced a relatively large family, and report marital disharmony (Brown, Harris, and Peto 1973).

Disharmonious, rejecting home backgrounds, parental loss, and broken homes are examples of *distal* life variables that are often linked etiologically to conduct and delinquent disorders (see Rutter and Giller, 1983) Figure 2 summarizes the most important influences. When the family fails the child

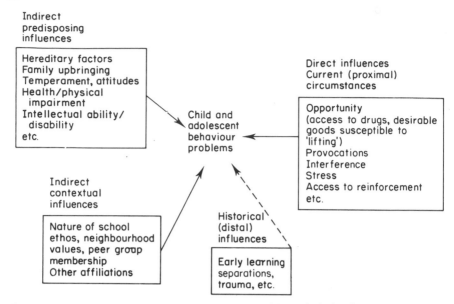

Figure 2   Levels and variety of influences on problematic behaviour

seems to be particularly vulnerable to the development of conduct and delinquent disorders, a fact reflected in empirical studies (e.g., West and Farrington, 1973). Achenbach's (1982) factor analytic and biographical study of multiple problems and symptoms (average 8.28) manifested by 300 children referred to a child psychiatry unit, showed that internalizers more often lived with both natural parents than externalizers, and their parents had fewer overt social problems. Parents of externalizers were more often rated as 'resentful' or 'indifferent'; parents of internalizers tended to be described as 'concerned'.

The factors that facilitate the development of moral awareness and moral behaviour include (see Hoffman, 1970; Wright, 1971):

(1) Strong ties of affection between parents and children.
(2) Firm moral demands made by parents on their offspring.
(3) The consistent use of sanctions.
(4) Techniques of punishment that are psychological rather than physical (i.e., methods that signify or threaten withdrawal of love and approval), thus provoking anxiety or guilt rather than anger.
(5) An intensive use of reasoning and explanations (inductive methods).
(6) Giving responsibility.

A variety of family conditions preclude the operation of these factors in the lives of some children. Typically, children with persistent conduct disorders come from families where there is discord and quarrelling; where affection is lacking; discipline is inconsistent, ineffective, and either extremely severe or lax; and supervision is inadequate; or where the family has broken up through divorce or separation. In addition, the children may have had periods of being placed 'in care' at times of family crisis (see Koller and Castanos, 1970).

Of course, these overinclusive concepts can be misleading. In the case of broken homes, for example, many factors must be taken into account (e.g. the sex of the lost parent, the cause of the loss, the age of the child at the time of the loss) if the circumstances of parental loss are to have any explanatory value. Rutter (1972, 1977) throws some light on this issue of moderating variables in his detailed study of the families of psychiatric patients with children of school age or younger. He found that a separation from both parents that had lasted 4 weeks or more was associated with antisocial problems in boys; however, this correlation held up only in homes where there was a very disturbed marital relationship between the parents. The effects on conduct disorder of such distal antecedents as separation from parents (see Figure 2) seem to have most to do with distortion of intrafamilial relationships before, during, and after separation.

The facilitation or disruption of social and moral training has much to do with disciplinary encounters between children and their caregivers over long periods of time.

Hoffman (1970) makes the point that all disciplinary encounters have a great deal in common. They all have three components: power assertion, love withdrawal, and induction.

Power assertion

There is a negative relationship between power assertion and various indices of moral behaviour, whatever the sex or age of the child. The evidence suggests that punishments which evoke anxiety are likely later to result in self-control, while those producing an aggressive reaction by-pass such subtleties. However, they may well make a child wary of being caught. For this reason, physical punishments are among the least effective as far as the development of the child's conscience is concerned. The normal reaction to any physical assault is anger and aggression, though the expression of anger may be inhibited by fear. Physical punishment may be confusing to the child. After all, he is probably being beaten by a parent whom he is normally expected to imitate but is now modelling the very behaviour for which the child has been blamed.

We know that, in general, extremely hostile and/or rejecting parents are likely to produce aggressive (and possibly delinquent) offspring (Feshbach, 1970). However, these child-rearing variables are influenced by moderator variables and cannot be considered in isolation. Within the *normal range* of parental behaviour, the value put on a particular punishment (or reward) depends on the overall emotional climate and nurturance in the home. What appears to be the same reward or punishment can occur under quite different overall conditions of nurturance, and therefore may differ in effectiveness. Conformity of behaviour to specific norms in particular situations is more likely to depend on sanctions attached to those particular situations than on the general parent–child relationships. *Love alone* is not enough in moral training; precise teaching has to be provided in seemingly endless moral learning situations, with great attention paid to the detailed consequences of transgressions on the part of the child.

Love withdrawal

These techniques take the form of parents expressing disapproval for undesirable behaviour by contingent removal of social reinforcers like affection, approbation, attention, company, verbal exchange, and other forms of social interaction. It is essentially a form of temporary exclusion of the child ('time-out') from social reinforcement or from 'love'. The commonly held view (see Wright, 1971) is that anxiety about threatened withdrawal of parental love is the major contributing factor to the child's internalization of parental values and *to making the child more susceptible to adult influence*. There is evidence that love withdrawal may contribute to the inhibition of anger (Hoffman and Saltzstein, 1967). The suggestion is that any action which threatens the withdrawal of the parent's love or approval provokes intense anxiety in the child as distinct from aggression. To be effective (it is hypothesized) any disciplinary technique must enlist already existing emotional and motivational tendencies within the child. In other words, a basis of affection must fuel the child's need for approval and hence his readiness to attend and heed what is being conveyed to him.

It can almost be considered a law of human nature that punishment leads to self-control only when the child is on the side of the person punishing. Since he loves his mother, the child is partly on her side. Because of this identification with her, he will join in her condemnation of himself. In learning theory terms, the closer the relationship between the child and his parents, the stronger his feelings of anxiety will be when the relationship is threatened, and the more effective the social conditioning will be. The converse of this is that if the relationship is weak or if the child is deprived of his parents, the child may be inadequately socially conditioned, for the threat of the withdrawal of parental love will not worry him very much. This is the explanation provided by social learning theorists for the finding that a very disturbed early home background is often associated with later delinquency.

Suffice it to say that social conditioning is most effective where sanctions are applied reliably and consistently. If many forbidden acts go unnoticed, the training process will take longer and might possibly go uncompleted. If misbehaviour is ever rewarded by giving it parental approval, it may become difficult, it not impossible, subsequently to condition feelings of anxiety to that particular undesirable act.

McCord and McCord (1964) observe that there is a constructive aspect in this development of inner controls; the child fears withdrawal of his parents' love and at the same time identifies with them. They observe that he wishes to emulate them.

Children who fear the loss of love develop the concept of 'must', but the 'ought' of behaviour comes only through identification with parents and other moral symbols. The McCords state that in a rejecting environment love, the central element, is absent, and because the rejected child does not love his parents and they do not love him, no identification takes place.

Induction

This involves pointing out to the child the effects of his behaviour, and giving reasons and explanations. It is postulated that the moral labels (or concepts) that the child is learning become capable through the processes of generalization and discrimination of evoking the anxiety that was previously conditioned to misdeeds that were externally sanctioned. As the child matures, the way in which he cognitively structures a situation will determine whether or not anxiety is elicited. This has a bearing on whether he inhibits the 'immoral' act or not. What happens then is that disapproved behaviours and the cues associated with the immediate antecedents of such behaviours ('impulses') come to elicit anxiety.

Parents may have, in a sense, a choice of whether they bring out to less or greater degree one or other of the attributes of guilt and resistance to temptation in their children. This will depend primarily on two things: the timing of the sanctions they administer for misconduct and the nature of the explanation they provide when they do so. There is evidence that suggests that punishment which immediately *precedes* a forbidden act (i.e., as the intention to transgress is forming and becoming explicit) maximizes resistance to temptation (Aronfreed, 1964; Aronfreed and Reber, 1965). Punishment has to be modulated. Above a certain optimal level of intensity, it produces a state of emotionality in the child which appears to interfere with learning. If discrimination of the punished choice is difficult, intense punishment is actually more likely to lead to transgression. A child must be able to distinguish what aspect of his behaviour is being punished if he is able to exercise control over the consequences of his actions.

There seems to be a subtle interaction, during the socialization process, between the child's cognitive structuring of situations, his ability to represent to himself punishment contingencies, and the extent of emotional arousal which is associated with his cognitions. The child's intellectual level, his verbal ability, and his ability to make a cognitive structure of the learning situation are important sources of control. They facilitate control by representing the potential outcomes of his behaviour and by enhancing the internalization of the social rules.

Socialization is particularly effective when training is presented in terms of a few well-defined principles. The use of inductive methods (explanations and reasons), especially when they elucidate a few clearly defined principles, enhances moral awareness and resistance to temptation. It is crucial that feelings of aversion are attached to general moral issues (e.g., 'stealing'). It is thought to be desirable that explanations are given in general terms as he gets older and can understand general principles. If a child steals from his friend's money-box his mother may simply say 'Don't ever do that again', in which case he associates the punishment with stealing from his friend's money-box. What the child needs to understand is that he is being punished for stealing and that all acts of theft are wrong. There is yet another process of moral development postulated by Hoffman (1970). This involves the individual's capacity to control his behaviour by considering its effect on the experiences of others, particularly the potential victims of proscribed behaviour. Little is known about the development of this capacity, empathy, although presumably it has some of its antecedents in parental statements involving explanations of the effects of one's behaviour on others. The capacity for empathy requires considerable abstract ability and represents a rather advanced stage in the development of moral behaviour.

The pursuit of altruism, idealism, and other moral virtues is explained by learning theorists in terms of instrumental learning. Because honesty and helpfulness have in the past been rewarded by parents, they become established habits; and since the concepts which structure such behaviour have also been associated with positively reinforcing experiences, the individual's recognition of his own honesty becomes rewarding. And, of course, strong habits of 'good' behaviour themselves have an inhibitory effect upon the corresponding but incompatible 'bad' behaviour. Hartshorne and May (1928–1930) found that altruistic behaviour on one test tended to be associated with similar behaviour on other tests and small positive association ($r = 0.33$) was found between overall measures of helpfulness and of honesty.

An extreme failure in socialization produces children whose character is distorted in ways that tend to earn them the label 'amoral' (see Wright, 1971). In the case of this amoral character temptation is never resisted out of obligation to a moral rule or out of concern for others; it is only resisted, if at all, out of self-interest. For example, the fear of the immediate and certain consequences of an act may be sufficient to inhibit it. Guilt feeling and self-blame are not in his repertoire, though misdeeds may be followed by action intended to avert punishment. Altruistic action, if it occurs at all, takes the form of advance payment for some future benefit — never for past benefits received or out of sympathy for others. Though he may be able to explain what the moral value of his society is, it has no real significance for him, and his reasoning on moral issues is dominated by the pursuit of pleasure and the avoidance of pain.

DELINQUENT MORALITY

A review of 15 studies (Blasi, 1980) supports the hypothesis that moral reasoning differs between delinquents and non-delinquents. Delinquent individuals tend to use developmentally lower modes of moral reasoning than do matched non-delinquents — as measured mainly by Kolhberg's scale (Kohlberg, 1976). It is often asked whether there are stages of moral development characteristic of delinquent adolescents. Kohlberg believes that the majority of adolescent offenders are preconventional in their moral reasoning, as compared with the mainly conventional reasoning of non-offending adolescents. The empirical findings are somewhat mixed and inconsistent and not easy to interpret or summarize. Several investigations in the Blasi review indicate that at least 80 per cent. of the delinquent group were at Kohlberg's Level 1 (Stages 1 and 2), where moral and self-serving values are not differentiated. Modes of reasoning are characterized here by the primacy of one's concrete self-interests; reward and punishment, pragmatism, relativism, and opportunism rule the day. These are preconventional moral attitudes normally associated with ages 4 to 10. But other studies found substantial numbers of delinquents who scored at Kohlberg's conventional Level 2 and where moral values are defined in terms of maintaining the social order. Social conformity, mutual interpersonal expectations, and interdependent relationships are emphasized.

However, Jurkovic (1980) concludes, following an extensive review of structural–developmental studies of moral immaturity in juvenile delinquents, that preconventional reasoning does not represent a necessary component in the development of delinquency; nor does conventional morality innoculate the individual against delinquency. Jurkovic (1980, p.720) states:

> On the most general level, it appears that adolescents who have failed to relinquish a premoral orientation in Kohlberg's framework at a time when their peers are moving to higher stages are at risk for behaviour problems, whereas those performing along more conventional lines may or may not be at a similar risk.

As pointed out earlier, moral judgement and moral behaviour intercorrelate in a complex manner; nowhere is the fact more apparent than in the conduct disorders and juvenile delinquency, where a plethora of situational variables and non-moral personality factors can be inculpated in the aetiology of the disorders. To the extent that premoral reasoning is conducive to delinquent actions, it is not clear whether preconventional delinquents are 'fixated' in their moral development or are progressing at slower rates than their non-delinquent peers.

Attempts to modify and enhance the moral maturity of juvenile offenders have produced ambiguous findings. Changes that have been brought about seem superficial. The methods used do not appear to stimulate a reorganization of moral reasoning at more advanced stages of sophistication (see Jurkovic, 1980).

Part II

The Assessment and Treatment of Conduct Disorders

Quidquid agas, prudenter agas, et respice finem. Whatever you do, do cautiously, and look to the end.

Gesta Romanorum

Introduction

The area of psychology most addicted to incautious assertion and speculation about cause and effect, and vagueness when it comes to goal-setting, is surely the field of psychological diagnosis and treatment. So little is incontrovertible about the nature of psychological problems that a cautious and open-minded approach is the only stance that can be justified. Having said this, the framework and ideas proposed here for assessing and treating children (i.e., in the next sections of the book) are done so in a spirit of humility and tentativeness which may not be as apparent on every page as they should be. Endless qualifications, in the end, produce a paralysis of thought and action. And *something* has to be done to help the parent and children of the kind we are discussing.

In spite of all the special provisions which exist, a substantial number of children with emotional and behaviour problems of one sort or another do not get specialized treatment, and parents and teachers have to cope as best they can. They have to fall back on their own ingenuity and knowledge of children's problems.

There are pressing reasons for attempting to modify the maladaptive behaviours of conduct-disordered children as soon as possible. This is not due to a belief that early experience exerts a disproportionate effect on subsequent development. Clarke and Clarke (1976) present evidence that early experience is no more than a link in the developmental chain, shaping behaviour less and less powerfully as age increases. What is probably crucial in the conduct disorders, with their poor prognosis, is that early (maladaptive) learning is continually reinforced and it is in this way that long-term effects appear. And there is also the possibility that some of the later deviance is the result of later reinforcement as well as original learning experiences. At whatever point in the child's development a therapeutic intervention is made, it is important that maladaptive learning processes are disrupted and prosocial actions encouraged in a manner that will persist over long periods of time. The therapeutic perspective is a long one. New adaptive behaviours need to become part of a child's life-style. We are *not* dealing, by and large, with transitory emotional disturbances.

3

Behaviour Modification: Assessment

THE ESSENTIAL ELEMENTS

Learning is usually defined as a relatively enduring change in behaviour which results from instruction or experience. All parents and teachers attempt to control and modify the behaviour of the children in their care by the application of informal theories of learning. Psychologists have discovered, as one of the more successful of their often-disappointing endeavours, a great deal about the nature of learning processes, social influence, and attitude formation. There is convincing evidence now accumulated (Kazdin, 1978, 1979a and b) that the application of this knowledge makes it possible to modify not only 'normal' behaviour and attitudes but also 'abnormal' phenomena.

Contemporary behaviour modification (or therapy) is defined as 'a process in which some observable behaviour is changed by the systematic application of techniques that are based on learning theory and experimental research' (O'Leary and O'Leary, 1972). The behavioural approach seems to offer what is both a theoretical and a practical framework for the treatment of a very wide range of childhood disorders (Bandura, 1977; Gelfand and Hartmann, 1975; Ollendick and Cerny, 1981) comprises a wide variety of techniques, but overall the aim is to bring about a systematic improvement in the child's environment so as to encourage or discourage particular forms of behaviour. To achieve this the therapist investigates the various influences impinging on the child, with special regard to his *overt* maladaptive behaviours.

An attempt is made to minimize speculations about causes based upon inference and interpretation. The therapeutic task is to remedy the problems by direct intervention. In its attempt to fulfil these desiderata behaviour modification focuses, particularly, on contemporary events — the here and now — rather than delving far back (as a major preoccupation) into the history of the child. It also concentrates on specific and observable behaviours. This concentration arises not from the naive delusion that there are no aspects of a child's problem behaviours which are determined by unobserved or unobservable factors, but from a conviction that a significant proportion of them are controlled by events — antecedent and consequent — that can be observed, measured, and modified. Knowledge of these events leads to *practical strategies* for producing change. It is acknowledged that while the social environment has a crucial role in shaping and maintaining human behaviour, so do inner cognitive events (Kendall, 1981).

The behavioural orientation espoused in this book makes room for such concepts as self-control, self-observation, observational learning, and cognitive mediation. It is the way in which these subjective phenomena are made explicit, operational, and modified in behaviour modification that differs radically from introspectionist or psychodynamic approaches (see page 290).

ASSESSMENT PROCEDURES

One of many available accounts of the assessment of problem behaviour and planning for its treatment is provided by the author (Herbert, 1981), who gives a conceptual framework in Figure 3 and Appendix B for the various stages before treatment is attempted: the identification and specification of the patient's problems; an analysis of the conditions controlling them; the ascertainment of the available resources; the selection and specification of therapeutic goals; and, finally, the planning of the treatment programme. Stress is laid on monitoring the assessment and treatment process throughout the contact with the client/s.

Behaviour therapists often refer to their assessment as a functional analysis (see the ABC terms, Figure 3). In essence they make use of direct observation and interview methods (Herbert, 1980b; 1987b) in order to specify those antecedent (A) and consequent (C) conditions under which behaviour (B) is manifested. A specific description of the child's behaviour is offered on the basis of the functional relationship between the behaviour and the conditions under which it occurs.

As described by Ollendick and Cerny (1981), 'the description is generally data based (rather than theory based) and is obtained from a "sample of the child's behaviour" (rather than inferred from a test "sign")'. Thus, from a behavioural perspective, a child who indulges in frequent, intense temper-tantrums would be observed in order to determine the specific circumstances and conditions in which the tantrums occur. Such conditions may involve antecedent organismic (O) and/or environmental stimulus events (A) which precipitate or set the scene for the temper outbursts and the consequent events (C) that maintain them. The functional relationship may be determined by:

(a) Operant conditioning Probably the best-known learning principle in

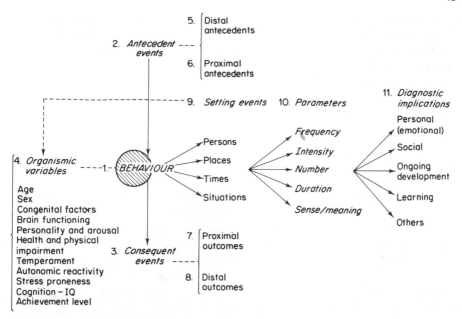

Figure 3   A conceptual framework for the assessment of individual cases of conduct disorder (adapted from: Herbert M. (1987) *Behavioural Treatment of Problem Children: A Practice Manual.* Academic Press/Grune & Stratton)

behaviour therapy is operant or instrumental conditioning. With operant conditioning the emphasis is on the response and consequent events (C). Behaviour is, to a large extent, a function of its consequences, 'favourable' or 'unfavourable', to the child. Thus, therapy involves the manipulation of reinforcement (rewards) and punishment (penalties).

(b) Classical conditioning   In the classicial conditioning model the emphasis is on the stimulus antecedent events (A.) The Pavlovian paradigm is well known. Counterconditioning treatments (e.g., desensitization and flooding) and aversive procedures (embodying escape, avoidance and punishment paradigms) are rooted in classical conditioning.

(c) Observational learning (modelling and imitation)   This is one of the fundamental means by which human behaviour is acquired, i.e., through modelling (imitation) or vicarious processes. A distinction is made between learning an action and the subsequent performance of the learned behaviour. Although observational learning can occur in the absence of response consequences, the nature of the consequences (e.g., reinforcement) to both the model and the child determine whether the modelled behaviour is performed or not.

(d) Cognitive learning   Perceptions and cognitions influence learning and behaviour in a systematic manner. Cognitive based procedures aim to modify

emotion and behaviour by influencing and changing the client's pattern of thinking and 'self-talk'. An attempt is made to modify specific perceptions, images, thoughts, and beliefs by the direct manipulation and restructuring of dysfunctional cognitions. Problem-solving skills are also taught.

These principles and their implications are elaborated on page 54. The steps to be taken in a functional analysis are listed below (and in more 'personalized' form in Appendix B).

(1) Identification and specification of the problem

The first step is to obtain information about all aspects of a child's behaviour which are considered to be problematic by his parents, any other persons (e.g., teachers), agencies (e.g., medical or educational), or the child himself. The process of labelling behaviour as deviant occurs in a social context (Kelly, 1955). In any group, be it a school, a family, marriage, or a work team, each member will have different perceptions of the 'real problem' in that system. It is not uncommon for workers (and parents) to focus on 'the problem child' as if the problem resides within him. For all intents and purposes he might be a small volcano erupting unpredictably. Behavioural (or social learning) theorists attempt to conceptualize the problem not as an encapsulated entity but as a process.

A longitudinal perspective is adopted which views the patient and his behaviours as part of a complex network of interacting social and learning systems, any aspect of which may have a bearing on his present troubles. Thus, in attempting to reach some kind of assessment and plan a programme of treatment, the unit of attention is far more broadly conceived; the focus of help is no longer simply on the child brought for assessment. Rather, attention, as Germain (1968) has put it, is on 'the whole human being within a fluid, real-life situation'. Treatment programmes are derived from a factual analysis of the current pattern of behaviour. The analysis is *functional*, in that it provides a description of the elements of a situation and their interrelationship (see page 55). It is based on the concept of a functional relationship with the environment in which changes in individual behaviour produce changes in the environment and vice versa.

Behavioural analysis

Difficulties, and indeed failures, in the treatment of children's behaviour problems can frequently be traced back to a lack of precision during the crucial assessment (or diagnostic) phase of a therapeutic contact. The analysis of a problem situation and the planning of a treatment programme probably require more knowledge and skill than any other aspect of the behavioural approach.

A behavioural assessment of conduct disorders is likely to encompass a broad spectrum of problems, ranging from legally definded delinquent acts to a variety of non-delinquent behaviours, including coercive or oppositional problems: commanding, screaming, crying, pestering, tantrums, negativism, and so on. (no. 1 in Figure 3).

(a) Aggression   Aggression is one of the more common complaints of adults who have to rear, care for, or teach a child with conduct problems. Such behaviour can include disruptiveness, destructiveness, physical attack, and verbal assault. Precise specifications of aggression in overt behavioural terms are a desideratum of research and therapy because of the possibilities of disagreement over inferential and abstract social definitions.

(b) Non-compliance   A major component of the conduct disorder syndrome, as we saw earlier, is serious non-compliance. On the one hand are those problems that involve an inability or unwillingness to conform to the values and rules of family and school life; on the other are those activities that constitute a disregard of society's laws and norms.

(c) Hyperactivity   This disorder is dealt with at length in Chapter 7. Here, some comment about the relationship between hyperactivity and conduct disorder is called for; their differential diagnosis raises formidable problems (Barkley, 1982). Children diagnosed as *conduct disordered* are frequently described as manifesting short attention span, overactivity, and restlessness. However, *hyperactive* children and adolescents are also characterized by brief attention span, overactivity, and restlessness in DSM-II. It is well known that a hyperactive child has a knack of generating very special learning and management problems at home and in the classroom. The findings of Stewart, de Blois, and Cummings (1980), based on a study of 126 boys attending the University of Iowa Child Psychiatric Clinic or Ward (and their parents), suggest strongly that conduct disorder is the primary problem of most children who are overactive and distractible.

Objective description

Granted that there is something called a 'clinical art', especially in the ingenuity and sensitivity with which a treatment programme is put into effect, nevertheless the major part of the clinical endeavour remains a scientific one. Scientists trying to explain a particular phenomenon will be at pains to bring that phenomenon into 'sharp focus' by describing and measuring it in all its manifestations as objectively as possible. They study its various parameters with as much precision as they can achieve *before* attempting to explain the phenomenon in causal terms. When they move to the formulation of explanatory hypotheses they are guided by the principle of parsimony, looking for simple or economical explanations which will accommodate the facts before they put forward more complex causal concepts.

48

Labelling

Sadly, what happens all too often in diagnostic conferences is an unwitting 'distancing' of the problem. This comes about, first of all, because of a tendency to describe the problem in global terms which are too vague to allow for the rigorous formulation of clinical hypotheses which can be put to the test. The unqualified use of descriptive trait or diagnostic labels such as 'aggressive', 'withdrawn', 'sadistic', 'affectionless', 'brain-damaged', or 'hyperkinetic' appear with monotonous regularity in clinical discussions or reports. Worse still, such labels are sometimes used as if they are explanatory constructs. The serious pitfall of using diagnostic labels is the illusory impression it gives the user of having explained the behaviour. What it usually represents is merely a *renaming* process. Take the child who is always on the go, inattentive, fidgetty, and difficult to manage. He is likely to be classified as hyperkinetic (or hyperactive). The inevitable question 'Why does the child have such poor concentration and why can't he ever sit still in his desk or listen to what I tell him?' receives the reply 'because he is hyperkinetic'. When asked to clarify this diagnosis ('How do you tell a child is hyperkinetic?') the clinician is forced to return to the observations he was asked to explain in the first place ('because he is overactive, inattentive, fidgetty, and non-compliant'). Many of the explanatory constructs used in clinical psychology and psychiatry are tautologies of this kind. They have the effect of short-circuiting prolonged and serious thought and empirical investigation of the problem.

A diagnostic label without descriptive, aetiological, therapeutic, and prognostic implications has no value. 'Minimal brain-damage' (a diagnostic label which is often linked with hyperactivity) lacks such implications (Herbert, 1964). Yet it is often put forward to 'explain' conduct and other disorders. Ross (1968) 'diagnoses' the preoccupation of psychologists with whether a given child is brain-damaged or not as the 'Rumpelstiltskin fixation'. As he puts it, this question and related questions of aetiology and classification often preoccupy psychological assessments and case conferences as if everything depended on that one answer. Ross urges psychologists and educators to repudiate these labels, thus ridding themselves of the mistaken notion that one of their tasks is to identify a disease from its signs and symptoms. He recommends that, instead, they get on with their real job of training, teaching, and rehabilitating the children who cannot cope successfully with aspects of their environment.

The fact is that there is often disagreement about what behaviours are covered by particular labels (Zubin, 1967). If we do not know what the *specific* behaviours are that define the label, we cannot specify in what ways a child's behaviours must be changed so as to make him less 'hyperactive' or less 'emotionally disturbed'.

Such semantic and conceptual devices encourage the sort of speculative 'free associations' about causes and remedies which are common at diagnostic or review case conferences, but which do not generate precise hypotheses and hence practical treatment strategies or the reformulation of treatment policies to replace failed interventions.

Specificity versus generality

There is a good deal of situational specificity to human behaviour. Mischel (1968), reviewing the evidence, concludes that assessment techniques designed to identify and gauge generalized trait variables in patients have poor predictive value. There is a danger of unreliability if a child's behaviour problem is not specified in terms of what happens, where, with whom, and when. Prediction is best from one situation to behaviour in similar situations (Bandura, 1969). The consistency that someone *perceives* in the behaviour of the 'other person' appears to come from conceptions of the perceiver rather than the person he is observing.

We have seen in Chapter 1 that conduct disorder is strongly influenced by situational factors with the result that the child's behaviour tends to be consistent within a given situation but variable across situations. Even the concept of morality is not unidimensional (Herbert, 1974); each of its facets is complex, and they do not intercorrelate in any simple way.

The classic study of some 12,000 subjects (ages 11 to 16) by Hartshorne and May (1930) demonstrated that there was very little correlation among situational cheating tests; children's verbal moral values about honesty had little to do with how they acted. The decision to cheat was largely determined by expediency. Even when honest behaviour was not dictated by concern about punishment or detection, it was largely determined by immediate situational factors of group approval and example.

Much weight has been given the development (or failure of development) of conscience, or the internalization of behavioural inhibitions and controls (Aronfreed, 1968; Hoffman, 1970). Our growing awareness of the importance of situational control and reinforcement of conduct disordered and delinquent behaviour does not necessarily contradict the theory of a central control 'mechanism'. Bowers (1973), following a review of empirical studies, concludes that both trait theorists and situationists have overstated their case.

A major source of error in the assessment and treatment of children in clinics or residential settings is the tendency to ascribe to the child properties which overemphasize the generality and invariance of personality traits and problem behaviour. In fact (as Rutter, Tizard, and Whitmore, 1970, found), there is very little overlap in the problems shown by children at home and at school. Patterson, Cobb, and Ray (1973) found that modifying children's behaviour problems in the home often does not solve behaviour problems in school, and vice versa. Mischel (1968) presents evidence which refutes the assumption that individuals harbour a constant amount of hostility, anxiety, dependency, or some other construct.

Yet reification continually undermines good assessment. The youngster is assessed in terms of what he *is* or *has* rather than in terms of what he *does* in particular situations. In the next stage the child is quite likely to be inferred to have 'a need for aggression'. From this point on, the distinction between what is observed and what is inferred, what is direct evidence and what is hearsay interpretation, tends to become blurred. For all the popularity of trait theories, practitioners make little use of the diagnostic information from personality tests in their conduct of treatment (Meehl, 1960).

The what question

The tendency at diagnostic conferences to leave the problem relatively unde-fined, or in the 'soft focus' of global terminology, leads directly to the *premature* formulation of cause–effect notions. To discuss causal factors before the 'to-be-explained' phenomenon is carefully specified and precisely de-scribed and measures is to reverse scientific method. Again, it seems to be much more interesting to try to solve fascinating 'why' and 'how' riddles in connection with behaviour problems than to wrestle with the more mundane 'what' questions. Graziano (1971) is quite clear that the key word in this phase of assessment is 'what'. He provides a list of the what questions that need to be asked. *What* is the child doing? Under *what* conditions are these behaviours emitted? *What* are the effects of these acts? *What* changes occur after they are emitted? *What* other behaviours might the child emit? *What* situations are being avoided? *What* acts may be encouraged and shaped up? These questions tell us about the specified problem and its effects (the pay-off) for the child. They also elucidate situational factors: the circumstances under which the problem occurs and those under which it does not. It is also necessary to know about the developmental level, abilities, and aptitudes of the child exhibiting the problem.

The problem (say aggressive behaviour) is specified in terms of observable responses which are accessible to other people (parents, teachers, the therap-ist) as well as the child. This includes what the child has to say (verbal behaviour), his self-perceptions and self-reports.

However, 'public events' such as his striking, pinching, or swearing at another person make for a more precise and consistent definition of the problem behaviour. They can be confirmed by the therapist and by other observers, and they provide tangible target behaviours for modification. After all, it is the *hitting* that hurts the victim and it is the *bullying actions* that in the end lead to the social isolation of the bully. Therein lie the problems. Many theorists would argue that to change the behaviour is to change the feelings in a way that is more sure and rapid than the reverse procedure (which is character-istic of the interpretive approach). In addition, a phenomenological or ex-periential approach to children's psychological problems is both difficult and of limited value (see Levitt, 1971).

What separates behaviours defined as 'problematic' from the aggressiveness, coercion, disobedience, and spells of exuberant activity shown by all children is the frequency, intensity, and persistence with which they are manifested, and the sheer number of problems with which they are associated (see no. 10 in Figure 3).

Obtaining information

Parents tend to report their children's problems in terms of rather vague and global labels such as 'tantrums', 'disobedience', 'rebelliousness', or 'aggressiveness'. These words may be used to refer to very different kinds of behaviour by different parents and, indeed, by the same parent on various occasions. The parent is encouraged to give descriptive examples of the problem, in other words to define what she means in specific and observable terms when she uses a particular label. A verbatim account of several examples of the problem behaviour provides not only an operational definition of what the problem is but also gives the context of antecedent and consequent events which will be useful during the next phase of the analysis. There follow two examples of a parent's complaint. The first is uninformative; the second provides a firm foundation for further assessment.

(a) Peter was playing with his cars when I asked him to get ready for school. Peter took no notice. I snatched away his toys and there was a scene. As a result, Peter had one of his tantrums and gave me a lot of abuse.
(b) Peter was playing with his cars. I told him it was already 7.30 and time to get washed, dressed, and ready to leave for school. Peter didn't answer or make a move. I told him the time again and repeated my instructions. Peter asked for a few minutes play. I said he was already late and told him to put the cars away. He now said 'No!' just like that. I snatched his cars away. He lay down, screamed, and kicked his legs on the floor for a few minutes until I smacked him. He then went to change, muttering that he hated me and would leave home. I took no notice. His father took no interest in what went on; he ignored the entire thing.

After an initial report from parents (or teachers) the therapist requires careful and controlled observation of the behaviours he or she thinks are important, as they are presently occurring. It is advantageous to observe what is happening currently in order to set realistic treatment goals or make plans for achieving them. It is important to confirm the parents' observations and especially those based on hearsay — e.g., what they have heard about their child's behaviour at school.

Parents who find their child's behaviour intolerable tend to overestimate the actual frequency of its occurrence. There are, on the other hand, parents who do not want to admit that their child has problems. They deny the frequency or intensity with which a behaviour is occurring. Not surprisingly, the results of objective observation and recording (made by the therapist and the parents) often differ markedly from the original estimates of those involved. From objective data, the therapist might refine the mother's complaint that 'he is always shouting and banging about', which is both inaccurate and vague, to: 'This boy has temper-tantrums, involving screaming, crying, hitting other children, and throwing property, lasting an average of 10 minutes on each occasion and occurring on average four times per day. They occur when he is thwarted such as when he is made to . . , etc., etc.' Given these difficulties, it is very important to make careful observations of the behaviours that are of concern by attempting to rate how intensely they are manifested and/or to count how frequently they occur.

Many practitioners maintain that behaviours which can be quantified and counted are easiest to change. Some would go so far as to claim that problem behaviours which cannot be observed and counted are not likely to be changed by the therapeutic agent. Unfortunately, most psychological tests and assessment tools do not sample the behaviour the therapist want to change. The therapist therefore needs to operationalize — often on an *ad hoc* basis — the target behaviours. By making them observable he ensures that they are amenable to behavioural counting or at least to more precise analysis of contingencies. Such a rigorous specification of contingencies is invaluable.

A useful question to ask is whether there are particular persons (grandmother, sibling, parent, uncle, friend) who get the 'best' out of the child, in the sense that he does not display his problem behaviour with them. If so, the interactions of those persons with the child are worth studying. There are several aids to observations: coding categories, instruction manuals for parents, and methods for keeping objective records by the therapist himself and/or by the parents, child, or some other person in the child's environment (see Appendix A).

When a problem requires treatment

A *high rate* (frequency) of emitting certain behaviours is one criterion of the seriousness to be attached to antisocial activities in children and therefore the appropriateness of a therapeutic intervention. The rare incident of stealing, bullying, or non-compliance may be overlooked; however, frequent acts of this sort are likely to be categorized as 'deviant'. Then, again, expressions of emotional and behavioural acts have certain allowable *intensity levels*. Very 'high' intensity responses (i.e. behaviours of excessive magnitude) which have unpleasant consequences for other people are likely to be designated as behavioural disorder. If aggressive children become destructive, sadistic, or harmful, their hostile behaviour tends to be labelled as 'pathological'. Even for the most philosophical of parents and teachers, emotional expressions and behavioural acts have certain allowable intensity levels. Above these, behaviours jar on the sensibilities and nerves of all concerned, and are called behavioural excesses or 'surplus behaviours'. There is an opposite extreme. A child may suffer not only because he is overaggressive or overanxious but because he is underaggressive and not anxious enough, or, indeed, because certain appropriate emotional responses or skills are entirely absent from his repertoire. These problems are called behavioural deficits. The complex issues of deciding when a problem requires treatment are discussed by the author elsewhere (Herbert, 1974).

(2) Identification of the conditions influencing the problem behaviour

In identifying controlling variables, two categories are generally considered: current environmental variables (antecedent and consequent events — see nos 2 and 3, Figure 3) and organismic variables (no. 4, Figure 3). For example, some problems are age related, influenced by the stage of development of the child and what some theorists regard as stage-associated life tasks and crises.

This phase of the behavioural assessment reflects the behavioural model of psychopathology in that it provides the data for a formation of explanatory hypotheses about the current factors which influence the initiation and maintenance of the problem. This emphasis reflects the importance attached to contemporary causes in the behavioural model. Secondly, it is the current form of the problem behaviour and the contemporary factors which initiate or maintain it that are mainly dealt with in treatment. A third consideration is the fact that very rarely can current problems be traced to specific past experiences with any degree of confidence.

Contemporary events

Many of the 'why' questions, in traditional psychotherapy assessments, are formulated in terms of an historical analysis of the client's life. Such a retrospective look at past events is often of interest (and occasionally of use), but essentially there is nothing that can be done to change history. An exclusive or predominant preoccupation in assessment with the child's history has the effect of 'distancing' the problem, keeping it vague because it remains at arm's length. It may alienate parents who are struggling with *current* problems in the child. There is a paradox that while most people are concerned with the present and are looking forward to the future, so many psychiatrists and psychotherapists spend their time delving into the child's (or adult patient's) past. Traditionally, the 'case history' has taken a 'vertical' form; it is an attempt to relate present troubles to past experience so as to see how they have evolved. 'We peer down the long avenue of the client's past life to see how the present event matured' (see Germain, 1968). This process, by producing insights, is thought to have therapeutic effects. The issue of how effective insight is in producing change and how relevant it is as a method for use with children is a continuing debate. Scepticism about interpretive, insight-giving methods of therapy gave behaviour modification its impetus.

The delinquent activities of adolescent youths provide a good illustration of the importance of current events in assessment work. Ryall's (1974) study of Approved School boys showed that an important characteristic of the deliquent behaviour of these young people is that it is not only habitual but also central to their self-image (see page 249).

It is one of the strengths of behaviour modification that treatment does not depend necessarily upon the discovery and understanding of the historical causes of the problem. The identification of the current problem behaviour and its contemporary causes may be assisted by information about the client's history, but this information is gathered primarily as a source of clues to these contemporary conditions rather than for more specifically therapeutic aims such as 'insight giving' or 'working through' of problems.

Current environmental influences

Once behaviour therapists have gathered all the information they can about the problem and its setting, they draw upon learning theory and experimental and clinical research for information which will help them to explain the breakdown that has occurred in the control (self and/or outward control) of this child's behaviour or in his understanding of the rules that make social life viable.

The basic elements of a stimulus–response or stimulus–control analysis of behaviour include the assumption (mentioned earlier) that most behaviour in the case of humans is learned. A study of stimulus functions concentrates simply and objectively upon the ways in which stimuli control behaviour: produce it, strengthen or weaken it, signal occasions for its occurrence or nonoccurrence, generalize it to new situations and problems, etc. . Behaviours are related to environmental (stimulus) events in two ways.

First, there are the respondents — those behaviours which are controlled by *antecedent stimulus events*. Respondents are those innate responses which are evoked naturally and regularly by particular stimuli. They are *elicited* automatically (unlike operants) without regard to consequences. Typically, this behaviour consists of relatively involuntary reflexes and responses mediated by the autonomic nervous system, including emotional reactions. A classical example of inappropriate antecedent events functioning as eliciting stimuli for maladaptive responses is the relatively innocuous object (e.g., a cat) or situation (e.g., leaving home) which evokes irrational fear (i.e. phobic anxiety). In the case of respondent (or classical) conditioning, a stimulus originally neutral with respect to a particular response (unconditioned response or UCR) is paired a number of times with a stimulus (unconditioned stimulus or UCS) eliciting that response, and the previously neutral stimulus (conditioned stimulus or CS) *itself* will also come to elicit that response (conditioned response or CR). The temporal relationship that must be controlled in order to produce effective respondent conditioning is the interstimulus interval time between CS and UCS. Recent evidence suggests that approximately ½ second is the best interval for conditioning.

Second, there are the operants; these are voluntary responses which are conditioned to stimuli by their *consequences*. Any consequence which strengthens a response is termed a 'reinforcer'. A consideration of consequences in a behavioural analysis often indicates inappropriate reinforcers which may be maintaining a maladaptive pattern of behaviour or the absence of reinforcement which might encourage prosocial behaviour. We know, to take one example, that aggression can be strengthened by reinforcement and extinguishes when reinforcement is withdrawn (Cowan and Walters, 1963). A reinforcer, then, is any event or any stimulus in the environment which affects the rate of a given operant.

Reinforcers can be *positive*, if the operant becomes more frequent following the occurrence of a stimulus, and *negative*, if the disappearance of the stimulus (called an 'aversive stimulus') results in the increased probability of the operant's occurrence. Because an operant is *instrumental* in procuring a reward or avoiding a punishment it has also been termed an instrumental response. In this kind of learning situation the individual can actively *change* his environment by 'operating' on it in some way to produce a reward, instead of passively anticipating events in this environment as in classical conditioning. In operant conditioning, then, the frequency of a chosen performance is altered by arranging suitable consequences (reinforcement or punishment), whereas in classical conditioning behaviour is altered by altering its antecedents.

Discrimination learning or training, as it is called, can result in a very high degree of stimulus control. The stimulus with which reinforcement is to be connected is called the discriminative stimulus (S^D). The stimulus with which reinforcement is not associated is referred to as S^Δ (ess-delta). When a desired response is more likely to occur in the presence of the S^D than in the presence of the S^Δ it is said that *stimulus control* has been established. Discriminative stimuli set the stage (so to speak) for operants; they mark the time or place when an operant will have reinforcing or punishing consequences.

Stimuli are vital because they direct behaviour. Put another way, it is crucial for the individual's survival that he learns to respond appropriate to stimuli. It is assumed that the social behaviours of persons in the child's world constitute stimuli whose occurrence is associated with changes in the probability of children's ongoing social behaviour (Patterson, 1974). The generic term 'controlling stimuli' is often applied to these events. Between input (stimulus) and output (response) various motivational states, cognitive processes, etc., can be inferred. A behavioural classification can be specified in terms of the following four components (see Kanfer and Saslow, 1969):

(a) *Prior stimulation* (S) These are the antecedent stimulus events which reliably precede the criterion behaviours. They may be functionally related to the response by setting the stage for them ('discriminative stimuli') or evoking them ('eliciting stimuli').
(b) *Organismic variables* (O) These include motives and the biological and psychological states of the organism.
(c) *Response* (R)
(d) *Consequent events* (C) Consequent events refer to the new conditions which the criterion behaviours were instrumental in bringing about. The

effects of these behaviours on the person's internal and external environment are crucial determinants of whether or not the behaviour will recur.

In teaching non-professionals how to make observations for a behaviour analysis a useful mnemonic for the classification above is the ABC (antecedents, behaviour, and consequences) of behaviour control used in Figure 3 (O'Leary and Wilson, 1975).

The elements of a behaviour analysis

It is possible to indicate the relative temporal relationships of the elements mentioned above as follows: S→O→R→C. The complete description of any behavioural sequence requires the specification of each of these influences and their interaction with the others. Jehu, (1972, p.76) summarizes the approach to the explanation of problem behaviour as follows:

> It is regarded as a function of somatic factors, previous learning experiences and contemporary events. The assessment of these events is directed towards the precise identification of the antecedent, outcome and symbolic conditions which control the problem behaviour . . . First, certain antecedent conditions may be eliciting or reinforcing problem responses, especially those of an emotional kind, while other such conditions may involve some lack of appropriate discriminative stimulus control over the client's instrumental responses. Second, there may be outcome conditions which either reinforce problem behaviour, or punish or extinguish desirable responses. Finally, any of these inappropriate forms of antecedent or outcome control may be operating in the client's symbolic processes, rather than in his external environment or physiological changes, or there may be an impairment of his problem-solving capacity.

Antecedent events (Figure 3, no. 2)

The literature on behaviour modification — as it applies to the conduct disorders — reflects a relative neglect of antecedent events. In their preoccupation with *consequences* of behaviour and, hence, operant procedures, behaviour modifiers sometimes overlook environmental controlling stimuli and the possibilities of restructuring the child's environment to produce antecedent control. It is no easy task to identify all of the stimuli that are functioning as S^Ds for a particular behaviour on the part of the child. They may involve persons, places, or times (see no. 9, Figure 3).

Certain respondents *in the individual* are called setting events (Bijou and Baer, 1961) and represent stimulus–response interactions which influence the occurrence of other patterns of behaviour. State factors such as hunger and fatigue may also constitute crucial intrinsic S^Ds for maladaptive acts. They may also consist of mood states. A child who feels tired and irritable is not as likely to manifest friendly or cooperative behaviour as a child who is not in such a bad mood.

Among the critical antecedents to behaviour — especially when one is considering non-compliant, rebellious behaviour at (say) school — are the rules. The particular rules which are set and the specific disciplinary techniques which are used are probably much less important than the establishment of some principles and guidelines which are both clearly recognizable and accepted as unambiguous and fair. For all that, rules are crucial. The pupil needs to attend to the consequences of his academic and social performance in order to make progress. One of the most important of these consequences is the feedback he receives from the teacher as to whether the answers he gives are correct or incorrect and in the case of behaviour, appropriate or inappropriate.

Cues (rules) inform pupils (and offspring) about what is required of them. The available evidence (Herbert, 1987 a and b) suggests that

(a) it is helpful to negotiate rules, to discuss the rules and the reasons for them, with children who are old enough to participate in such a process. Rules are more likely to be obeyed if they are perceived as fair and seem to have a purpose. Compliance is likely to be facilitated if adults engage young people in the formulation of their classroom (or home) rules.

(b) It also helps to work out classroom (home) objectives and clarify the part played by rules in facilitating these objectives.

(c) To be effective, rules should elicit responses which children or teenagers are capable of making. It is also important

(d) to emphasize rules that offer beneficial outcomes for appropriate actions,

(e) to select a few essential rules only — ones that can be enforced, and reinforced, and

(f) to praise children who follow the rules, identifying the precise grounds for the praise.

(g) Rules alone are unlikely to be effective. Group and/or individual reinforcers (privileges) might be built into an intervention.

Organismic variables (Figure 3, no. 4)

We have already touched upon transitory organismic influences on behaviour emission. There are other factors to be taken into account. Genetic or congenital factors may limit the individual or predispose him to certain behavioural styles, but they do not *cause* specific behaviours, i.e. shape the content of particular problems. For example, the minimally brain-damaged child may suffer from difficulties such as short attention span, restlessness, and other difficulties which have a parallel with the deficits of the child with poor ego-control. These difficulties are not sufficient, of themselves, to cause behaviour problems; rather it is their *interaction* with the environment which causes the problems.

Too often, clinicians explain away behaviour problems in simplistic terms of genetic or congenital factors. Nevertheless, these factors are important, and information about the maternal pregnancy and delivery and the child's early and later development is required at some stage in the assessment. The therapist needs to be alert to physical and intellectual limitations such as short-sightedness, deafness, epilepsy, slow learning and low IQ, and the referral services available for dealing with these disabilities. Information about genetic or congenital factors aids the fuller understanding of problem behaviour, as does comprehensive data about the family history and present family environment.

The uncertainties about the taxonomy of the conduct disorders makes correlations with organic (and other) factors doubtful. Pasamanick and Knobloch (1961) suggest that there is convincing empirical evidence of correlations between complications of pregnancy and birth and behaviour disorders in children; the latter constitute part of what they call a 'continuum of reproductive casualty'. While they are aware that many influences besides abnormalities of pregnancy and childbirth produce behaviour disturbances, they report that an analysis of the medical histories of children with behaviour problems reveals more complication of pregnancy and a great incidence of prematurity than occurs in a control group of matched subjects. Such complications are especially evident in confused, hyperactive, and disorganized children, and suggest some *organic influence* at work.

The findings, however, of multivariate studies (e.g. Paine, Werry, and Quay, 1968) show no correlation between conduct problem disorder and organic indicators.

What it is possible to speak about with some conviction as a potentially significant factor in the development of behaviour problems is a *temperamental or congenital factor* in the child which has powerfully modified the parents' interactions and the manner in which they have reared him. This influence can range from the trivial to the height of significance (see Sameroff 1975). He states that breakdowns in the parent–child relationship may take a great variety of forms. To quote Sameroff (1975, p.275):

> The most heavily researched and carefully documented of these transactional failures relates to the inability of parents and their children to work out an interactional style which both guarantees the child a reasonable margin of safety and satisfies the child's basic biological and social needs. This is the issue of child abuse. Physical abuse is dramatic evidence of a disorder in the parent–child relationship.

In the case of this kind of breakdown and other less dramatic problems in parent–child relationships, environmentally orientated theorists tend to be rather one-sided in their downgrading of the child's individuality.

Where difficulties arise, parents are usually presumed to be somewhat at fault. It is often forgotten that the parent–child relationship is a two-way process, and some children *are* consistently more difficult to rear than others (Bell, 1971). These may include a significant proportion of *physically handicapped* children, in respect of whom it is necessary to be aware of their possible adverse effect upon their parents (Graham, Rutter, and George, 1973).

The results of research surveys indeed suggest that as many as one child in seven with a physical disability is further handicapped by significant psychiatric disorder; in addition, the incidence of behavioural disturbance is highest among those children with neurological disorders (Rutter, Tizard, and Whitmore, 1970). The family which contains a physically disabled child has many problems to cope with: not only the fact of having a child who is handicapped and therefore, probably, demanding, but also depressing doubts and uncertainties about the future. The parents' dilemma is that they have to manage the day-to-day practical difficulties (e.g., attendance at clinics, special schooling, and transport) and make important decisions on the child's behalf, even though they may be uncertain about what should be reasonable expectations for the child. What allowances must they make for his handicap? To what extent can they go on the 'norms', as they understand them, of child-rearing practice in society at large? The parents may have to cope with feelings within themselves of guilt, anxiety, hostility, and the wish to make amends to the child, which put constraints on their intuitive and spontaneous approaches to child management.

At least physical handicap is recognizable and can be identified as a good reason for making allowances for the child and parents when difficulties arise. Less obvious are the disabling consequences of certain kinds of temperament in the child. Parents are less likely to receive sympathy when the child 'looks normal' but they find him difficult if not impossible to manage (Thomas and Chess, 1977).

It seems clear that the stress resulting from a mismatch between the mother's temperament (including her annoyance threshold) and the child's *behaviour style* sets the stage for discord, conflict, nervous exhaustion, and eventual feelings of inadequacy as a parent. Frustration, guilt, anger, rage, despair, and worse are likely outcomes.

The investigation by Thomas et al. (1968) showed that a group of children who developed behaviour disturbances as they got older had received significantly higher scores on activity level in their first year of life. Findings such as these and others interested the author in the possibility of detecting 'vulnerable' children, that is to say, children 'at risk' of developing behaviour problems, with a view to doing preventive work with them.

In the author's opinion (Herbert, 1986) toddlers who for one reason or another have excessively high 'demand' characteristics, if they are not dealt with firmly and consistently by competent, resourceful, and tolerant parents, do not emerge from the negativistic stage described on page 21. In a sense their mothers (and fathers) are defeated by the strong-willed oppositional behaviour of their child, particularly if they already have special sensitivities towards him or uncertainties about child rearing. If they live in a semi-detached house with thin partitions their deference to the neighbours peace of mind may also cause them to 'give in' to their child's wilful tantrums and screaming. A confrontation with the child is avoided or faced up to only sporadically, with inconclusive results or a humiliating retreat. Inevitably the parents lose confidence in their effectiveness as parents; they feel that the child is beyond their control and is manipulating them. They are also likely to be exhausted (there are usually sleeping problems) and in despair about the feelings of rejection and violence towards the child.

The studies published by Thomas and his colleagues provide a longitudinal perspective on the development of behaviour problems in their sample. In the course of the 10-year contact with the research team, 42 were identified as manifesting psychological disorders. Children with psychological disorders thus represented 31 per cent. of the total study population. This figure, it should be remembered, is high because it represents the prevalence of disorders over a 10-year span.

The children who put such heavy demands on mothers that they came to be known as 'difficult children' were characterized by the following elements:

(1) Irregularity in biological functions (especially eating and sleeping)
(2) Negative and aversive responses to new stimuli (new foods, bathing, going out, coming in, etc.)
(3) Slowness in adapting to changes, as in the examples just given
(4) A high frequency of negative moods
(5) A high intensity of reactivity

Compared with children with easier temperamental characteristics, the 'difficult children' were far less likely to grow up without behaviour problems. Approximately 70 per cent. of the temperamentally difficult children are reported as having developed such problems. Case analyses indicated quite clearly that the parents' attempts to cope with their offspring represented in part their reaction to a particular kind of child and also their *own* highly individual behavioural styles.

Thomas et al. (1968) are at pains to point out that a given combination of behavioural styles in a specific child does not in and of itself lead to behaviour problems, but that it is the interaction between these stylistic characteristics and the child's environment which can eventuate in clinical referral. They regard individual behavioural style not as an inevitability that must be fatalistically accepted but as a condition which, once recognized, gives both parent and child logical means of coping with individual differences. It is an intriguing question whether the incidence of behaviour disorders among 'difficult children' can be reduced by educating parents to accept their child's individuality and helping them to adapt to his behavioural style so that the child in turn can adapt to the successive demands of socialization.

Sex is yet another organismic variable of significance in the conduct problems. Throughout the age range we are considering, and with regard to all the specific, so-called externalizing (conflict with the environment) behaviour problems that make up the conduct disorder constellation, boys show a higher incidence than girls. Achenbach (1966) suggests that the socialization process — which includes the stereotyping of gender roles — plays an important part in determining whether a child becomes an externalizer or an internalizer.

Consequent events (Figure 3, no. 3)

The analysis of outcome controlling factors includes an assessment of why, when, and how parents (and others) reward the child. This means finding out whether rewarding the child is contingent on his behaving in a certain way, whether rewards are applied indiscriminately, or whether there is any consistency in the pattern of rewarding. Indeed, do the parents remember occasionally to reward (approve of or praise) good behaviour? Timing of the rewards is also crucial, and knowledge of what is rewarding to the child is important for the design of a treatment programme. The same assessment is made of the use of sanctions and punishments.

(3) Assessment of the resources for treatment

The third component in a behavioural analysis concerns the potentialities and limitations of the child or adolescent and his family for coping with treatment. First, it is necessary to consider the child's and/or his parents' capabilities; they will determine the programme level. Parents usually come to a clinic with a mental set for discussing the negative aspects of their child's behaviour. There are advantages in asking them to talk about and observe (by monitoring at home) those areas in which his behaviour is socially appropriate. They may be surprised at how much prosocial behaviour they have overlooked. This may increase their own self-esteem as parents and also help them to establish a more balanced view of the child's behaviour. If parents focus their attention more on the positive behaviour, even if of rather poor quality (see page 148), this behaviour is quite likely to increase and therefore leave less time for antisocial behaviour. There are also various family attitudes to assess. How do they see the behavioural methods which have been explained to them? What is their attitude to the child and the work (and possible stress) a therapeutic intervention may involve? How realistic are parental (or teacher) expectations of the child and of the therapy?

Motivation for treatment is a significant factor in the successful outcome of a therapeutic intervention, so the assessment of resources explores the child's (and his parents') personal attitudes, competencies, and limitations with regard to treatment. In the case of the child, these might include his degree of motivation, capacity for self-regulation, and any skills which might be capitalized on for treatment purposes. In the case of the younger child, there is the question of how much he should be directly involved in the intervention.

There is also the issue of how intensive treatment should be. This will depend, in part, on the severity of the problem and current parent and child resourcefulness, and also on the availability of personnel in the treatment agency. Other significant persons in the family, such as grandparents or siblings, can be an aid (and sometimes a hindrance) to the implementation of a programme. These matters must be calculated. Part of the calculation must take into account the fact that behavioural treatments are not like fixed items on a medical prescription to be implemented in an inflexible manner.

4

Behaviour Modification: Treatment

There is a creative element to the planning of an overall treatment programme and a human (and therefore fallible) component in its application.

I like to think of behaviour modification as a craft. Each art has its technical side (e.g., the potter) and each science has its creative or imaginative element. The most fruitful communication of those who work primarily with symbols (the artists) and those who work with sensed data (the scientists) occurs in some of the crafts. The application of science — applied psychology — to complex human problems requires imagination and sensitivity; it has all the hallmarks of a craft.

Decision to intervene

Given that we are dealing with social rather than medical criteria for what is problematic, it is important to look not only at the immediate consequences of a child's behaviour but also at the longer-term implications (distal outcomes) (see no. 8 in Figure 3). What are the likely consequences of non-intervention in the problem for the child and the family? There are essentially two issues to be resolved at this stage of a behavioural assessment: (a) the diagnostic issue, that is, is the problem sufficiently serious to merit an intervention; and (b) the ethical issue, that is, is it ethically right to intervene so as to produce changes in the direction of Goals X, Y or Z?

One of the simplest ways to uncover a therapist's implicit or latent definition of mental health is to ask about the therapist's criteria for successful termination of a therapeutic case. The other side of the coin, of course, is to ask how he or she decides that treatment is actually required. Problem behaviours are called thus because they have a variety of unfavourable short- and long-term outcomes. They are therefore referred to as maladaptive actions; they are inappropriate in terms of several criteria that are assessed by the therapist. The diagnostic criteria are listed as medium- or long-term outcomes (under no. 11 in Figure 3) with regard to social, personal, developmental, and learning implications. Ultimately, the professional judgement of a child's behavioural/psychosocial status is made in individual terms, taking into account the child's particular circumstances as well as the consequences that flow from his or her specific behaviours and general life style, with particular reference to personal and emotional wellbeing, social relationships, ongoing development and maturation, ability to learn academically, and accessibility to socialization. All are gravely affected in the conduct disorders (see Rutter, 1978). Behaviour problems, especially the conduct disorders, are more common in children who are retarded in reading skills (Rutter, Tizard, and Whitmore, 1970; Varlaam, 1974) than those who do not manifest such deficits. Given the relationship between underachievement (deficits in academic skills, especially reading difficulties) and conduct problems, it is an argument for intervention to find that in such areas as arithmetic, spelling, and reading, performance has been improved by the use of principles of reinforcement (Felixbrod and O'Leary, 1973; Lahey, McNees and Brown, 1973). The same applies to social skills, self-esteem, and self-efficacy.

Definition of treatment goals

Once the problem is precisely specified the therapist and others (including colleagues, the parents, and, if he is old enough, the child) decide whether the allegedly problematic behaviour ought to be changed. They need to know how different it is from what is normal for a child of that age and sex, and in that situation. Other decisions concern the direction which the change should take. Then again, how far should the changes go? The *total* elimination of anxiety or (in a 3-year-old) of tantrums as a treatment objective would be extreme, unrealistic, and unattainable. Because behaviour modification is very directive and often quite powerful, it should only be employed as a specific treatment or management procedure after full and careful consideration of the desirability of the proposed changes. The objectives are decided primarily on personal, social, and ethical grounds. The clinician has a special responsibility of acting, in a sense, as an 'advocate' for the child. This is especially the case with the younger child, who cannot speak for himself and defend himself against the sometimes unreasonable demands made of him.

If a behaviour is defined as part of the treatment goals but is not functional for a child, in the sense of being rewarding and having survival value, then a treatment programme may produce only a transitory effect. When the therapeutic procedures are withdrawn there may be nothing to maintain the behaviour and it will extinguish. Ayllon and Azrin (1968) propose a guideline: 'Teach only those behaviours which will continue to be reinforced after training.' The therapist's aim in using behaviour modification procedures is to introduce the child to behaviours which are either intrinsically reinforcing or which make reinforcements available to him which he was not previously experiencing. For example, an illiterate delinquent youth might be encouraged in the initial stages of a remedial reading programme by the use of extrinsic incentives, but it would be hoped that once the skill was established its use would be sufficiently functional for the boy to continue reading himself, being able to enjoy books and to collect interesting information, etc. The continued application of extrinsic rewards would thus be rendered superfluous.

Once the goals have been identified, they are ranked according to the negotiated consensus about what are priorities. The behaviours the parents most want to see changed usually become the focus of the first interventions, but there may be disagreement on the part of the therapist as to what *are* appropriate (and manageable) target behaviours for initiating the programme. Balanced against the proposition that treatment must begin with the most troublesome behaviours is the proposition that the client's first intervention attempts should hopefully be successful. Maximizing the chances for success may be more important than beginning with the client's first choice, because she may already have a sense of failure in dealing with the child. If she experiences failure at the beginning of treatment, such an experience is likely to reinforce the sense of despair and helplessness which caused her to seek professional help in the first place. Patterson et al. (1975) argue for tackling *all* the child's problems concurrently, and there may be a case for this when they share a common basis, (e.g., attention seeking). In order that goals can be pitched at a realistic level and the effectiveness of any intervention strategy evaluated, present behaviour is assessed individually with regard to the child's behavioural repertoire and degree of responsiveness. Assessing the child's prosocial behaviour (assets) also enables the therapist to set a realistic level for planning a treatment programme. If concerned with academic goals or self-help skills, this may then be done using objective standardized tests. If concerned with social behaviour, assessment may be made through observation.

A serious difficulty which often arises in treatment is due to the tendency for therapeutic goals in some therapies to be conceived in vague 'global' terms rather than specified as measureable targets. This makes it difficult to measure success or failure and thus to validate or invalidate one's way of working. The goals of treatment are specified as publically observable responses occurring in defined settings. Otherwise, when improvement does not follow treatment it is rather too easy to scapegoat the parents and their children by using labels which exculpate the therapist.

Furthermore, failure to improve can be attributed to the shortcomings of the clients rather than to the therapist's lack of skill. Granted that clients do sometimes fail to cooperate, keep appointments, or keep to the agreed arrangements for the programme, it is important not only to specify the goals of treatment very precisely in terms of the responses to be produced and the conditions under which these should occur, but to decide the expectations of both sides in fulfilling them. Any objective must contain five elements: who will do what, with whom, to what extent, and under what conditions? These are usefully made explicit in a verbal or written contract with the clients.

PLANNING TREATMENT

There are several broad considerations, with regard to the choice of therapeutic agent and setting of treatment, that determine the precise details of the treatment plan. For example, there are three main settings in which behavioural work with children takes place. Therapy based on the dyadic (one-to-one) model tends to take place in the clinic; treatment on the triadic model (using significant caregivers or teachers as mediators of change) takes place in the home *or* in the school.

The treatment of 'neurotic' and stress disorders is likely to occur in the clinic, although there is nothing absolute about such a demarcation. These problems tend to be of relatively *short-term* duration (Herbert, 1974). Although the distinction between treatment and training is, at times, indistinct, the treatment model is most appropriate to the 'emotional' (or 'personality') disorders of childhood.

There is insufficient space to do justice to the significant behavioural work (with *long-term* objectives) carried out with mentally handicapped and autistic children and youngsters with learning disabilities. Excellent reviews on these subjects are available by Weatherby and Baumeister (1981), Schreibman and Koegel (1981) and Lahey et. al (1981) respectively. Such children often display conduct problems and we shall concentrate on these. The training model of behaviour modification, involving the teaching of caregivers and teachers (as well as children) in behavioural analysis and/or techniques, is particularly applicable in both these areas. Not surprisingly, parents figure significantly in the therapeutic programmes, not least because of their major contribution to the evolution of such problems. Training in the principles and application of learning theory encourages parents to think about behaviour sequentially (in ABC interactional terms). They learn to monitor behaviour, often with the aid of a chart or diary. Some children and parents improve during the baseline period. Certainly, baseline phases of assessment are not usually therapeutically 'inert'.

AB and ABC designs are the ones predominantly in use in clinics orientated primarily towards service-delivery. The AB design, involving as it does a simple comparison of the occurrence of the problem behaviour under pre treatment baseline conditions and under conditions of a treatment programme, allows us to determine only whether a change in the level of the behaviour has occurred, and the approximate magnitude of that change. The ABC design entails a comparison of baseline conditions and two different treatment programmes (see Appendix A).

The next step is to relate the hypotheses about the behaviour problem and its controlling factors to the tentative treatment plan. Parents are invited to a discussion or case conference (which occurs, on average, after some 2 weeks of baseline work). Here all concerned discuss and analyse the plan of treatment, and draw up a working contract. Once the participants have arrived at a broad but clear outline of the treatment plan, they work on the 'nuts and bolts' (the fine detail) of the programme which the parents initiate with a good deal of practical, techinical and moral support from the therapist.

CHOICE OF METHODS

Procedures are chosen on the basis of knowledge of their therapeutic effects and acquaintance with the literature on the modification of particular problems (see Chapters 7 to 12). The choice of therapeutic approach will depend not only on the nature of the target behaviour to be modified and the stimuli which maintain it, but also on the circumstances under which the child manifests the problem behaviour and the aspects of the environment which are subject to the therapist's influence. There are two basic learning tasks that are commonly encountered in child therapy:

(a) the acquisition (i.e. learning) of a desired behaviour in which the individual is deficient (e.g., compliance, self-control, bladder and bowel control, fluent speech, social or academic skills);
(b) the renunciation (i.e. unlearning) of an undesired response in the child's behavioural repertoire (e.g., aggression, temper-tantrums, stealing, facial tics, phobic anxiety, compulsive eating) or the exchange of one response for another (e.g., self-assertion in place of tearful withdrawal).

Each of these tasks may be served, as we have seen, by one or a combination of four major types of learning: (a) classical conditioning, (b) operant conditioning, (c) observational learning, and (d) cognitive learning. Furthermore, they can be analysed (and a therapeutic intervention planned) in terms of antecedent events, consequent events, organismic and self variables.

5

Therapeutic Procedures

A treatment programme may include various combinations of antecedent and outcome procedures, as well as both environmental and self-control methods. There is no generalized formula or simple recipe approach to the choice of treatment procedures such as X methods for Y problems. The planning of a therapeutic intervention is based upon a strategy which is adapted to fit a given situation, so in behaviour therapy learning principles are combined into an adaptable strategy according to a behavioural analysis. A programme once initiated may continue or be adapted according to its progress or lack of progress or unexpected practical difficulties.

One criterion for selecting procedures is based upon whether the problem is conceptualized as representing a deficit or excess of behaviour. Broadly speaking, the therapeutic task with deficit problems is (1) to increase the strength of a particular behaviour (response increment procedures) or (2) to aid in the acquisition of new behaviour patterns (response acquisition procedures), whereas with excess behaviours the therapeutic task is (3) to eliminate them or reduce their strength (response decrement procedures).

(1) RESPONSE INCREMENT PROCEDURES

(a) Contingency management

Contingency management is the name given to methods that involve the manipulation of reinforcement. Positive and negative reinforcement are distinctive procedures that serve to maintain, strengthen, or increase the likelihood that a behaviour will be emitted. The general principle of reinforcement

— that responses which have contingent reinforcing consequences are likely to occur more frequently in the future — is fundamental to many procedures for the acquisition of behaviour. Reinforcement is defined solely by its effect on behaviour. If the behaviour increases in frequency, it is being reinforced; if it does not, it is not being reinforced.

Positive reinforcement involves the *presentation* of a stimulus (a rewarding event or object) after a response (operant) is emitted; it has the effect of increasing the strength of that response. Circumstances are arranged so that the correct performance of an act (or an approximation of it) is followed closely in time by what are thought to be rewarding consequences. A mother wants her child to say 'Please' when he makes a request, so she says 'Good boy!' as soon as he asks for something in the polite manner. The words of praise act as a social reinforcer or reward. She will add to the potency of the training situation if she only gives him what he wants when he says the word.

Removal of an aversive stimulus can be made contingent upon a required behaviour, a procedure known as *negative reinforcement*. Like the application of positive reinforcement in operant conditioning, it tends to increase the required behaviour. Thus the mother says: 'If you don't say "please" when you ask for something I'll slap your hand.' If the rate of saying 'please' on appropriate occasions increases, the slap on the hand (that is to say, the avoidance of it) has acted as a *negative reinforcer*.

Positive and negative reinforcement procedures generate four training methods: reward training, privation training, escape training, and avoidance training. The procedures (all of which strengthen behaviour) involve the following characteristic statements: reward training: 'If you make the response, I will present a reward'; privation training: 'If you don't make the response, I will withdraw a reward'; escape training: 'If you make the response, I will withdraw a punishment'; avoidance training: 'If you don't make the response I will present a punishment'.

In order to improve, increase, or maintain a child's behaviour, three crucial elements must be present: choosing a reward that is really effective for the youngster, delivering the reward on a precise and scheduled basis when he manifests the desired behaviour and ensuring that a reward is possible — i.e. that the behaviour (or an approximation) is within the repertoire of the child. But how is the clinician to know what is rewarding or reinforcing to the child? Children find different things pleasurable or aversive. After all, they have different kinds of physical constitution and unique reinforcement histories (Baron, 1966). The answer to this question is essentially an empirical one. Reinforcers have to be determined by investigation, observation, trial and error, or by asking parents.

Rewards' such as praise, attention, words of encouragement, smiles, affection, privileges, free time, food, sweets, games, money, and so on, which tend to be positively reinforcing for a wide variety of behaviours and a large cross-section of children, are known as *generalized reinforcers*. The tokens used in token reinforcement programmes tend to have these properties (see

Walker and Buckley, 1974). Noxious or aversive stimuli which strengthen behaviour when their withdrawal is made contingent upon the emission of the response tend, in 'real life', to involve shouting, scolding, disapproval, smacking, and other sanctions, whereas in therapeutic work, time-out, response cost, and procedures of this kind are most likely to be used. These, too, depend upon an empirical test of effectiveness. Although some positive reinforcers are more effective if a person has been temporarily deprived of them, others continue to be reinforcing no matter how often an individual has been exposed to them.

Some reinforcers which are commonly in use (e.g., stars, tokens, points, etc.) are neutral of themselves, but through frequent pairings with primary reinforcers (food, for example) or other strong reinforcers (praise or privileges) come to assume reinforcing properties. They are referred to as 'conditioned reinforcers'. 'Social reinforcers' such as the giving of attention, approval, and the like, are presented by other individuals within a social context. The main contingencies or consequent events naturally available within classrooms are social reinforcers, activities, and punishment (Becker, 1971). Social reinforcement covers a variety of interpersonal responses to behaviour, including teacher attention and praise. Becker claims that probably 85 per cent. of behavioural problems can be brought under control by social reinforcers, and the results of many studies give support to this claim. Social reinforcement provided by teachers and parents can be supplemented or replaced by peer group reinforcement, and this has been demonstrated in a number of studies (e.g. Patterson, Shaw and Ebner, 1969; Solomon and Wahler, 1973).

Therapists have made use of the principle that the opportunity, or privilege, to engage in preferred activities can reinforce activities or behaviours that are less popular. In other words, high probability behaviours can act as contingent reinforcers for low probability behaviours. The value to a child of reinforcing activities can be estimated by observing the frequency of behaviours in a free-choice situation. Homme et al., (1963) observed that running round the room, screaming, pushing chairs, or doing jigsaws were high probability behaviours in pre-school children; the authors used these as contingent reinforcers for less preferred activities such as attending to the teacher. Some authors call this principle informally 'Grandma's rule'. It states that 'first you work, then you play' or 'you do what I want you to do before you are allowed to do what you want to do'. Clearly this notion, like so many other learning principles, has been known and practised by succeeding generations of child rearers as simple common sense. However, it has been enshrined as a formal principle — the *Premack principle* — defining one type of reinforcer, following Premack's research into the problem of response probability and his search for an index that would predict between response preferences for a wide variety of topographically dissimilar behaviours (Premack, 1965). Danaher (1974) offers a comprehensive review and critique of this work.

A child's behaviour is affected by much more than the particular nature of reinforcements or goals. As Rotter (1966, p.1) notes, the effect of reinforcement is not a simple stamping in process but 'depends on whether or not the person perceives a causal relationship between his own behaviour and the reward'. This perception may vary in degree from individual to individual and even within the same individual over time and different situations. A significant influence on behaviour is also provided by the person's *anticipation* ('expectancy') that his goals will be achieved. Such expectations are determined by his previous experience.

This principle attempts to deal with the question of how the individual, in a given situation, behaves in terms of potential reinforcers. The assumption is that a concept dealing with anticipation of reinforcement is important in accounting for behaviour directed at specific goals. In short, one needs a concept other than simple value of reinforcement to account for human behaviour. The development of a notion about the workings of behaviour-reinforcement contingencies is a particularly important influence as a growing child learns appropriate social and personal behaviour.

There is a positive relationship between the number of reinforced trials used in the learning phase of an experiment and the number of responses made during the extinction phase when reinforcement is removed. Other things being equal (as can be made the case in the laboratory situation), the greater the number of reinforcements that are given during the learning phase the greater is the number of responses made during the extinction phase. This is an important principle: the strength of an association between a stimulus and a response is, in part, a function of the number of times that the association has been reinforced. This is not, however, the entire story about the stability of learned responses; other things are not equal outside the laboratory. Immediate reinforcement is more effective in establishing a conditioned response than delayed reinforcement. Furthermore, responses that are reinforced on a partial or intermittent basis (the pattern of learning for most organisms in the natural environment) prove to be more resistant to extinction than reinforcement that follows each correct response, the so-called *continuous* schedule. To establish new behaviour as promptly as possible it is reinforced immediately on each occasion. In order to encourage a child to continue performing a newly established response pattern with few or no rewards, the frequency with which the correct behaviour is reinforced is gradually and intermittently decreased.

Reinforcement schedules can be categorized along two dimensions: the interval between reinforcements may be a function of either time elapsed or the number of responses made. These intervals may be either regular or irregular. This classification gives four basic schedules: *fixed ratio*, in which reinforcement occurs after a fixed number of responses; *fixed interval*, in which reinforcement follows after a fixed time from the previous reinforcement; *variable ratio*, in which reinforcement occurs after a variable, possibly randomly, selected number of responses; and *variable interval*, in which reinforcement follows after a variable, possibly randomly selected number of responses.

A further consideration in judging the potential of reinforcement procedures concerns the concepts of *satiation and deprivation*. If a subject has so-to-speak 'had his fill' of a particular reinforcing stimulus (satiation), then the stimulus loses its strength in eliciting the desired response. Deprivation may have the opposite effect, increasing the potency of the reinforcement (the thirsty child is more interested in doing a task for a glass of lemonade than the child who has just had a drink). Therapists might offer a variety of reinforcing stimuli so as to avoid reinforcer satiation (see Bijou and Baer, 1966); some make use of the 'reinforcing event menu' which allows children to make a choice of reinforcers.

Indications for the use of positive reinforcement

A variety of studies suggest that positive reinforcement as a method of change is indicated when (a) a new behaviour is to be incorporated in the child's repertoire, (b) when the strength of an already acquired behaviour pattern is to be increased, and (c) when by increasing the strength of a particular behaviour the effect will be to cause an undesirable incompatible response to diminish in strength. Parents often make use of a mixture of punishments and positive reinforcers on the 'stick and carrot' principle.

Contracts

Reinforcement contingencies can be made explicit in the form of behavioural contracts (or 'agreements') between the individuals who wish for some behaviour change (e.g., parents, teachers, nurses) and those whose behaviour is to be changed (children, students, patients) (De Risi and Butz, 1975; Sheldon, 1982). A contract is signed by both parties to the negotiated agreement indicating that they accept the terms. The contract specifies the relationship between the behaviours desired by (say) the parent who has requested a change in the child's behaviour and the consequences of such a change, i.e. the reinforcers desired by the child or adolescent.

Contracts can be used to restore a 'profit' in mutual relationships. Agreements (whether written down or verbal) have the effect of structuring reciprocal exchanges. They specify who is to do what, for whom, and under what circumstances. Reciprocal contractual agreements are not unnatural to most people; they exist in families and other groupings, whether explicit or implicit.

In some family exchanges there is, sadly, very little cooperation, not much in the way of kindly, mutually rewarding actions or words in evidence. Rather there is an excess of mutual criticism, recrimination and threat ('If you do X I will pay you back with Y', or 'Until you listen and do Z, I will continue to do Y'). The harmony and 'give and take' of affectionate, thoughtful family life have been put to flight.

In such circumstances it is usually more fruitful to attend to *family* relations *per se*, rather than to the resentful parents alone *or* only to the adolescent, who is allegedly 'at odds' with everyone.

Contracts are potentially valuable because:

(a) They necessitate discussion.
(b) They encourage communication about personal and family goals.
(c) They involve negotiation, thus teaching the art of compromise.
(d) They provide an agreement about rules of conduct which cannot be changed unilaterally.

Ideally, contingency contracts contain five elements (Stuart, 1971a). First, a contract details the conditions and privileges each side expects to gain from the contract. For example, parents may want a child to complete his homework and attend school regularly. On the other hand, the child desires more free time with friends, pocket money, or later bedtimes. Second, those target behaviours chosen for the child to fulfil must be readily observable. If the parents or teachers are unable to discern whether an obligation has been met, they cannot grant a privilege. Not surprisingly, some behaviours do not satisfactorily fit into the contract system. Parents cannot always check, for example, whether their adolescent daughter visits certain undesirable friends, so it would be inadvisable to incorporate an agreement not to do so in a contract. Third, the contract imposes sanctions for a failure to fulfil the agreement. The child is told precisely the conditions for failing to meet the terms of the contract and what penalties will be incurred. The sanctions are decided in advance (i.e. agreed to by both sides) and are applied consistently. There can be no arbitrary unilateral tinkering with the arrangements. Fourth, a contract can provide a bonus clause so that extra privileges, special activities, or allowances of free time are available as rewards for consistent performance over a prolonged period. Consistent performance often goes unreinforced in everyday life. It often gets overlooked because adults *expect*, of right, such behaviour* ('Why should I reward him for what he should be doing anyway?') Finally, a contract should have built into it a means of monitoring the rate of positive reinforcement given and received. The records are kept to inform each participant of the progress (or lack of it) of the programme. Behaviours that occur in settings that are not easily observed by the parents or teacher (or whoever is acting as contingency manager) can be monitored by others in those settings. Observations are then reported (by phone, checks on a card, etc.) to the contingency manager, who subsequently provides appropriate consequences.

Contracts are sometimes drawn up between the therapist and the mediator of treatment (e.g., parents) to specify the mutual obligations required of them. Penalty clauses and 'bonus' arrangements (to reinforce the reinforcer/mediator) can be included. These may involve termination of treatment, on the one hand, or a treat (dining out for the parents) or reimbursement of a portion of the fees or return of a deposit (where payments are involved), on the other hand.

*This is often a sticking point for adults in the use of positive reinforcement, when the dreaded word 'bribery' comes up — a delicious irony given our economic philosophies and work ethics (see O'Leary, Poulos, and Devine, 1972).

Token economies

Positive reinforcement can be applied as a group-management procedure, or, as it is called, a token economy programme (Ayllon and Azrin, 1968). The token economy is, in a sense, a work-payment incentive system. The participants receive tokens when they manifest appropriate behaviour and, at some later time, they exchange the tokens for a variety of potent back-up reinforcers — items and activities. These have a prearranged exchange rate. The system parallels the way money is used in society and the economy at large. Kazdin and Bootzin (1972), after a review of the evidence on token economies, list the following advantages: (a) they allow the consequences of any response to be applied at any time, (b) they bridge the delay between target responses and back-up reinforcers, (c) they can maintain performance over extended periods of time when the back-up reinforcers cannot be administered, (d) they allow sequences of responses to be reinforced without interruption, (e) the reinforcing effects of tokens are relatively independent of the physiological state of the individual and less subject to satiation effects (see page 72), and (f) they permit the use of the same reinforcers for individuals with preferences for different back-up reinforcers. Of course, a token economy depends upon the learning theories and behaviour principles which support it. Token reinforcement procedures are not applied in isolation; they are usually supplemented simultaneously by rules, extinction, praise, and response-cost.

An important study entitled 'How to make a token system fail' (Kuypers, Becker, and O'Leary, 1968) suggests important procedures for preempting the things that go wrong. As they remark: 'a token system is not a "magical" method to be applied in a "mechanical way" '.

(b) Stimulus control

Something of a preoccupation in the literature — over the past years — with consequent events, has been most marked in special education, in the case of the development of token economy systems (Bijou, 1973; O'Leary and Drabman, 1971). The major drawback of this focus on outcomes is to do with generalization which is often disappointing and limited. The analysis of antecedent and setting events (stimulus control) offers another (though not necessarily) a separate approach.

Stimulus control has to do with 'the extent to which the value of an antecedent stimulus determines the probability of occurrence of a conditioned response' (Terrace, 1966, p. 271). A frequent complaint from parents is that their child 'won't listen' or 'knows what to do but just won't do it!'. These are examples of faulty stimulus control. The child has a behaviour in his repertoire but will not perform it at the appropriate time, i.e. when the would-be directing stimulus is presented. The therapist has to reinstate stimulus control. The fundamental rule for correcting faulty stimulus control, as for establishing initial stimulus control, is to get the behaviour (or some approximation to it) performed while the child is attending to the stimulus which is to control it. There are several ways to reinstate the discriminative stimulus.*

Differential reinforcement in discrimination training

When a young child is to be taught to act in a particular way under one set of circumstances but not another (in other words, to develop new behaviour), he is helped to identify the cues that differentiate the circumstances. This involves clear signals as to what is expected of the child and it presupposes unambiguous rules. To achieve stimulus control the appropriate behavioural response is repeatedly reinforced in the presence of the S^D, but never in inappropriate circumstances (S^Δ). This process is called *differential reinforcement.*

When the desired response is more likely to occur in the presence of the S^D than in the presence of the S^Δ it is said that *stimulus control* has been established. Discrimination learning or 'training', as it is called, can result in a very high degree of stimulus control. This has implications for the treatment of behaviour problems. The knowledge of these principles can also be used to teach even seriously mentally handicapped children to make very fine discriminations.

Learning always involves knowing *what* to do (the appropriate response) and *when* to do it (under what stimulus conditions the response is appropriate). The acquisition of new behaviour is taught using reinforcement and shaping procedures; it is conditioned to occur appropriately through the application of reinforcement *and* stimulus control techniques. They are not necessarily either/or approaches.

If the child never or only very rarely emits some desired behaviour and if this low rate can be attributed to a deficit in the child's repertoire rather than inadequate incentives, then cueing, prompting, instruction, putting through (sometimes called 'passive shaping'), or modelling should be used so that the behaviour can occur and be reinforced.

Cueing

In order to train a child to act at a specific time it is necessary for him to respond to cues for the correct performance just before the action is expected, rather than after he has performed incorrectly. Thus a child with hostile impulses is helped to respond to signals from his incipient 'feelings' by training him to identify them and the situations in which they occur, and then taking him through self-control procedures rather than letting him know he has gone

---

* Any stimulus that marks a time or place of reinforcement, positive or negative, being presented or removed, is a discriminative stimulus. A discriminative stimulus marks the time or place when an operant will have reinforcing consequences; it does not elicit a response!

wrong after he has lashed out at another child. There are intrinsic and external cues.

The external cues are not always clear. Parents do not always give the child unambiguous signals. They may ask the child to do something, or not to do something, after much soul searching and interior debate. The net effect is prevarication and, even then, the 'command' is likely to be given in a vague uncertain manner or in a voice apprehensive with the expectation of defeat.

Prompting

Prompting is a general term referring to any one cue presented prior to behaviour which increases the probability that the behaviour will occur. It may sometimes be necessary to use prompts in training the child in the sense of giving a child special cues that direct his attention towards the task the adult is trying to teach him. They may also involve showing him what to do or say. For example, the observant mother or teacher may notice that the child is getting white with anger, clenching and unclenching his fists, and draws his attention to his autonomic and central nervous system signals, reminding him to 'count up to ten'. She may be required to help the child verbally and physically through the behaviour of self-control, encouraging him to unclench his fists, holding him back, or in other ways giving him prompts or verbal instructions. Attention is crucial to the establishment of stimulus control. A child will neither learn, nor have the stimulus control, if he does not pay attention to the cues being used to direct his behaviour. Having established stimulus control, a special procedure is still required to maintain stimulus control under changing stimulus conditions. To get a previously taught response to occur to a new signal (cue) the previously taught cue is used as a prompt and then is faded out.

Fading is a procedure for gradually decreasing stimulus control. It is essentially a process of slowly changing the cues in the child's environment, i.e. the gradual removal of discriminative stimuli (S^D) such as cues and prompts. If cues are withdrawn (e.g., prompting the child less and less) the procedure is called *fading out* cues. If new cues are gradually introduced this is called *fading in* cues. A basic objective in therapy and education is the goal of having learned behaviour emitted spontaneously (in response to cues present in the natural environment) rather than always as a response to a specific 'therapeutic' prompt or cue. In order to produce generalization of treatment effects (see page 285), the therapist gradually fades out tangible reinforcers putting reliance eventually upon the more naturally occurring social reinforcers.

(2) RESPONSE ACQUISITION PROCEDURES

(a) Shaping

The process of shaping makes possible the building of a new response, viz. by making reinforcements contingent upon successive approximations of the final behaviour. The use of reinforcement in this context requires a much more sophisticated approach than anything described so far; it involves the use of differential reinforcement and a shifting criterion of reinforcement. In order to encourage a child to act in a way in which he has seldom or never before behaved, approximations to the correct act are rewarded. The successive steps to the final behaviour require an increasingly rigorous criterion of the approximation to be reinforced. The therapist does this by working out the successive steps the child must, and can, make, so as to approximate more and more closely to the desired final outcome. This last element, called 'shaping', or the principle of 'successive approximation', is an important one in behaviour modification; it involves taking mini-steps towards the final goal. The therapist starts by reinforcing very small changes in behaviour which are in the right direction, even if somewhat far removed from the final desired outcome. No reinforcement is given for behaviour in the 'wrong' direction. Gradually the criteria of the individual's approximation to the desired goal are made more rigorous.

(b) Modelling — observational learning

In order to teach a child a new pattern of behaviour the child is given the opportunity to observe a person performing the desired behaviour and the consequences of his actions. The application of modelling to bring about change can be used effectively in at least three clinical situations: (i) acquiring new or alternative patterns of behaviour from the model which the child has never manifested before (e.g., social skills, self-control); (ii) the increase or decrease of responses already in the child's repertoire through the demonstration by high prestige models of appropriate behaviour (e.g., the disinhibition of a shy withdrawn child's speech and social interactions, or the inhibition of learned fears — e.g., phobias of dogs — or the suppression of impulsive, antisocial behaviour); and (iii) the increase in behaviours which the observing child has already learned and for which there are no existing inhibitions or constraints.

With regard to the acquisition of alternative behaviours the following principles provide a useful guide for the therapist: (1) the conditions maintaining the deviant actions should be assessed; (2) the agents of change (e.g. parents) are taught the nature of the changes required to produce a successful outcome in terms of the child's behaviour; (3) alternative socially approved actions have to be modelled (i.e. demonstrated); (4) there is supervised practice of these behaviours; (5) the range of skills relevant to alternative behaviours is widened; (6) successful outcomes of these alternative actions are deliberately arranged for; (7) the child is given constant feedback concerning his performance; (8) the alternative actions will have been arranged and presented in order of difficulty; (9) the newly acquired actions are generalized by eliciting and rewarding them in as many different contexts as is possible (Bandura, 1973).

Some models exert more influence over a child than others, although the reasons why they do so are not adequately explained in the literature. It is usually possible to identify individuals in the child's peer group (or adults) of significance to the child whose behaviour is likely to be imitated because of the *prestige* they have, either for the patient alone or for the entire group in which he interacts (e.g., the popular child at school). The problem in the case of the delinquent youth is that his reference group and his 'heroes' are so often models of deviant behaviour. *Similarity* is another important factor determining imitation. There is evidence that student observers who perceive or who are told that they have some characteristics or qualities similar to the model (e.g., sex, age, and physical attributes) are more likely to imitate other responses of the model than are students who do not identify such similarities (Rosenkrans and Hartup, 1967). Therapists can facilitate imitation by pointing out areas in common between the model and the client. A behaviour is more likely to be modelled if its complexity is not too great or too rapidly presented for assimilation and if the child perceives that it has some components which he has already mastered.

As the observation of exemplary models can influence the acquisition (and the instigation and maintenance) of behaviour — prosocial and antisocial — it follows the prosocial behaviour may be encouraged at the expense of deviant actions by providing models of the former kind. The *consequences* of modelled behaviour are an important determinant of imitation in the child; therefore it is useful to arrange for him to observe models of prosocial behaviour to whom rewards accrue for their actions and to provide models of deviant behaviour who incur aversive consequences.

One of the most obvious methods of facilitating behaviour modification available to the classroom teacher is that of modelling by demonstration. The teacher may, for instance, show a child how to carry out, stage by stage, a particular academic task and then expect the child to imitate his actions. Teachers (like parents) commonly expect children to imitate their own behaviour modelled in areas of personal conduct such as manners. Other modelling strategies include role-play (Boies, 1972) and behaviour rehearsal (Lazarus, 1966).

(c) Cognitive methods

Cognitive learning includes the encoding of information, the postulating of hypotheses, their evaluation, and inductive and deductive reasoning. This category of learning has been neglected in behavioural formulations of childhood deviance, although there are signs of a growing interest in training children in problem solving and cognitive control (see Hobbs et al., 1980; Kendall, 1981; Spivack and Shure, 1973).

One of the objectives in a therapeutic programme may be *cognitive restruc-*

turing (e.g., Masters, 1970). This involves changing the person's characteristic ways of organizing his experiences and producing alternatives. What a person tells himself about his experience affects his behaviour. For example, one youth may tend to *attribute* the causes of what happens to him to forces beyond his control, while another may see himself as having a major influence and say on the unfolding events of his life (see page 248).

Most treatment programmes combine elements of each of the types of learning enumerated above. Thus, in treating a hostile, aggressive child a therapist might attempt to associate calm and relaxation with the anger-provoking stimulus, while also modelling non-aggressive behaviour under provocation and reinforcing any exhibition of pacific behaviour by the child.

(3) RESPONSE DECREMENT PROCEDURES

When a particular behaviour occurs with excessive frequency, intensity, or magnitude, or where a response is emitted under conditions a child's environment considers inappropriate, the therapeutic task is to bring the behaviour within a range that is more socially acceptable. Unlike the child with a behaviour deficit, who has to learn a response that is not in his repertoire, the child with excess behaviour has to learn to modify existing responses. To facilitate this, the therapist has a choice among a variety of techniques which she can use singly or in combination.

(a) Skills training

Many children, because of tragic and depriving life experiences, lack some of the crucial skills required to cope with life in a satisfactory manner. Consequently, they may behave problematically in response to a variety of stresses, frustrations, and humiliations (see page 250). Parents, too, may be taught skills by means, inter alia, of role play. Here is a brief account of how one mother tackled her social isolation at the Centre. The words are hers:

> The hardest problem to deal with was my self-doubt and isolation. Being depressed for several years and feeling an inadequate failure had eroded my self-confidence and produced a profound dislike for myself. It was necessary to change that before I could look up and outwards.
> Dr. H. asked me to role-play as a means of learning new ways of coping with my fears and suspicions of people. I started by writing a self-portrait. (Rereading it recently I was struck by its negative qualities.) Dr. H. took each point and changed it to some extent. Where I was serious, introverted, careful, I was to be rather more spontaneous and impulsive, even a little frivolous — without 'overdoing' it. I was to think and act like an attractive woman; in fact we created a different 'persona' and role to my usual ones, but not too far removed (he said) from reality to make the task impossible.

The next step was not easy. What I had to do was go out and live my role daily. Privately I thought Dr. H. was probably insane! It was certainly very difficult at first. You feel like a second-rate actor with severe stage-fright. But the remarkable thing was how it gradually became easier; and when the results were good I felt elated. I discovered casual conversations with local mothers, in the park or at the shops, soon unearthed common interests and I gradually developed new friendships with women in similar circumstances to myself, all with children for Tommy and Claire to play with. For the first time since Tommy's birth we were making regular visits outside the immediate family. Social skills are like any other. The more practice you get the better you become. As my confidence grew with each success so Tommy also relaxed and he began to look forward to these visits eagerly. Over a period of 2 months Tommy made amazing strides — from short visits to new friends where he would hardly leave my side, to attendance at a state nursery school for 2½ hours daily, where he showed no nervousness at being left at all. Now 8 months on he attends nursery school all day and stays to dinner, has a large circle of friends, and happily attends parties and outings with me.

Socially skilled children tend to be able to deal with provocative situations by compromise actions, persuasion, humour, and other appropriate verbal responses, which not only reduce the provocation but also preserve self-esteem without resort to extremes. By contrast, children who lack social and verbal skills have few choices when it comes to dealing with aggravations and are likely to become aggressive more easily. Thus, they may profit greatly from training in non-aggressive ways of coping with interpersonal conflicts.

There are programmatic texts available which are designed to develop *problem-solving* skills in children (see Spivack and Shure, 1973). Behaviour therapists use role playing as an effective technique to help a person learn new skills through behavioural rehearsal under the direction of a therapist (Lazarus, 1966). A child may be explicitly asked to perform a normal role which is not normally his own, or asked to perform a normal role but not in a setting where it is normally enacted. The method is used to teach youths very basic skills, to help them become more effective in their interactions, and to help them to become more effective when extremely anxious (e.g., through enacting scenes such as using the telephone, going to an interview with an employer, or dealing with provocation). Role playing has been used to help persons effectively interact in situations where they are too anxious. Scenes with increasing degrees of anxiety provocation are enacted in such cases. A variation used with children is emotive imagery (Lazarus and Abramovitz, 1962).

(b) Changing discriminative stimuli

It may be possible to eliminate a behaviour by removing or altering the discriminative stimuli signalling reinforcement or cues signalling punishment.

Stimulus change is the process of changing the discriminative stimuli — the environmental cues — which have been present when problem behaviour has been reinforced in the past. Stimuli associated with rewarded undesirable behaviour are removed — a technique commonly practised by teachers. For example, if a child continually talks to the student next to him the teacher generally moves his desk away. By moving the desk, the teacher is changing the setting that brought about the talking. Otherwise, stimuli that signal the likelihood of punishment for manifesting that behaviour or of reinforcement for alternative (appropriate) behaviour can be provided. Stimulus change has the short-term effect of reducing unwanted behaviour. A return to the original stimulus events is likely to produce a renewal of the problem behaviour. It simply gives the teacher or parent time to encourage some alternative and more appropriate behaviour by using positive reinforcement.

(c) Correcting faulty stimulus control

Guthrie (1935) gives the following illustration of faulty stimulus control and the method used to stop a child being untidy. The behaviour of the child was used to reinstate the S^D:

> The mother of a ten-year-old girl complained to a psychologist that for two years her daughter had annoyed her by a habit of tossing coat and hat on the floor as she entered the house. On a hundred occasions the mother had insisted that the girl pick up the coat and hang it in its place. These wild ways were changed only after the mother, on advice, began to insist not that the girl pick up the fallen garments from the floor but that she put them on, return to the street, and re-enter the house, this time removing the coat and hanging it properly (p.18).

As we saw on page 75, the child must be made to perform the required act while he is attending to the stimulus which is to control it. In the Guthrie example the mother had been getting the response out in the presence of the wrong stimuli. The stimuli which were meant to control the response were those present immediately after the child entered the house. What was going wrong was that the 'tidy' response was being repeatedly evoked in the presence of a stimulus such as the mother saying 'Please pick up your coat'.

(d) Reducing aversive stimuli

Problem behaviour may be instigated in the child by a large variety of aversive stimuli: by bullying and by teasing of a painful, threatening, or humiliating nature, and by deprivation of the proper nurturance, rights, and opportunities that are his due. Reduction of such aversive stimuli may be accompanied by a reduction in the undesired behaviour — a proposal easier to make on paper than to meet in practice. The bleak reality of the lives of many delinquent youths makes the possibilities for the reduction of stress and temptation very limited. A helpful technique involves the defusing of aversive stimuli by diminishing their power to arouse anger in the child. This may be achieved by desensitization procedures or by demonstrating to the young person the value of humour in fraught situations.

(e) Desensitization and relaxation

Relaxation is thought to be incompatible with emotional behaviours such as fright, anger, or frustration. It may be possible to teach a child how to relax when he becomes frustrated, agitated, or angered. In 1938, Jacobson introduced a method for obtaining muscular relaxation which has since been incorporated into many treatment procedures for adults. They have also been used for children.

Relaxation has the advantage that it can be taught like any other skill. If the relaxation exercises have been well practised, the person becomes relaxed when he says to himself, 'relax'. The anger responses which sometimes facilitate aggression might be reduced by desensitization.

(f) Promotion of alternative behaviour

Reinforcement, which is so crucial to the acquisition of behaviour, is also useful in eliminating unwanted responses. For example, the therapist can strengthen (by reinforcement) alternative acts that are incompatible with, or cannot be performed at the same time as, the maladaptive response. Indeed, there are very few occasions where it is desirable only to eliminate a given behaviour without at the same time training the child in some alternative prosocial act.

Principles of operant conditioning are applied to strengthen socially acceptable alternatives. In the case of the so-called hyperactive child (to take one practical example) it is assumed that both environmental and internal stimuli have become conditioned elicitors of classroom behaviours such as squirming, getting out of the seat, walking about the room, looking around, pinching, tapping, and being generally disruptive. The basic approach has been to follow a counter-conditioning paradigm, supplanting hyperactive behaviour by strengthening alternative, incompatible, on-task (attending) behaviour. Positive reinforcers may be administered in accordance with the procedures of the *differential reinforcement of other behaviour* (DRO) or of the *reinforcement of incompatible behaviour* (RIB).

Differential reinforcement of other behaviour (DRO)

In the case of differential reinforcement of other behaviour it is necessary to arrange for reinforcing stimuli to be contingent upon the occurrence of any responses other than the unwanted target behaviour. In addition, the latency between the occurrence of one of these desirable responses and the occurrence of the reinforcing stimulus must be very short.

DRO is indicated in circumstances in which it is desirable to discontinue reinforcement for an undesirable response but it is unwise to decrease the overall quantity of reinforcement the child receives. This is particularly pertinent in the case of conduct-disordered children who so often have been deprived of reinforcing approval. One of the advantages of DRO procedures is that they are relatively simple to use. On the other hand, the problem with DRO methods is their 'sledgehammer' properties. The fact that *any* behaviours other than the undesired one are equally reinforceable gives rise to the possibility that unwanted behaviours may be unwittingly encouraged.

For instance, that hyperactive child we referred to earlier may have failed to perform some required academic task during the specified observation period, but because he is not out of his seat, shuffling his desk, or pinching his neighbour he remains eligible for reinforcement. This complication might be avoided by putting other patterns of undesirable behaviours on a DRO regime as well as hyperactive behaviour. Hopefully there will be enough intervals which merit reinforcement to allow the programme to work. Another problem in the use of a DRO regime is the so-called *behaviour contrast* effect. If hyperactivity is being dealt with by DRO procedures in one situation (say at school) but is rewarded in another situation (at home), then while it decreases under DRO conditions it may actually increase in the rewarded circumstances.

Reinforcement of incompatible behaviour (RIB)

This procedure consists of positively reinforcing a particular class of behaviour which is inconsistent with, or which cannot be performed at the same time as, the unwanted activity. The advantage of this approach is the possibility of choosing a competing behaviour of a prosocial kind to strengthen, while reducing the occurrence of the undesirable behaviour. The process may occur fairly slowly, and it may be helpful to attempt to accelerate the programme with a time-out or response-cost procedure (see pages 90 and 93). It is likely that DRO and RIB are more often beneficial than either punishment or extinction procedures because the net rate of reinforcement the child receives is not diminished and, indeed, may even increase. There are less likely to be the side-effects of protests and rebellion sometimes observed in the case of punishment and extinction procedures because they involve deprivation of reinforcement.

(g) Punishment

Basically there are two punishment procedures. One involves the delivery of some form of aversive stimulation, perhaps a frown, reprimand, or smack, as a consequence of unwanted behaviour. The second consists of following such behaviour by the withdrawal of some reward such as pocket money, television viewing, or a play opportunity, as in the procedures of time-out, response-cost, and overcorrection which are described later.

Punishment is defined as the process of following a response with a stimulus which results in a *decrease* in the rate of responding. Only if a particular stimulus weakens or terminates the particular behaviour on which it is contingent is the process called punishment; spankings are obviously not punitive for some conduct-disordered children because they do not produce a reduction in the non-compliant behaviour which they follow. However, in general it can be said that both withdrawal of positive reinforcement and contingent presentation of an aversive stimulus tend to decrease target behaviour.

Punishment, in one of its forms, obviously requires an aversive stimulus. But what is aversive? However noxious it may seem from a cultural or even physical standpoint, a stimulus is not defined by its *intrinsic* qualities; the effect of the stimulus on the preceding behaviour may appear 'paradoxical', as when scolding by a teacher increases disruptive behaviour in some children rather than decreasing it (Hall et al., 1968). Nowhere in the mythology of child rearing are the legends more potent or misleading than in the area of punishment. As always, the soothsayers of child rearing take up their extreme positions, glowering at each other across the great divide of common sense. 'Spare the rod and spoil the child!' says the one side; 'You are teaching him to fear and hate you when you punish him' replies the other. The trouble is that punishment always seems to be equated with hitting or hurting when, in fact, it involves much more complex issues. Even the most permissive of parents, intentionally or unintentionally, punish their children in the course of bringing them up. To quote Walters, Cheyne, and Banks (1972, p.14):

> If virtue is its own reward, the acquisition thereof is fraught with inherent punishment. Parents not only whip, spank and beat children, they scold, shout at, isolate and withdraw love from their children, sometimes at the slightest provocation. Many permissive parents who would never dream of beating or otherwise hurting their child may frequently utter a harsh word or send the child from the room for misbehaving. Such actions may cut as deep or more deeply than all but the most violent of thrashings.

In child-rearing practice, punishment usually refers to any intentional action by one individual which has aversive emotional consequences (such as anxiety, fear, embarrassment, guilt, disappointment, pain, and so on) for the child, and which he is subsequently motivated to *avoid*. The problem with this definition is that some people may seek punishment, for example, if it terminates feelings of guilt.

The popularity of punishment as a means of modifying behaviour for parents and teachers may be due (to some extent) to the fact that is often reinforced in the user by the immediate (if temporary) cessation of the child's misdemeanour. The more general and, indeed, long-term consequences of punishment in everyday life may not be constructive. It is likely to be applied in the heat of the moment, which may mean that it is extreme and retaliatory. It may be ill-timed and inconsistent, on the other hand, because it is done in 'cold blood' when father comes home or threatened but not carried out.

Punishment, if fierce, tends to preclude the choice and encouragement of more acceptable substitute behaviours. Punishment alone tells a child what he cannot do but not what he can do. Several researchers have urged caution in the use of punishment with children (be it withdrawal of positive reinforcement or the use of aversive stimuli). Aggressive adult behaviour might provide an undesirable model for the child and in addition it may lead to the adult losing his own reinforcing value. Frequent and intense punishment may stimulate escape behaviour such as running away and truancy.

Skinner (1953) concludes that the consequences of punishment on a target behaviour are short-term and he describes three effects: arrest of the target behaviour; a conditioned autonomic response, emotionality; and a conditioned skeletal-motor response, escape or avoidance. He suggests that these could give rise to undesirable side-effects such as hesitancy and indecisiveness caused by approach-avoidance conflict, and possibly fear, anxiety, rage, and frustration which may interfere with normal social functioning. Mowrer's (1960) view is that punishment does not lead to extinction of a learned deviant response because it does not constitute a reversal of the learning process by which it was acquired. Rather it represents the learning of an additional response incompatible with the maladaptive response, thus leading to its suppression. Withdrawal of the aversive consequence may lead to the re-appearance of the target response. Punishment in this view is a fear-conditioned process.

A review (Marshall, 1965) of the research on the effects of punitive consequences such as blame, reproof, failure situations, and the word 'wrong', as well as the removal of positive reinforcers, but *not* physical punishment on children reveals that, in general, such negative reinforcers tend to improve learning and performance of various school tasks. There is no simple, clear-cut relationship between negative reinforcement and performance. Other factors found to influence the consequences of punishment include intellectual and achievement level; the complexity of the task, delay of reinforcement, instructions, the subject's and experimenter's personality, the atmosphere in the home or classroom, and so on. The fact that so many factors interact in a complex fashion explains the inconsistent results of various experiments on punishment.

Aversive stimulation

The effectiveness of aversive stimulation in instrumental conditioning is dependent on its severity. If the stimulus is severely aversive, a fear response may be elicited which incapacitates the organism to such a degree that it is unable to emit the response which will allow it to escape the aversive stimulus. Learning is incompatible with strong anxiety. On the other hand, a very mild aversive stimulus may be insufficient to provoke an escape, i.e, it is indiscriminable. This principle was established by Yerkes and Dodson (1908) through animal experimentation and is known as the Yerkes–Dodson law, which can be stated as follows: the optimum level of aversive stimulation in the control of learning is at some moderate intensity, lower and higher values being less effective.

Apart from ethical misgivings about applying aversive stimulation to a child there are a number of adverse side-effects commonly attributed to the use of punishment. One of these, as we saw above, is that punishment may increase anxiety or aggressiveness, because it constitutes an aversive experience. The latter is most likely because the punishing adult models aggressive means of dealing with provocation which the child may imitate. This would be most invidious in the case of the already aggression-prone conduct-disordered child. The risk of this occurring can be minimized by using a punishment procedure involving withdrawal of reinforcement rather than the delivery of aversive stimulation, and by combining this with the reinforcement of alternative behaviour.

Extinction (withdrawal of reinforcement)

Extinction is the term used to describe the relatively permanent *unlearning* of a behaviour (the elimination of a behaviour from a person's repertoire). It also applies to a procedure by which reinforcement that has previously followed an operant behaviour is discontinued. For example, to stop a child from acting in a disruptive attention-seeking manner, conditions are arranged so that he receives no reinforcement (attention) following the maladaptive act. It is thought essential that the behaviour *should occur* in order for extinction to take place, for only then are the internal motivating factors truly weakened. So no restraint is put upon the child.

Rimm and Masters (1974) observe that according to this theoretical model severe punishment tends to *suppress* behaviour rather than extinguish it. The behaviour is only likely to be performed a very few times, perhaps only once in the instance of intense punishment, before it ceases entirely. The prediction is that punishment will be ineffective because suppression behaviours tend to recur while extinguished ones do not. Such theorizing has led to the present emphasis upon the encouragement in the child of alternative behaviours that are mutually exclusive to the undesirable ones which are being punished. The training of these behaviours may take place during the period of suppression that follows punishment.

Thus, what we generally have in the design of a programme of extinction is the careful assessment of the contingencies currently operating to maintain deviant behaviour and the planned elimination of such contingent reinforcement. Often these contingencies involve social reinforcement, and the reinforcing agents (parents, teachers) are requested to offer their attention, responsiveness, and smiles contingently upon behaviours *other* than the undesirable one, and to 'grit their teeth' but look away, leave the room, or divert their attention to someone else when the maladaptive behaviour occurs.

Children tend, when it comes to attention, to be like that actress who said she would rather have bad publicity than no publicity at all. Nagging may be a poor thing but at least it *is* attention. Thus an interesting point about the maintenance of deviant behaviour is that much unwanted behaviour is unwittingly reinforced by parents and teachers because they pay attention to the child (even though it be scolding or nagging) when he acts in that way. The mother often ignores her child when he is behaving well but interacts with him as soon as he begins to cause trouble. One way or another she may be providing a form of reinforcement. This sequence of events is probably widespread and may account for much of the maladaptive behaviour on the part of children attending clinics, especially those who are emotionally deprived.

Patterson (1971) has reported, on the basis of 10 hours of observation of each of seven families, that the parents of deviant children provided attention, interest, approval, and positive physical contact as a consequence of behaviour such as shouting, hitting, and non-compliance. The positive reinforcement was sufficient to offset any aversive consequences, which (in the form of nagging, scolding, or threats) were usually mild *if* at all noxious. Studies (e.g. Wahler, 1969a) have consistently demonstrated that when parents change their approach so that the child's desired behaviours receive reinforcement from them while undesirable behaviours are ignored or punished, his behaviour changes in desired directions. Often this change is dramatic.

Teachers are also likely to attend to pupils when they are difficult and rowdy. Walker and Buckley (1973), for example, found that 18 per cent. of a teacher's attention to 'non-problem' children was for inappropriate behaviour while 89 per cent. of her attention to 'problem' children was for undesirable classroom behaviour. Furthermore, 77 per cent. of the attention given to all the observed children was bestowed on the disruptive children. The same pattern is seen in institutions for the mentally subnormal, where a child exhibits some form of undesirable (say self-injurious) behaviours and attendants terminate the behaviour by restraining the child. Such *attention* — a commodity which is very precious in an institution where stimulation, affection, and self-esteem are sometimes in short supply — may reinforce the self-mutilation.

The process of withholding reinforcements such as approval, attention, and the like, which have previously and inappropriately been contingent on the production of inappropriate responses, provides the therapist with a potent therapeutic method to extinguish or decrease the frequency of such responses. When this approach is combined with methods that promote alternative patterns of behaviour that are considered socially acceptable it can achieve enduring changes in prosocial behaviour. For extinction to be effective it must be used consistently. It also requires persistence. This presupposes that the maintaining reinforcers of the maladaptive behaviour have been identified. A point worth noting is that the choice of punishment procedures rather than extinction — when it *is* possible to identify inappropriate reinforcers of deviant behaviour — is probably doomed to failure. To achieve their full impact the aversive consequences of punishment would need to equal or exceed in strength the maintaining reinforcers already present.

To withhold reinforcers appears easy in principle. However, as therapists have found out to their cost (and the cost of their neat and tidy therapeutic programmes), people other than parents or teachers often provide the offending reinforcement. So it may be difficult in practice, in the untidy and unpredictable world outside the laboratory, to gain contingency control. The therapist has to assess whether she is in a position to arrange for the crucial reinforcers to be withheld. There are obvious problems; a deviant act may provide intrinsic satisfaction and pleasure (self-approbation) over and above the external reinforcement inherent in the adult paying anxious attention to it. If a child plays up in the classroom the child may still obtain reinforcement from his peers although the teacher ignores his behaviour. Then again, some behaviour is so disruptive of others, or so destructive, that it just cannot be ignored in the hope that it will eventually extinguish. In some cases it has proved necessary to supplement extinction by procedures designed to short-circuit these difficulties, Carlson et al. (1968) reinforced classmates for ignoring certain aspects of the client's behaviour. Kubany, Weiss, and Sloggett (1971) reinforced the peers contingent upon his improvement.

Characteristically, when a behaviour no longer results in reinforcement, the child will increase the frequency and/or intensity of the behaviour in an attempt to reinstitute and guarantee reinforcers (the so-called 'extinction burst'). And he may go to some lengths to bring them back. It is therefore advisable to warn parents or teachers that the child's behaviour which they are expecting him to abandon with extinction may temporarily increase in frequency after reinforcement is withdrawn. Otherwise they may mistakenly conclude that the procedure is not working and abandon it prematurely. Persistence with the withdrawal of reinforcement (given an accurate clinical formulation) usually results in extinction.

Training alternative prosocial behaviours while maladaptive ones are being extinguished may provide one way of countering the child's disconcerting intensification of problematic behaviour in response to decreased reinforcement.

Sometimes the unwanted behaviour which has been successfully extinguished returns, to everyone's dismay, after a period. This may occur when the child returns (say) to his classroom after a holiday. In learning terms this is referred to (paradoxically, for the clinician) as 'spontaneous recovery'. Extinction procedures are most suitable for the reduction of behaviours whose temporary continuance and (possibly) exacerbation before extinction can be tolerated. This would exclude high-intensity assaultive and self-injurious acts. Another consideration is the possibility of imitation by other children. If this is a major concern then extinction *alone* is probably not an appropriate choice of treatment procedure.

We saw (on page 71) that the rate at which behaviour is extinguished is a function of the schedule of reinforcement by which the behaviour was acquired and/or maintained. The optimal situation for therapy is when the target has been consistently reinforced; extinction then tends to occur relatively swiftly. Ratio schedules produce behaviour which is resistant to extinction. There is a tendency for behaviour to persist at a high rate but to reduce fairly suddenly when it is about to extinguish. Interval schedules of reinforcement are particularly resistant to extinction and removal of reinforcers may result in a continuation of responses at a low but rather persistent rate. Knowledge of the reinforcement history of the child's maladaptive behaviours could provide a helpful appreciation to the therapeutic difficulties that lie ahead. It may be advisable in some cases to put the unwanted behaviour (and it obviously depends on the kind of behaviour) on a continuous schedule of reinforcement so as to take advantage of the 'contrast effect' when extinction is begun.

When extinction procedures have been decided upon, there are cogent reasons for providing positive reinforcement (e.g., praise) contingent upon alternative behaviours. For example, if the performance of the deviant behaviour being extinguished occupies a fairly substantial amount of time before it is completed, the youth obviously has to find *something* to do during the time previously taken up by carrying out the offending behaviour. If this activity can be channelled into socially acceptable lines, it could become the object of the reinforcement formerly contingent upon the unwanted behaviour. This would be a timely opportunity to model or shape appropriate alternative behaviours in the child. It is probably too much to hope that the youngster will necessarily and of his own accord turn to socially desirable actions once the target problems are extinguished.

As with punishment procedures, extinction methods on their own do not indicate to the child the kind of actions that should replace the unwanted ones. The alternatives could indeed be as problematic, including aggression or absconding. At the best of times, ignoring inappropriate behaviour is a particularly difficult thing for some parents and certainly for most hard-pressed teachers to do. Here then is a further reason for trying to facilitate the extinction process by combining the procedures.

The possibility of obtaining reinforcement by other means may hasten the renunciation of deviant behaviour. Sadly, some children do appear to get worse rather than better when their parents ignore deviant behaviour and attend to more appropriate behaviour (Birnbrauer, 1985; Herbert et al., 1973; Sajwaj, Twardosz, and Burke, 1972). Why should this be? Several explanations have been put forward. It may not be certain that attention by caretakers was definitely the reinforcer for the disruptive behaviour of the child observed. Thus it is feasible that removal of the parent's or teacher's attention following the deviant behaviour does not really constitute extinction. Even where it is considered unnecessary to introduce additional procedures in order to maximize therapeutic control over reinforcement, it is likely that residual minor sources of reinforcement for deviant behaviour may go unnoticed after withholding the more powerful reinforcers. These leftover low-potential reinforcers continue to subvert attempts to extinguish behaviours. There is still

90

obviously a need for further research to make it possible to use combined extinction and reinforcement regimes with greater discrimination and effectiveness.

Time-out from positive reinforcement (TO)

TO provides another means of reducing specified actions by the withdrawal of reinforcement — a classical penalty system. TO is a period of time during which the child is prevented from emitting the problematic behaviour (say a tempertantrum) in the situation in which it has been positively reinforced in the past.

This procedure, then, is intended to reduce the frequency of an undesirable behaviour by ensuring that it is followed by a reduction in the opportunity to acquire reinforcement, or rewards. In practice one can distinguish three forms of time-out:

(a) 'Activity time-out', where a child is simply barred from joining in an enjoyable activity, but still allowed to observe it — e.g., being required to sit out of a game, having misbehaved;
(b) 'room time-out', where the child may be removed from an enjoyable activity, not allowed to observe it but not totally isolated — e.g., standing outside a classroom having misbehaved;
(c) 'seclusion time-out', where the child is socially isolated in a situation from which he cannot voluntarily escape.

In practice 'activity' or 'room' time-out is generally to be preferred (as a *least intrusive* method) to any form of 'seclusion' time-out. TO periods rarely exceed 15 minutes and are usually a lot shorter than this.

A critical determinant of the effectiveness of TO is the extent to which the youngster actually enjoys the situation from which he is removed. If that situation is positively frightening, anxiety provoking or boring it is possible that the TO procedure might involve removing the child to a less aversive situation and thereby actually *increase*, rather than decrease, the frequency of the inappropriate behaviour.

Not unnaturally, some non-compliant preschool children strongly resist TO initially. For instance, TO can lead to tantrums, crying, screaming and physical assault, especially if the child is taken by force. Warning children of the contingencies (e.g., 'If you have a tantrum whilst on TO you will remain in TO longer') does not necessarily decrease the resistance to TO.

Another problem encountered with TO (Forehand and McMahon, 1981) is that if TO is mastered early, children's problem behaviour may well be reduced, but without the concomitant use of the so-called phase I skills (in which parents *attend differentially* to acceptable and unacceptable actions) the parent–child interaction can remain a somewhat negative one.

The child removed for misbehaving, may or may not continue to display the tantrum in the TO room; the point is that it is being ignored. However, TO differs from extinction. In the case of extinction, the reinforcers which are withdrawn are those specifically *identified* in terms of their maintaining function with regard to the deviant behaviour. TO, in contrast, involves the temporary withdrawal of *most* of the reinforcement currently available to the child. In a sense, extinction by socially ignoring disruptive behaviours constitutes a focused TO.

The TO room (sometimes referred to as a quiet room) is made non-reinforcing by being cleared of its entertainment value (Leitenberg, 1965). The child is warned in advance about those of his behaviours that are considered inappropriate and the consequences that will flow from them. It is essential that the child sees that the consequences of his maladaptive behaviours are predictable and inevitable. The mother must be consistent and timely with her use of the procedure. Herbert and Iwaniec (1981) have found it important to spend time in the home supervising the programme (especially in its early stages) and, when necessary, prompting the mother. The use of dolls or puppets combined with role-plays helps the child (and parents) to understand the contingencies and sequencing of TO.

It is generally considered advisable not to threaten at length but to carry out the removal consequence after failure to comply with a signal which is used as soon as, and every time, the deviant behaviour occurs. This requires a clear specification of the rules before the behaviour occurs. A stimulus associated with and discriminative for TO can acquire conditioned punishing properties, and thus lead to behaviour suppression. If so, the full TO sequence may not have to be administered in some instances. The presentation of the pre-TO stimulus which might consist of a verbal warning ('Stop that, or you'll have to go into time-out'), a warning look, or a gesture may be enough to suppress the target behaviour. Verbal warnings frequently give rise to an argument over whether a TO is justified. So parents are advised not to get into reinforcing disputations with the child. Some non-verbal stimulus may be suggested; a special 'watch out' hand signal is handy to use and only requires that the parent attract the child's attention. TO is made contingent — and promptly so — upon the child's ignoring of the signal and persisting with the maladaptive behaviour. The child is told (or made) to go to the TO room for a defined period of time. (The author has found it useful to get the mother to set a kitchen timer so that she, and usually the child, receives a signal when the time is up.)

For younger children the time may be 3 to 5 minutes, for children of perhaps 8 years and older, longer. Periods of 10 to 15 minutes are usually felt to be the maximum desirable duration. Ten-minute TO's are typically used in classroom situations.

Although a minimum period of exclusion is usually specified, if the child continues to act in a maladaptive manner during TO, then TO is persisted with (in the Centre's practice) until the disruption ceases. The purpose of such extensions is to avoid the possibility of release from TO acting as a reinforcer for the continuation of the unwanted behaviour, Johnston (1972) points out in his review of the effects of punishment on human behaviour that various criteria have been used for scheduling release from TO: (a) when the punished response terminates, (b) after the end of some undesirable behaviour plus some predetermined additional time interval, or (c) following the occurrence of some appropriate response. One possible problem with the use of (c) is that the TO may lose its aversive properties for the child who learns that he can be released nearly immediately from TO should he quickly begin to behave in an appropriate fashion. Is he free simply to return immediately to the original situation having experienced no more than a very mild and probably ineffective punishment? Some therapists have made release from TO, following a specified minimum period, contingent upon the child stopping his disruptive behaviour (e.g., Sachs, 1973). Other studies (e.g., Hamilton, Stephens, and Allen, 1967) have used a TO of constant duration not contingent on the patient's behaviour during TO. Hobbs and Forehand (1975) compared the effects of contingent and non-contingent release procedures on disruption during TO and non-compliance outside of TO. Contingent release yielded better results in twelve children aged from 4 to 6½.

Mothers almost invariably state that they have tried (and often failed) with a version of TO. Sending a child to his room for unspecified periods of time is not TO, especially when the procedure is undermined by the presence of entertaining books and toys and (most important) the absence of clear-cut contingency rules. Nor is TO the unethical practice of confining him in a dark and frightening place. O'Leary (1972) points out that teachers have long used the procedure of placing a child at the side of the room, in the back of a room, in a corner, or in days gone by on a dunce's chair. Such a situation has a number of counterproductive effects for the child. He is in the limelight, possibly acting the buffoon and therefore still the centre of attention. Or he is getting out of doing some unwelcome scholastic task. A lightweight screen for use in the classroom may overcome both these difficulties.

Obviously TO has to be carefully planned and its implications in a particular setting thought through. The drawback with TO, if prolonged, is that isolation suppresses *all* activity, including desirable alternative behaviours. It thereby reduces opportunities for encouraging more desirable behavioural change through positive reinforcement. TO sometimes arouses tantrums or rebellious behaviour such as crying, screaming, and physical attacks, particularly if the child has to be physically taken to a quiet room. With older, physically resistive children the method may not be feasible for the last-named reason. Most children, in the author's experience, are prepared (surprisingly) to stay in TO, although a door may have to be locked. Very rarely are children destructive, but, if so, precautions have to be taken in the choice and preparation of the TO room. In some homes there just is no such room! Additional difficulties to be aware of are the possibility that the child may adapt to the TO situation by acquiring new means of obtaining reinforcement, such as self-stimulation or fantasy, and the possibility that adults who have initial reservations about TO are likely to use the procedure tentatively and inconsistently.

Where it is difficult or counter-productive to remove the child himself, an equivalent of TO may be instituted by removing the primary sources of reinforcement from him. So if the mother is a major source of reinforcement she could be advised to remove herself, together with a magazine, to the bathroom, locking herself in when her child's temper-tantrums erupt and coming out only when all is quiet. This method is especially helpful when the behaviour to be eliminated is an extraordinarily compelling one that all but demands attention (reinforcement) from those present or when TO is difficult to administer because the child is a strong and protesting boy and the procedure calls for isolating him against his will.

Response-cost (RC)

Parents often withhold love, approval, and privileges when their children are 'naughty'. This is an informal use of RC which essentially refers to the withdrawal of specified amounts of reinforcement from the child contingent upon his displaying unwanted behaviours which have been specified in advance. In effect the child pays a penalty for violating the rules; the withdrawal of reinforcers constitutes the 'cost' of the maladaptive action. RC is thus another penalty procedure which seeks to reduce the future probability of a response. The method — in the form of loss of points, money, tokens, privileges, etc. — is applied in token economy programmes in the classroom (McIntyre, Jensen, and Davis, 1968) in institutions (Burchard and Barrera, 1972; Kaufman and O'Leary, 1972) and in home settings (see Kazdin, 1972).

Points or tokens are easier to withdraw than primary reinforcers and, as they are used for rewarding desirable behaviours, their withdrawal for incorrect behaviour makes for a convenient and effective symmetry in treatment. A study by McIntire, Jensen, and Davis (1968) illustrates the method at work. They used a RC procedure in an after-school programme for elementary and junior high school boys. Each child had a counter on which a teacher could either add or subtract points. The child gained points for correct answers and lost points for disruptive classroom behaviour. Whenever disruptive behaviour occurred, the instructor would turn on the counter associated with that student's name and allow the counter to continue to subtract points until the instructor felt that that student had corrected himself.

Gottman and Leiblum (1974) suggest that in order to put a RC contingency into effect:

(a) Some level of positive reinforcement must be administered to the child (so that there will be something to withdraw if necessary).
(b) The value of conditioned reinforcers such as tokens, points, or money have to be established for use in the programme.

As with other behavioural methods there are individual differences in the reactions of children to RC procedures (Burchard and Barrera, 1972). Their results support the notion that the actual aversiveness of TOs and RCs appears to be a function of the child's interactions, within a particular social context, the way in which they are implemented, and his reinforcement history.

It is obviously essential to determine the reaction of each individual child and adapt the treatment programme accordingly. As with other procedures containing a punitive element it is necessary to make clear to the child in advance precisely the 'cost' (in the form of fines, etc.) for each unwanted behaviour. Consistency, immediacy, and knowledge of results (feedback) are crucial to a RC programme. The child has to learn that his maladaptive acts will be consistently punished; this involves applying the cost immediately after the unwanted act has occurred. Feedback means ensuring the child has information about which of his actions produced the consequence of a penalty.

If costs become too high and the reinforcement rate too low, or vice versa, the programme is likely to fail. It is common practice for prompts to be arranged. For example, in the classroom situation a card on the child's desk is used to list the deviant behaviours and the points he will lose if he emits them. In addition, the child may receive information about his performance, i.e. consistent and immediate feedback about the consequences of his behaviour.

In the use of RC, there is no time restriction before reinforcement is available as there is with TO. For example, a child may have to pay a fine for disruptive behaviour in the classroom. Having been fined, there is no fixed period of time during which positive reinforcers are beyond the reach of the child, as is the case if he is placed in a room for 10 minutes for the same maladaptive behaviour. Another difference between the RC and TO procedures is the amount of reinforcement lost. A *specified* amount of the reinforcers is withdrawn in the case of the former, whereas *all* reinforcers are withdrawn (for a specified time) in the latter.

There is a paucity of evidence regarding the proper use or effectiveness of the RC method. In particular there is little information concerning the relative effectiveness of RC and TO. Burchard and Barrera (1972) carried out a study to analyse the effectiveness of several values of TO and RC and, additionally, to compare their relative effectiveness in suppressing undesirable behaviour. A further aim was to analyse the conditions under which TOs or RCs become effective. A group of mildly retarded adolescents with high rates of anti-social behaviour was exposed to two parameters of TO and RC within the context of a programmed (token economy) environment. The results indicated that both types of aversive control are similarly suppressive, even when the opportunity to emit a TO offence is controlled. From a practical point of view, there were at least two advantages favouring the use of a RC. One is that RC does not remove the subject from the opportunity to engage in desirable behaviour. From that stand-point, any time spent in TO (as we saw earlier) is, in a sense, wasted time. Because a RC does not remove the subject from the ongoing situation it avoids this particular problem. The second advantage is that by not removing the child from the situation which is unfolding and which involves choices about whether to behave or misbehave, the child is provided with a more realistic learning situation. He is given the opportunity either to continue to perform the behaviour and be punished, or not persist in the undesirable behaviour and experience no punishment, or preferably some reinforcement. By placing the subject in TO, the opportunity to make such a decision is taken away from him and thus the control is less self-directed. The mother, by placing the child in a quiet room, has made the decision for him and by the time he returns to the scene of combat the provocative aspects of the situation are likely to have dissipated. The distinction between allowing the subject the opportunity to control his own behaviour and removing the opportunity to engage in additional unacceptable behaviour is analogous to what is referred to as internal *versus* external control (Aronfreed, 1968).

Comparisons have been made between RC and other methods with favourable findings for the RC approach. The persistence of punishment effects depends upon several carefully investigated variables (Azrin and Holz, 1966). The variables controlling the longevity of effects when reinforcers are withdrawn (RC or TO) have been less thoroughly studied. However, laboratory studies show that reinforcer withdrawal is often superior to the presentation of a negative reinforcer in controlling behaviour (McMillan, 1967; Tolman and Mueller, 1964). In studies using RC, behaviours which are abandoned do not always reappear when the contingency is withdrawn. In two of three RC studies reported by Phillips (1968, Expt. I, V.) the behaviour of pre-delinquent boys did not deteriorate when fines were lifted for 30 days. There is some evidence (Kaufman and O'Leary, 1972) that the use of RC does not produce undesirable side-effects, even when used with particularly vulnerable children, and that RC does not lead to an increase of disruptive behaviour. Even though children could have removed themselves from the situation (in the former study) to avoid a fine for inappropriate behaviour they did not. Like TO procedures, RC can be combined in many situations with positive reinforcement for pro-social behaviour.

Overcorrection

Another form of response-cost or penalty recently investigated is referred to as *overcorrection*. With overcorrection we have a method combining positive reinforcement and aversive control, which is used to discourage inappropriate or disruptive behaviour. Two types of overcorrection have been described (Foxx and Azrin, 1973). The first, *restitutional overcorrection*, requires the youth to correct the consequences of his misbehaviour. The person who has engaged in the inappropriate behaviour not only remedies the situation he has caused, but also 'overcorrects' it to a better-than-normal situation. He makes restitution by performing some work as a penalty for maladaptive behaviour; he is required to restore the disrupted situation to a better state than existed before the disruption. For example, a violent child in a residential establishment who overturns a dining table might be required to set all the tables in that refectory after the meal. Setting the table that was overturned corrects the situation that the violent behaviour disrupted; setting all the other tables is the 'overcorrection'.

The second component of overcorrection is an extensive rehearsal of the correct forms of appropriate behaviour (Foxx and Azrin, 1972). This is called *positive practice overcorrection* and it requires the individual to practise correct behaviours contingent upon episodes of misbehaviour. For example, in the case of stealing, the thief is required to give extra items to the victim; with aggression, the aggressor is required to comfort the victim. This kind of approach could seem vindictive to the child. To defuse it of that possibility, the teacher explains to the student that the additional practice is needed only because the student had not yet learned the proper skill.

Overcorrection is an aversive stimulus. It requires effort to complete the overcorrection. Also, the child cannot engage in other (possibly disruptive) behaviour while he completes the overcorrection task. Here is another function of the overcorrection procedure: to bring to an end any inappropriate rein-forcement (e.g., attention) associated with the deviant behaviour. Stealing results in the thief acquiring goods he desires; turning over a table might get a child attention and concern from the peer group or from an otherwise busy ward staff. The thief is made to return the stolen goods to the shop and make some restitution; the violent child must set *all* the tables. In addition, the overcorrection procedure itself is often educative, in that the process of restoring the original situation generally requires the individual to engage in appropriate behaviour. This can be positively reinforced.

SELF-CONTROL TRAINING

Self-control and external control can be conceptualized as opposite ends on a *continuum* rather than absolutely distinct procedures. Self-control techniques involve an important assumption — namely, that mediational processes oper-ate in human learning (Mahoney, 1972) and that these internal actions obey the same laws or principles as external actions do. Thus, a child can be encouraged to reward himself either covertly (by engaging in very positive self-thoughts and self-statements) or overtly (by indulging in a favourite activity). The sources of antecedent and outcome control may be in a person's own symbolic processes rather than his physiological changes or external environment, and the therapeutic endeavour thus becomes concerned with the manipulation of these symbolic sources of control. While arguments will continue about the use of the term 'self-control', there is general agreement that self-controlling behaviours are a product of the same principles of control as are publicly accessible behaviours.

Bandura (1969) and others have reviewed many research studies that generally support this assumption. The assumption of a correspondence be-tween internal and external action opens the door to a great variety of covert self-rewards and self-punishments. The self-control procedures which have been applied to clinical problems are (a) covert sensitization, (b) contingency management, (c) self-punishment, (d) self-reinforcement, (e) contract management, (f) self-confrontation, (g) self-administered behavioural analysis, (h) self-monitoring, and (i) altering the discriminative stimuli for the target response.

The choice of therapeutic strategies is a wide one. They are derived mainly from principles of respondent, instrumental, and observational learning and they incorporate methods of self-regulation and cognitive restructuring. The point is that they are applied systematically to produce change in some observable behaviour. This process is monitored throughout as rigorously as possible so as to indicate whether the treatment objectives are being reached or not.

Skinner (1953) maintains that the behavioural processes involved in a person's control of himself are the same as those one would use in controlling the behaviour of others. We have seen that the ability to delay gratification is one expression of self-control. The individual has free access to reward, but does not partake of it until he has performed some desired response. Self-reinforcement, then, becomes an important therapeutic issue in the operant approach to self-control. Bandura and Perloff (1967) have been able to demonstrate that self-reinforcement can alter the likelihood that a person will behave in a certain manner.

Most self-management programmes combine techniques that involve standard-setting, self-monitoring, self-evaluation, and self-reinforcement (which also involves self-specification of contingencies and self-administration of reinforcement). Before a child can be taught to reinforce himself for a behaviour pattern, he must learn to evaluate his behaviour correctly. To teach a child to properly evaluate his own behaviour, he must be taught to use some sort of standard by which he can measure his own behaviour. He also needs to attend to his own behaviour, monitoring it accurately. For example, he will have to learn to 'read' the signs of his own feelings (for example, hostility) and to label them correctly. If he hits out at another child, he will require a standard for evaluating his act as antisocial and therefore as grounds for criticizing (i.e. punishing) himself. Or, if he desists from lashing out, praising himself (reinforcement) for showing self-control.

The reliability of self-monitoring, when compared to independent measures of the same behaviour, varies widely in different situations (Kazdin, 1973). While some researchers have reported high correspondence between self-monitoring and independent observations, others have found that subjects vary greatly in the accuracy of self-monitoring. As an assessment instrument, therefore, self-monitoring may be useful only when independent observations are used to check on the client's reports. Self-monitoring does not only provide the clinician and client with a baseline record of target behaviour for treatment purposes; in some instances the observed behaviour may actually change in a favourable direction. Clinical practice has therefore attempted to utilize self-monitoring as a therapeutic technique.

Broden, Hall and Mitts (1971) describe two examples of self-recording with problem children. In one, a girl tallied her own on-task during lecture periods and later presented her records to a counsellor (not the class teacher) at a weekly meeting. The counsellor praised her if the record was good. Observation showed a significant increase in on-task behaviour even though the class teacher did not participate in this part of the experiment. In the second experiment, a boy recorded his calling-out behaviour, but did not show his results to anybody. Although there was an initial decrease in the disruptive behaviour, this trend was not sustained, suggesting that self-recording without additional reinforcement such as praise was insufficient to maintain desirable behaviour change. Glynn, Thomas and Shee (1973) used random intermittent taped signals in a self-record programme. When children heard the signal they recorded their behaviour of the previous 5 seconds as on- or off-task. Free time was awarded as reinforcement for on-task behaviour. Observer checks were made of the children's self-evaluation; it was found that the mean accuracy was 76 per cent., and the 24 per cent. mean inaccuracy was composed of 15 per cent. too lenient assessments and 9 per cent. too harsh.

Self-control of antecedent conditions

These procedures involve the manipulation of those eliciting, reinforcing, or discriminative stimuli in the youngster's symbolic processes which influence his maladaptive behaviour. There are popular fallacies concerning self-control. Many people seem to be of the opinion that the 'badge' for self-control has to be earned by being able to resist any and all temptation. (And, indeed, resistance to temptation is an aspect of self-control.) However, the therapist does not conceptualize the task as a sort of moral struggle between will-power and the forces of self-indulgence. For her, the test of self-control is in the ability (and inclination) to minimize temptation by the early interruption of behavioural sequences which end up in the transgression of some self-imposed standard. When behaviour is under stimulus control it should be possible for a youngster to eliminate or weaken unwanted behaviour and increase desired behaviour by modifying his environment in certain ways.

The adolescent girl with a weight and eating problem might make a rule never to eat anywhere but at her place at the table and then at specified times, and to remove herself from food stimuli whenever possible, by avoiding the kitchen and by asking her siblings not to eat cakes and sweets in front of her. There are several methods of stimulus control which involve building in appropriate stimulus–response connections. One such method is the technique of cue strengthening. This requires that conditions be made favourable for the person to practise the response in a specific situation where previously it was not associated strongly to any set of environmental cues. Take the student whose study behaviour is virtually absent. He might be encouraged to study in a certain specified location so that stimuli associated with that location come to connote study behaviour. Another method involves narrowing or tightening stimulus control. An overall pattern of behaviour may be especially maladaptive because it is practised in a wide variety of situations. Some obese children have acquired the habit of eating while watching television, reading or playing. Narrowing means restricting the behaviour to a limited set of stimuli. For example, as we saw above, eating might be limited to the dinner table at certain times of the day, with the television off.

Self-instruction

This provides another antecedent control procedure. The effects of self-instruction were investigated by Luria (1961), who found that children with a particular brain dysfunction could not press a balloon when an external signal such as a light was flashed. When the children were taught to instruct themselves (to say 'press' as they pressed the balloon), they could press the balloon without errors. Luria's research with children, has led him to propose three stages in the verbal control of the initiation and inhibition of voluntary motor behaviours. During the first stage, the speech of others, usually adults, controls and directs a child's behaviour. The second stage is characterized by the child's overt speech becoming an effective regulator of his behaviour. Finally, the child's covert or inner speech comes to assume a self-governing role.

There is a strong case with older children and adolescents for using more cognitively orientated methods (see Abikoff, 1979; Meichenbaum and Burland, 1979) including self-control training (assertion and relaxation training, desensitization of anger, role play, behaviour rehearsal), problem-solving skill training (see Dong, Hallberg and Hassard, 1979; Urbain and Kendall, 1980) and social skill training (see Goldstein, 1978; Herbert, 1986). A technique that is used with hyperactive, impulsive children is *self-instruction training* — the development of children's skills in guiding their own performance by the use of self-suggestion, comments, praise, and other directives (see Kendall, 1977; Snyder and White, 1979).

Stress-inoculation training has been used successfully (Meichenbaum, 1973; Meichenbaum and Cameron, 1974) in the self-management of phobic anxiety, anger, and pain. Children are provided with a set of skills and defences so as to deal with future crises. The training programme has three stages:

(a) *Education*   The child is provided with a conceptual framework for understanding the nature of his problem
(b) *Provision of coping strategies*   A number of behavioural and cognitive coping skills, arising from the conceptual framework, are rehearsed by the child in the 'safety' of the home or consulting room
(c) *Practice*   The opportunity is provided for the child to practise his coping skills while being exposed to a variety of real stresses and/or practice by means of imagery and behavioural rehearsal.

Meichenbaum and Cameron (1974), on the basis of Luria's hypothesized developmental sequence, evolved a treatment paradigm for training verbally mediated self-control (cognitive self-instruction). They use a procedure consisting of fading a set of prompts and instructions from an overt (spoken aloud), external (verbalized by a model) condition to a covert, self-produced target response. Since the individual is the source of behavioural control within the verbal mediation paradigm, response maintenance and transfer of training effects should be facilitated.

Most self-instructional procedures focus on problems associated with deficits in self-control (e.g., Camp et al., 1977). The outcomes of these studies are generally positive (see Kendall, 1981), but not all efforts have been entirely successful.

Over the past decade, there has been growing interest in interpersonal problem solving among those involved in clinical and developmental issues. This interest was stimulated in part by the attempts by Spivack Platt, and Shure (1976) to identify, measure, and enhance a set of thinking processes which theorists have come to call interpersonal cognitive problem-solving skills. A recent review of problem-solving interventions (Urbain and Kendall, 1980) identified methodological shortcomings but also identified some encouraging results.

Kendall and Braswell (1982) investigated 27 non-self-controlled problem children (8 to 12 years old) who were randomly assigned to a cognitive-behavioural treatment, a behavioural treatment, or an attention-control condition. All subjects received 12 sessions of individual therapist contact focusing on psychoeducational play and interpersonal tasks and situations, with the cognitive-behavioural treatment including self-instructional training via modelling and behavioural contingencies and the behavioural treatment involving modelling and contingencies. The cognitive-behavioural intervention improved teachers' blind ratings of self-control, and both the cognitive-behavioural and behavioural treatments improved teachers' blind ratings of hyperactivity. Parent ratings did not show that treatment produced improvement. Several performance measures (cognitive style, academic achievement) showed improvements for the cognitive-behavioural and behavioural conditions, whereas only the cognitive-behavioural treatment improved children's self-reported self concept. Naturalistic observations in the classroom were variable but off-task verbal and off-task physical behaviours suggested the effectiveness of treatment.

Normative comparisons and 10-week follow-up provided additional support for the efficacy of the cognitive-behavioural treatment, whereas 1-year follow-up data did not show significant differences across conditions. The data nevertheless provide support for the inclusion of the cognitive component in the cognitive-behavioural intervention.

Modification of false beliefs

If irrational cognitions (such as hypochondriacal thoughts) which elicit maladaptive behaviour are corrected, then the associated anxiety may be reduced as well as instrumental avoidance behaviours. This may be achieved by methods designed to help the client to become aware of his maladaptive self-statements and to modify his actions through discussion, explanation, and by education, persuasion, and encouragement.

Counter-conditioning

Positive counter-conditioning which involves the use of emotive imagery and aversive counter-conditioning involving the use of covert sensitization (Cautela, 1967) are two more antecedent control procedures which may be helpful in reducing those stimuli in a child's psychological processes which are eliciting problematic responses. Studies have indicated that imagined aversive consequences may be as effective as physical punishment in reducing the frequency of behaviours (Bandura, 1973). Aversive imagery has been successfully used as self-punishment for behaviour problems (Davison, 1969). A young boy was taught to imagine his father acting in an extremely aggressive fashion. The boy then successfully used this aversive image as a punishing stimulus to reduce confrontations with his father. Covert sensitization is perhaps the most commonly used self-punishment technique of this type. In this procedure, the person first imagines the behaviour to be reduced and then vividly imagines a very aversive consequence such as feeling extremely nauseous or being punished.

Self-control of outcome conditions

During treatment youngsters can be taught to rearrange contingencies that influence behaviour in such a way that they experience long-range benefits, even though they may have to give up some satisfactions or tolerate some discomforts at first. This involves, first, a precise analysis of the behaviour to be controlled (and, as with any other behavioural analysis), its antecedent, and consequent conditions. Second, it is necessary to identify behaviours which enhance appropriate actions as well as behaviours which interfere with the undesired inappropriate responses. The third stage involves identifying positive and negative reinforcers which control these patterns of behaviour. Finally, reinforcement is applied to alter the probability of the target behaviour (see Stuart, 1967).

There is evidence, as we have seen, that children may be able to modify or maintain their own behaviour by administering rewards or punishments to themselves in a contingent manner. Those consequences may occur in the child's environment or in his symbolic processes. The self-administered rewards and punishments may be overt (see Homme, 1965) or covert (see Davison, 1969). Sometimes a point system is very effective in instituting a programme of self-reward. A youngster can provide himself with a point immediately after a response, and that point in turn can be exchanged for a variety of reinforcers. Bolstad and Johnson (1972) have demonstrated that disruptive schoolchildren can learn to reward themselves for not acting inappropriately (e.g., for not talking, running around, or being physically aggressive). Points could be exchanged for a variety of school materials, such as pencils, erasers, and note-pads.

The self-managed outcomes may be covert and punitive. A young person with (say) compulsion to shoplift might be treated by using covert punishment, self-administered. First he is instructed to imagine punishing consequences to stealing, that is, being in a shop having the urge to steal and then imagining the manager is watching him or that he has been caught. He then has to go into shops and practice imagining the managers are watching him as he shops. To increase the power of the aversive consequences, he is instructed systematically to imagine a list of negative repercussions of stealing, such as being caught, the police being called, being handcuffed, being put in the police car, being booked, standing before the judge, and his parents being called.

Thought-stopping is a variation of negative self-punishment. Instead of using criticism or aversive imagery, the person is trained to shout the word 'stop', first aloud, then softly, and finally quietly to himself, immediately after having an undesirable thought. In positive self-punishment, the person voluntarily removes some positive event in response to the problem behaviour. Thus, positive self-punishment is a type of 'time-out' from reward. This method of self-control is closely related to the 'response-cost' method, in which a person fines himself for engaging in the behaviour to be reduced. (For example, 'Every time I go out to play instead of doing my homework, I lose 30 minutes of free time to read for pleasure or watch television.')

PEER GROUP THERAPY

There is a variety of methods which uses a *group* modality for therapy rather than the more usual individual-based approach. The following studies provide some idea of the methods that have been tried.

(a) Clement (1976) suggests that *tailormade peer therapy* groups can be helpful when children have difficulties with their peers (e.g., impulsive, aggressive behaviour). This procedure illustrates the use of group contingencies with peers recruited from the child's class or neighbourhood.

Typically, the peer therapy group is formed by the child's parents or teacher, who recruit three to five peers from the local neighbourhood or the classroom. The parents generally invite the parents of the other children over to their house for coffee and an explanation of the procedure is given by the therapist. The parents are told that their children are not to receive therapy themselves but to act as therapeutic agents for the target child.

The tailormade peer group usually meets for an hour a week in the large playroom at a mental health clinic. In a gamelike atmosphere, one child is chosen at random to be 'chief' and to wear the headdress that contains a bug-in-the-ear device. The therapist observes through a one-way mirror and coaches the chief as to when to give tokens to the other children. These tokens are redeemed at the end of the session for material rewards from the therapist's store. Tokens are awarded whenever the children play cooperatively with one another. The chief receives the same number of tokens as the child earning the most tokens for that day.

Another procedure involves having the 'chief' record points for the group on a points counter whenever the therapist's pocket programmer goes beep. The therapist actuates the beep whenever the target child is playing cooperatively with one or more of the other children. Videotape feedback, live modelling, and behavioural rehearsal are also common techniques used in these group sessions. At the end of a session, the therapist often asks the children to practise their group behaviours during the coming week in the natural environment. Teachers and parents are also often given behavioural prescriptions for the next week.

Clement has found that, with a little persuasion and explanation, parents are generally willing to 'loan' their children for such a purpose. The approach can be used to modify the behaviour of hostile/aggressive, bizarre/psychotic, shy/withdrawn, and immature/scapegoated children. Clement also reports success with tailormade groups formed with siblings rather than peers. The major rationale for using peers or siblings as therapeutic agents is to enhance the generalization of treatment effects from the treatment setting to the home and/or classroom environments.

(b) Henderson and Silber (1976) make use of behavioural techniques to treat five to eight preadolescent children in an *open-ended group*. The group meets for 1½ hours a week. Sitting in a circle, for the first 45 minutes they set up or discuss the contracts they will work on at home during the next week. Parents and/or teachers are sent a copy of the contract and asked to record daily the presence or absence of specific problem behaviours, such as not hitting a brother. Group members earn tokens not only for setting up and fulfilling their contracts but also for specific prosocial behaviours during the activity period of the session. Thus, while playing a table game, a boy might earn a token for playing by the rules of the game, or ignoring provocative teasing of others. Refreshments are served at the end of the session and then the boys go to the co-therapists' 'store' either to bank their tokens or to exchange them for concrete rewards, like candy, models, and radios. Most disruptive behaviour in the group is handled by ignoring it or paying attention to the desirable behaviour of another child. Excessive aggressiveness, such as kicking or fighting, is dealt with first by placing the boy in a corner for 5 minutes of quiet time. If this proves unsuccessful, the boy is sent to a separate isolation room until he can remain quiet for 5 minutes. The parents of the boys attend separate bimonthly groups for instruction in behavioural and child management principles.

(c) Dannefer, Brown, and Epstein (1975) combine both activities and verbal interactions in one group session. During the activity session, a short discussion session is held that maximizes the effectiveness of both verbal and active group therapy. The group assigns each boy specific tasks related to his problem.

An aggressive boy, for example, might be assigned the task of playing cooperatively with another boy. If he does well at his task, the boy receives a gold star: if he does not do well, he is given a blue star; and if he lies to the group, he is assigned a red star. Whenever a boy forgets his task, he not only receives no star but is also rebuked by the group (e.g., 'This group is only for guys who want to change'). At the end of each month, the boy with the most gold stars is given the 'Most Improved Player' trophy. To uncover a boy who is lying, the group play a 'detective' game, in which they look for missing facts in a boy's story or a logically incoherent report. Once a month the boy's parents are invited to observe the group through a one-way mirror.

Rose (1974) has provided a comprehensive review of the advantages and disadvantages of group therapy.

BIBLIOTHERAPY

Bibliotherapy (see a review by Turvey, 1985) refers to the use of any literary work, including fiction, in the treatment of physical or emotional problems. An important subset of bibliotherapeutic materials includes self-help treatment programmes that present readers with a specific set of instructions for therapeutic use. This approach may be supplemented by so-called *minimal contact*. The model of 'minimal contact bibliotherapy' obtains where there is some contact with a therapist (for instance, a weekly visit) but the clients rely primarily on a written programme.

There are also therapist-administered programmes — regular meetings to clarify or elaborate on the information in the manual. These methods compare with therapist-directed conditions in which therapist contact constitutes the sole treatment and no books are used.

Glasgow and Rosen (1978) draw attention to the relevance of cost-effectiveness of bibliotherapy which allows potentially effective treatments to reach a greater number of clients without involving the expense of a professional adviser's time. Self-administered programmes may be preferred by parents even if they are somewhat less effective than a professional's intervention.

Patterson and Gullion's (1968) manual *Living with Children* has been widely used and modest changes in children's behaviour have been reported when parents are exposed to the book alone (Patterson and Reid, 1973). However, Patterson and Gullion (1971) suggest that professional assistance *is* necessary in order to make a substantial impact on family behaviour.

Baker et al. (1976) have developed ten minimanuals for teaching parent skills. Parents were assigned to self-administering, minimal-contact, or therapist-administered bibliotherapy; therapist-administered group meetings with home visits or to a no treatment control group. All treated groups were found to be generally equivalent and superior to the no-treatment group on behavioural and self-report measures. The results auger well for the bibliotherapeutic method with a reduced input required from the therapist. Although the initial effect of bibliotherapy has been studied there is little evidence as yet for the post-termination persistence effects of parent-training procedures. Although there is moderate support, the case for parent training by means of bibliotherapy is far from proven and requires further investigation (see Patterson and Fleischman, 1979, for a discussion of follow-up data).

Consumer satisfaction with a treatment strategy or approach is likely to be an influence in the ultimate effectiveness of the intervention as well as its generalization. Christensen et al. (1980) found that satisfaction with treatment outcome was greater for mothers and fathers in individual and group conditions than in a minimal-contact bibliotherpay condition. But the costeffectiveness of minimal-contact bibliotherapy may counteract such disadvantages.

6

Parent Training

The traditional treatment of problem behaviour takes place in a clinic or a hospital. Parents bring the child to the professional (a psychiatrist, psychologist, or social worker) who works primarily with the child as the 'target' patient with 'target' problems to be modified. The setting for the therapy is the consulting room and the so-called dyadic model obtains: the expert 'treats the patient'. This is a situation far removed from the child's experience of life and occupies a miniscule proportion of it. Frequently, therapists are unable to see parent–child (or teacher–child) interactions in their natural settings and, indeed, they may not even observe directly, in the artificiality of their consulting room, the problem behaviours for which the child was referred.

Although parents may discuss family matters, report the child's progress, or be reported to, their involvement seldom extends to an active engagement in the assessment process or to giving them specific behaviour change skills (see Berkowitz and Graziano, 1972).

Griest and Wells (1983) in a special series on child behaviour therapy have stressed the importance of examining family variables when assessing and modifying child behaviour problems. And parents in particular have been a prime focus for this work (e.g., Berkowitz and Graziano, 1972; Herbert, 1985b).

The simpler forms of behavioural therapy are reductionist and linear: assuming a direct link between cause and effect, between stimulus and response, where people are seen as passive reactors to environmental forces impinging on them. Contrasted with this model is the *systems* version of family therapy. The perspective, influenced by a general systems or cybernetic paradigm, embraces the concept of circular/reciprocal causation. What we have is a recursive sequence in which each action can be considered as the consequence of the

106

action preceding it and the cause of the action following it. No single element in the sequence controls the operation of the sequence as a whole because it is itself governed by the operation of the other elements in the system.

Thus any individual in a family system is affected by the activities of other members of the family, activities which his or her actions or decisions (in turn) determine. An individual's behaviour is *both* stimulus and response. Such considerations have influenced the way in which casework is conceptualized by contemporary behaviour modification — especially that brand that finds its intellectual sustenance in social learning theory (Bandura, 1977).

Systems theorists in contemporary behavioural practice — those who work within a behavioural modality — are agreed in focusing not only on the individual but on the system of relationships in which he acts out his life. Whereas the traditional treatment model tended to identify the nominated client or patient as the unit of attention (for example, the child referred to the child guidance clinic), the focus of assessment in the light of this interactional frame of reference is far more broadly conceived. Thus the focus of help is not necessarily prejudged as (say) the child who was referred to the psychologist, alone.

The unit of attention may now be defined as the family (or one of its subsystems). It goes beyond the kind of 'lip service' which treats the child 'in the context of his family'. Workers who adopt a behavioural orientation also attempt to conceptualize problems in a horizontal (rather than the traditional vertical–historical) manner. They view the client as part of a complex network of interacting social systems, any aspect of which may have a bearing on his present predicament.

Behavioural and systems approaches to family therapy are often viewed as being incompatible. Despite their epistemological differences there are several significant similarities. Both approaches

(1) focus on interactional rather than intrapsychic causation, i.e., how the problem behaviour of one person fits with the behaviour of others;
(2) seek to discover regularities or repetitive sequences in interpersonal processes;
(3) emphasize observable behavioural events rather than unobservable subjective events;
(4) view the presenting problem as representative of broader classes of interactional patterns;
(5) utilize behavioural interventions aimed at changing dysfunctional patterns of interpersonal behaviour.

The variant of behaviour modification, the behavioural casework approach, is anchored in the natural environment, the family and the community. The triadic model, whereby the psychologist or social worker acts as consultant to the clients (say parents) who constitute the main mediators of change, fits well with community psychology and social work purposes and tasks, whether the setting is a residential unit or a natural home (Jehu et al., 1972; Herbert and Iwaniec, 1981, 1985; Hudson and Macdonald, 1986).

The systematic and successful involvement of parents, particularly mothers (Johnson and Katz, 1973; O'Dell, 1974; Forehand and Atkeson, 1977), is now well-established. The advantages of training parents are notably, primary prevention (Hawkins, 1972; Yule, 1979), therapeutic effectiveness (O'Dell, 1974), and cost-effectiveness (Johnson and Katz, 1973).

The common goal of behavioural work in home settings is to develop in the parents an awareness of their own importance in producing and maintaining desirable and undesirable behaviours in their children. In contrast to the clinic-based intervention, the natural environment approach seeks to utilize the ongoing and intensive influence of those in closest everyday contact with the client in attempting to alter problematic behaviour and teach new strategies of child management, coping with stress, and so on.

The triadic model gets around the problem of generalizing change from clinic-based sessions to the child's real world, and is geared to the only people — parents — who can intervene often enough, and long enough, to produce the long-term changes in what are often (in the case of the more serious conduct problems of childhood) matters of faulty socialization. After all, the parents are 'on the spot' most of the time to initiate and consolidate social learning experiences; they are likely to facilitate therapy (or what is better called an educative exercise) because of their emotional significance to the child. Help is therefore most logically directed to the modification of that environment rather than withdrawing the child from it.

Because the intervention involves the active application of social learning principles, it tends to have 'face validity' for parents; they are all in the business of behavioural change, utilizing informal 'principles' of learning (modelling and operant ones, in particular) to attain the objectives they set for their offspring.

As behaviour is currently viewed as a function of the total environment, behaviour modification is not only about changing the undesirable behaviour of 'problem children'. It is also about altering the behaviour of the persons — parents, teachers, and others — who form a significant part of the child's social world. Such assumptions about behaviour change lead inexorably (Tharp and Wetzel, 1969) to the proposition that maladaptive behaviour can most effectively be changed if parents themselves are provided with what knowledge psychologists have, in order to cope better with their child. This is not the prescriptive, detailed 'do this . . . do that . . .' formula of the past; rather it is the application of principles of learning (firmly anchored in social and developmental psychology) to the treatment and, increasingly, the prevention of personal problems. The fact that this approach has been taught to parents more often than other more traditional approaches may be due to certain advantages that behaviour modification is assumed to have:

(a) persons without a considerable amount of psychological knowledge can grasp the concepts;

(b) many persons can be taught at one time;
(c) a relatively short training period is needed.

Gardner (1976) describes different levels of parent training. The applicator is able to apply specific behavioural techniques under circumscribed conditions to solve particular problems; the technician is able to apply a broader variety of techniques but still under limited conditions to solve specific problems. The generalist has the know-how to apply theory and techniques to a wide spectrum of problems with a minimum of supervision. Gardner considers the generalist level to be the most common level for training parents. Indeed, it may be a necessity for parents dealing with multiple and fairly chronic or resistant childhood problems (e.g., conduct disordered, mentally subnormal, or autistic children).

Herbert and Iwaniec (1981) stress the importance of the following casework skills: clarifying problems, listening sympathetically, and indicating empathetic understanding and acceptance. Alexander et al. (1976), in examining therapist skills, found that relationship skills (affection, warmth, and humour) and structuring skills accounted for approximately 60 per cent. of the outcome variance in treated cases, relationship skills being of greater significance.

The therapist should (it is claimed by Johnson, 1980) adopt a positive attitude to change in discussing a person's problems. In this way they become more clearly defined. An important factor to consider is the stability of the problem implied by the explanation. People feel less demoralized when they attribute their problems to unstable causes. Explanations in terms of inappropriate attitudes, learned habits of thinking and behaving, or environmental stresses, all imply instability. Attributions of difficulties to fixed personality traits or to a malignant destiny imply stability. As Johnson (1980, p.71) puts it: 'All too often demoralized people fear that their personality make-up has a permanent defect. Others feel that they have been singled out and fated to endure a painful existence. Neither of these attributions lead to change and health'.

Many of the problems dealt with in families with conduct disordered children are unstable, i.e., capable of modification. Parents of deviant children display a significantly greater proportion of commands and criticisms and high rates of threats, anger, nagging, and negative consequences than parents of non-referred children (Delfini et al., 1976; Lobitz and Johnson, 1975). There is frequently a lack of contingent consequences among the distressed family members. The probability of receiving a positive, neutral, or aversive consequence for coercive behaviour seems to be independent of the behaviour — a gross inconsistency. Indeed, there may be positive consequences for deviant behaviour and punishment for those rare prosocial actions (Patterson, 1977; Snyder, 1977). Patterson and Fleischman (1979) hypothesize that the disturbed social interactions among the members of the family induce powerful feelings of frustration, anger and helplessness, and low self-esteem.

Parent-training programmes thus include methods designed to reduce confrontations and antagonistic interactions among the family members, to increase the effectiveness (and moderate the intensity) of parental punishment. We return to this issue later.

This approach has provided encouraging evidence of the ability of parents to help themselves and their problematic children over a wide range of problems, ranging from conduct disorders (Herbert, 1980; Holmes, 1979); developmental disorders such as enuresis and encopresis (Herbert and Iwaniec, 1981), child abuse and failure-to-thrive (Iwaniec, 1983; Iwaniec and Herbert, 1985), to maternal rejection (Gambrill, 1983; Herbert and Iwaniec, 1977) and mental handicap (Dean, 1976). It has been pointed out (Forehand and Atkeson, 1977) that psychologists have moved beyond the broad question of whether parent training is effective to the specific parameters within which it works. As with the history of systematic desensitization, the main thrust of research is to refine the triadic approach so as to discover the active therapeutic ingredients in what are usually multi-element treatment packages (see Horton, 1982).

The need to train parents of non-compliant children to give clear instructions has been well documented in the literature (e.g., Forehand, 1977). The focus has been on the content of what is said, and also on the non-verbal aspects of instruction giving. The non-verbal elements of (i) distance from child, (ii) body orientation of mother, (iii) eye contact between mother and child, (iv) tone of voice, and (v) mother's orientation towards objects involved in the instruction are all related to child compliance.

It would appear that the involvement of fathers in parent-training programmes is important (see Lewis, 1986, on the paternal role). Self-control training for mothers increases the likelihood of temporal generalization of beneficial change (Wells, Griest, and Forehand, 1980).

It is necessary to find out the most economical and effective techniques for changing maladaptive behaviours, and to elucidate a coherent theory of practice. The question of why some families fail to respond needs answering. The maintenance of change (temporal generalization) remains a formidable technical problem; so does the difficulty of working in single-parent homes and with parents who enjoy (or suffer) powerful theories/ideologies about child rearing (Holmes, 1979). We still need to know what range of problems can be tackled by this approach. It is safe to say that it is particularly promising for parents with chronically handicapped children who are likely to need a strategy for coping with novel problems, or at least a succession of teaching tasks, in the future.

An unresolved issue that remains is how best to train parents (see O'Dell, 1974). Walder et al. (1969) describe three broad approaches to parent training. In the *individual* consultation approach, the parent complaining of specific problems is instructed in how to behave towards the child under various contingencies. Individual instructions can range from enabling parents to carry out simple instructions in contingency management to a full involvement as co-therapists in all aspects of observation, recording, programme planning, and implementation. The level of skill to which parents need to be trained in order to cope effectively with their child's problem is still a matter of debate.

The controlled learning environment, another variant of parent training, involves highly structured individual instruction, with the consultant directly shaping or modelling parent–child interactions. Sophisticated signalling and feedback devices are used while the parents work with the child.

Another means of training parents is within *educational groups*. Courses vary in duration, intensity, and structure. Various aids to learning such as lectures, guides, manuals, role playing, videotape feedback, modelling, discussion, and home exercises have been used. Parents have been successfully trained in groups (e.g., O'Dell, Flynn, and Benlolo, 1977) and, not unnaturally, this approach has been compared for its cost-effectiveness with the other models of training.

The *consultation format* in which parents receive reading materials and attend films, lectures, and demonstrations (e.g., Cobb and Medway, 1978) has had its successes as has the individual training approach (e.g., Iwaniec, Herbert, and McNeish, 1985; Zeilberger, Sampen, and Sloane, 1968). But there appears to be only one study (Christensen et al., 1980) which has directly compared these three formats. Although parents in all three approaches perceived their children as significantly improved at the end of treatment, parent recorded behaviour observations demonstrated that the individual and group formats were superior to the consultation-only approach.

Parents found the individual treatment format most satisfying. This format was most costly in therapist time. There are advantages and disadvantages in all of these approaches.

Rose (1974) found that group sessions were more cost-efficient than either individual or family sessions, a finding not confirmed by Mira (1970) or Kovitz (1976).

Ollendick and Cerny (1981) conclude from an excellent review of the evidence on content and formal aspects of parent training that although training in basic behavioural principles may not significantly increase parents' intellectual comprehension of child management techniques in the behavioural modality, or their attitudes towards parent training, a grounding in these principles does seem to facilitate the implementation and generalization of the newly acquired child management skills in non-training situations. They are of the opinion that it is cost-efficient to include in parent-training packages education in *general principles* of behaviour change as well as training in the modification of specific behaviour and problems.

Initially, there were euphoric claims for the effectiveness of the behavioural approach in general; clinicians could be forgiven if they were seduced by the literature into believing that a panacea for all child problems had been discovered. The excessive optimism was founded on sometimes fragile data, derived mainly from single subject descriptive case studies. Research methodology since the late 1960s has become more sophisticated, critical, and rigorous. Fortunately, much of the enthusiasm (properly tempered by caution) was not misplaced. Kazdin (1979), in a special issue of the *American Psychologist* entitled *Psychology and Children: Current Research and Practice*, concluded, on the basis of his review of the evidence, that 'for many problem areas, effective treatments have emerged that can be applied in naturalistic or treatment settings. For other problem areas, research has yet to make the necessary progress' (p.987).

The failure of some treatment programme has been attributed to problems between parents and to other conflicts within the family. At the Centre for Behavioural Work with Families we have found that marital problems and stresses of single-parent family life weigh heavily against the successful application of a programme — which involves the need for mutual practical and moral support from partners, and additionally the burdens of increased consistency, patience, and sheer hard work. The social isolation of many of these families — also reported by Wahler and Fox (1980) — has led to the formation of self-help parents' groups (Herbert and Iwaniec, 1976). These groups have proved useful not only for their experiential and social functions, but also for the didactic and training purposes to which they are put.

There is evidence that parental motivation, parental perceptions, and family characteristics can influence the outcome of treatment (McAuley, 1982). In planning an intervention strategy it is important to take such variables into account. To summarize:

Families who fail to engage in successful treatment tend to be of low socioeconomic status, have poor educational attainments; many are single parents. They tend to have frequent contacts with the helping professions. Their social interactions are frequently experienced as unpleasant or aversive. Not surprisingly they are somewhat isolated socially. The explanations they offer for such isolation in the community tend to be vague and blame-oriented. Failure appears to be associated with an inability to report or track children's interactions objectively and specifically. In particular, these families find maintaining initial treatment gains extremely difficult. McMahon et al. (1982) noted that parents at poverty level who also suffered depression tended to drop out of parent-training programmes. Griest et al. (1979) found that parents who drop out tend to have distorted perceptions of their children.

Patterson (1982) reports that, given a problem child and two siblings, an American mother might expect an average rate of one aversive event per minute. Research by Seligman (1975) shows that repeated unsuccessful attempts to avoid/escape from aversive stimuli produce a state in which, despite the clear possibility of escape, the individual has great difficulty in learning to do so. Patterson (1981) hypothesizes that a mother's repeated inability to avoid conflict or escape from the aversive nature of her child's problem behaviour will generate just such learned helplessness, anxiety, depression, and low self-esteem.

The classical early work in the triadic mode was conducted by Tharp, Wetzel, and Thorne (1968):

In the triadic (consultant-mediator-target) model, a consultant familiar with behaviour modification technology assists a mediator (anyone in the environment who controls reinforcers for the youth) in modifying the behaviour of the youngster. Tharp and Wetzel, in their behaviour research project, studied cases treated by 'behavioural analysts' whose role was that of behavioural consultants or counsellors to parents and teachers. The counsellors trained 77 parents to manage their own children — 6- to 16-year old youths referred by local schools in the Tucson area. While the type of acting-out problems treated varied somewhat over the course of the study, the nature of the sample was reasonably well spelled out so that replication might be possible. The counsellors were not required to see target children except when they were involved in initial assessment observations and in cases of emergency. The 'mediators', so-called, were parents and teachers.

On referral each case was assigned to a counsellor, who visited the home and the school and explained the behaviour research project services. If the parents agreed and signed a 'permission form' assessment began. The duration of the assessment phase was generally between one and three weeks, and involved interviews with parents and teachers, supervized observation by parents and teachers or by the counsellor, and an interview with the target child by another counsellor. The aims were to specify problem behaviours and record a baseline of their frequency. In addition, antecedent and consequent events were analysed where possible. A reinforcement hierarchy for the target child was established by interviewing the mediator and by eliciting the responses of the target child to a thirty-four item sentence-completion questionnaire designed to elucidate his reinforcers and the persons who controlled them.*

Upon completion of assessment an intervention phase was drawn up by the counsellor and his supervisor, sometimes in conference with other staff members; this specified target behaviours and the contingencies and mediators to be involved in change. The counsellor then visited the mediators concerned and discussed the plan; negotiation and alterations might follow before implementation. During implementation he kept in very close touch with the mediators, often by telephone, supervizing progress and liaising between home and school (or within school) as necessary. Implementation included a full explanation of the programme to the target child; this constituted one source of prompting, but the mediators also carried on informal prompting as part of their normal interactions with the child. Contingency management, involving material and social rewards, was a crucial element in the programme. Shaping of behaviour was also used (reinforcing approximations to desired behaviour already in the child's repertoire); modelling was not used, except in the sense of altering the behaviour of mediators to make them more acceptable natural models.

The criterion data consisted of global ratings of improvement by counsellors, parents, teachers, and daily records of targeted problems. Mediators were asked to obtain measures of target behaviours during baseline and treatment phases. Of 163 behaviours assessed, measures on 135 provided sufficient data

* This included such items as, 'I will do almost anything to get . . .' and, 'the only person I will take advice from is . . .'

to allow evaluation. Treatment levels of 120 of 135 behaviours showed substantial improvements over baseline levels. The data that were available suggested substantial improvement in many of the families. This was a massive and admirable effort to train lay personnel and to employ multiple criteria in the evaluation of outcomes. Unfortunately, the absence of assessments of the reliability of mediator observation makes these data difficult to interpret. In addition, no information was given on staff-time requirements; and systematic follow-up data are also lacking.

Part III

Therapeutic Work with Particular Problems

The golden rule is that there are no golden rules.
GEORGE BERNARD SHAW
(*Maxims for Revolutionists*)

Introduction

Any division of the conduct disorders into separate problem areas such as non-compliance, hyperactivity, aggression, disruptive behaviour, and so on, is somewhat arbitrary. It makes for a neat organization of Chapter headings but belies the frequent overlapping of problems. Such overlap is seen in some of the case-histories provided in this section. They should illustrate most of the behavioural methods applied to conduct problems in the home, the classroom, and other settings.

To this purpose, at least, one detailed case-history has been included in each problem area to indicate the 'rough edges', the unexpected difficulties and failures which (for lack of space and an understandable desire to publish one's successes) do not always get into the journals. An attempt has also been made to include a representative (rather than exhaustive) cross-section of reports on therapeutic methods in use. Although the therapeutic research on conduct disorders is relatively sparse compared with the work on other problems, there are still far too many studies to do full justice to them in the space available. However, references are given to some of the work that cannot be detailed here, so that the reader can follow up particular interests.

It is a difficult and premature task to evaluate the effectiveness of behaviour modification in the treatment of the conduct and delinquent disorders. Research in this area is still in its infancy. There are several critical reviews available which provide tentative evaluations of the progress made by behaviour modifiers with these problems (Gelfand and Hartmann, 1975; Ollendick and Cerny, 1981).

Much of the evidence, as will become apparent, comes from detailed studies of a few cases at a time, although the rigorous methodology of some allows one to relate changes in behaviour with some confidence to particular behavioural interventions. This is because of carefully specified time–event relationships. There are only a few control group studies which compare the behaviour modification of conduct problems with other treatment methods or with no intervention at all. We need to know a great deal more about the generalization and persistence of beneficial change which has been brought about by this method.

Each problem is discussed from a developmental and aetiological point of view prior to a review of therapeutic interventions. Specific information about particular problems which could not be covered in the general outline of Chapter 2 is provided in each chapter.

7

Non-compliant Behaviour

Non-compliance to parental requests is one of the most common forms of behaviour problems of childhood, comprising, in one normative study nearly one-third of children's deviant behaviour (Johnson et al., 1973). In Chapter 2 we discussed some of the developmental aspects of compliant, non-compliant, and oppositional (negativistic) behaviour. Those who have worked with children with severely problematic behaviour frequently point to a fairly general tendency among many of them to be extremely antagonistic to requests and commands. So intense is the resistance that at times it becomes quite clear that the child is not merely failing to comply, but is doing precisely the opposite of that which is desired of him. This pattern, while present in the behaviour of many children to a mild degree, may be so severe as to seriously handicap learning in many areas, and therefore to take on clinical significance.

Johansson et al. (undated) made a study of the social and behavioural correlates of compliance and non-compliance in 33 'normal' children of 4 to 6 years of age and their families. The children and their families were observed in their homes on five separate occasions for 45 minutes on each occasion. The behaviour of the target child and that of any family members who interacted with him was recorded with the use of a behavioural coding system designed for rapid sequential recording. It was found that there was significant consistency in children's compliance and non-compliance to their mothers and fathers. The generality of compliant behaviour was a central question posed in this investigation. Generality was analysed by relating the compliance ratios to the occurrence of other deviant behaviours and by relating the compliance ratios with regard to one person with those to another. The authors found consistent evidence of a negative relationship between children's compliance ratio and the display of all other deviant behaviours; this suggests that non-compliance may be related to a more general tendency towards deviant activities. They suggest that, although this finding provided some evidence for a general deviancy 'trait', the magnitude of the correlations is quite small. Again, although the correlations relating children's consistency of compliance across agents provided evidence for the generality of compliant behaviour, the correlations were at a low level.

Cowan, Hoddinott, and Wright (1965) investigated oppositional behaviour among 12 autistic children. The children all had severe speech and language deficits. They were requested to solve various discrimination problems such as picking tiles with particular shapes and colours. The experimental design allowed the researchers to determine whether or not a child actually knew the solution to a problem so that they could differentiate failure to comply based on inability from a failure to comply of the kind that stemmed from negativism. Of the 12 children, 10 not only selected tiles incorrectly, but did so below the level of accuracy which could be expected by chance alone. In other words, these children were not merely guessing but were deliberately selecting the tiles which were contrary to adult instructions. The researchers employed reinforcement techniques, using popcorn as a reinforcer, in an effort to counteract resistance. It is of significance that they could, in this manner, modify the pattern in some of the children, getting them to comply with directions. There were six 'compliers' and six 'resisters' at the end of the project, with some indications that the compliers might be functioning at a somewhat higher level in terms of general ability. The authors comment that this high degree of negativism may partly explain the great difficulty in language development of autistic children. Since the learning of a language is so dependent on early imitative skills, children who refuse to imitate can hardly be expected to develop a large verbal repertoire. (The broader implications of this for the non-compliant and often educationally retarded conduct-disordered child and adolescent are discussed in Chapter 11).

NON-COMPLIANCE AS THE EXERCISE OF COERCIVE POWER

What we are referring to in this chapter in discussing oppositional or negativistic behaviour will be a relatively broad and general tendency in children to refuse to comply with most requests, or actually to do the opposite of what is requested. It should not be confused with the refusal to comply with a few specific requests, which, after all, might well be a legitimate act of asserting personal integrity.

The display of seriously disobedient behaviour is often accompanied by a display of temper-tantrums and aggression. The oppositional child, if coerced by his parents or teacher, often turns on a breathtaking display of hostility, which, in its turn, is highly coercive.

Patterson (1975) suggests that applications of pain control techniques (e.g., crying and screaming) by infants may be innate. Their yelling when in distress has obvious survival value in providing a method by which babies (in a sense) train their mothers in some of the necessary caretaking skills. We have discussed some of the individual differences in 'demand characteristics' of infants and we shall be looking at other variations such as crying tendencies in babies (page 142). Patterson states that by the age of 2 most toddlers have advanced to the point of possessing an important range of verbal and motor strategies to replace their more coercive responses of former times (see also page 21). He traces the developmental history of coercive behaviours. They display a steady decline in performance rates from a high point in infancy down to more moderate levels at the age of school entrance. The highest rates of negativistic-disruptive behaviours occur before the age of 3, followed by a steady decline through to the age of 4½ years (Reynolds, 1928). Hartup (1974) also noted a significant decrease in aggression from the age of 4 through to 8 years in his study of classroom behaviour. The identified 'aggressive' boy, according to Patterson, displays coercive behaviours at a level commensurate with a 3- to 4-year-old child and, in this sense, is an exemplar of arrested socialization.

With increasing age, certain coercive behaviours are no longer acceptable to parents (see page 21). The behaviours then become the target for careful monitoring and punishment which in turn is accompanied by reductions in their rate. A study (Patterson, 1974) revealed that 2- and 3-year-olds display the highest rates of whining, crying, yelling, and high frequency behaviours, as well as high rates for most other coercive actions. By the age of 4, there are substantial reductions in negative commands, destruction, and attempts to humiliate. By the age of 5, most children used less negativism, non-compliance, and negative physical actions than younger siblings.

CONTEMPORARY INFLUENCES

Johansson et al. (undated), in the study quoted earlier, found a consistent positive relationship between the parents' rate of reinforcing compliance and the amount of obedience received by the parent, but this relationship was significant only for fathers. In addition, the consistency between parents in reinforcing obedience was positively related to compliance in the child. It was found that parents responded more positively to obedience and were more negative and neutral to disobedience. Fathers were significantly more discriminating than mothers in delivering positive consequences for compliance and non-compliance. In fact, children who were more disobedient to their fathers were also more deviant in other respects.

The display of non-compliant behaviour is often associated with temper-tantrums and aggression. The oppositional child if coerced by an adult in authority is quite likely to react with rage. The child tends to escalate the aggravation. A vicious circle is thus set in motion. If the tantrum is intense or persistent enough the parent or teacher may concede to the child. Giving in to the child's non-compliance tends not to occur on every occasion, producing what is, in effect, an intermittent schedule of reinforcement for non-compliant tantrum sequences of behaviour. Such schedules, as we saw earlier, produce deviant patterns which are highly resistant to change.

Johnson et al. (1973) demonstrated that there is a fairly high correlation between overall parental negativism and child deviance. In an investigation of some of the processes involved, Johnson and Lobitz (1974) were able to provide conditions (by instruction) in which parents in twelve families could manipulate the deviancy level in their children (aged from 4 to 6) according to prediction. They did this by increasing their rate of ignoring or commanding their offspring, and of being negative, restrictive, disapproving, and non-compliant.

In another study by the same researchers (Lobitz and Johnson, 1973) it was found that the best discriminating factor between 'normal' children and children referred for psychological treatment was a parental negativeness score. There was also a clear trend for parents of referred children to give more commands. Interestingly, there was a great deal of overlap in the distributions of deviancy rates in the referred and non-referred children, although the former showed significantly higher rates.

CONTINGENCY MANAGEMENT

There have been several case-study reports of the successful modification in home settings (and other natural environments) of non-compliant-oppositional behaviour (e.g., Forehand. Cheney, and Yoder, 1974; Goetz, Homberg, and Leblanc, 1975; Zeilberger, Sampen, and Sloane, 1968). They vary in the sophistication of their methodology (i.e., the extent to which they provide rigorous designs,* precise base-line measurements and data, observer reliability figures, follow-up data, etc.) and the extent to which the parents participate fully in the programme. All used differential reinforcement: positive reinforcement plus extinction or time-out procedures.

In one of the first case-studies of a treatment programme conducted by parents in a home setting, Williams (1959) described the elimination of a 21-month-old child's coercive behaviour. The boy, Jimmy, had required special care during a serious illness in his first year and a half of his life. Not surprisingly, on recovery, he continued to demand the parents' undivided attention with intense tantrums and crying spells, especially at bedtime. When put to bed he would scream until the adult returned to his bedroom. Williams instructed the parents in the application of a simple extinction procedure in relation to the severe bedtime crying. They were advised to put him to bed pleasantly, leave the room, and remain away regardless of his screaming. On the first evening, he raged for 45 minutes before going to sleep. The duration of the unrewarded tantrum behaviour dropped markedly and ceased altogether within 10 days. The child no longer created a scene at bedtime, but instead played happily until he dropped off to sleep. The importance of consistency in

*See Appendix A.

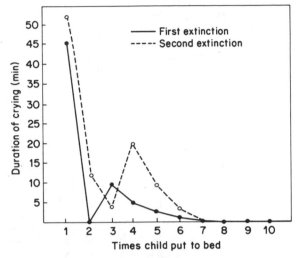

Figure 4 Length of crying in two extinction series (Williams, 1959)

implementing a programme based on extinction is well illustrated by this programme. A week later the tantrum behaviour was reinstated because the child's aunt complied with his demands to remain in the room after being put to bed. Jimmy cried for 50 minutes before going to bed. A second extinction booster produced complete and enduring remission of the tantrums in 9 days (see Figure 4). At 3 years 9 months of age Jimmy still went to bed without bedtime tantrums. He seemed a friendly outgoing child who had experienced no ill-effects from his problems or their treatment.

Zeilberger, Sampen, and Sloane (1968) examined the effectiveness of time-out, extinction, and differential reinforcement in reducing a 4-year-old boy's aggressive behaviour and in increasing his willingness to follow instructions. They successfully modified his severe screaming, fighting, negativism, teasing, and 'bossy' behaviour. Treatment was conducted at home with the mother as therapist. The authors trained the parents in the home, using daily 1-hour sessions, showing them how to apply differential reinforcement. The procedures consisted of ignoring maladaptive behaviour, putting the boy in time-out, and giving social rewards paired with food or special toys for compliant behaviour. The parents did not have responsibility for making observations and recording data. Observations were made and recorded by two observers in the home. Their training was apparently limited to specific techniques for dealing with the presenting problems rather than a broader theoretical framework which would allow them to deal with any subsequent problems in the child of their own accord. The authors incorporated a design for reinstating baseline conditions to demonstrate that the behaviour was in fact under the mother's control (see Figure 5).

Wahler (1969b) reported two cases involving the contingency management of oppositional behaviour. This study of non-compliance in a 5-year-old boy

124

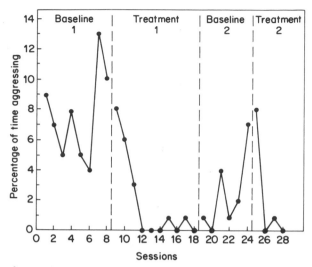

Figure 5 Rate of agressive responding during treatment periods when positive reponses were rewarded and injurious actions were punished by brief social exclusion. The figure shows the reductions in physical agression achieved by a mother in her 5-year-old son (Zeilberger, Sampen, and Sloane, 1968)

and study behaviour in an 8-year-old boy is of interest because it compares what was happening in the home with what was happening at school. Figure 6 presents the results of a contingency-management programme for treating the oppositional behaviour of the 5-year-old boy. At first, the parents were trained to give attention to cooperative (non-oppositional) behaviour and to utilize time-out procedures contingent upon oppositional, argumentative behaviour in the home. By the ninth session it may be seen that there was a great increase of cooperation at home, but no change at school. When the changed contingencies and time-out procedures were removed, the behaviour reverted to baseline. Finally, however, when both home and school became the setting in which contingency management occurred, cooperative behaviour increased in both settings.

Scarboro and Forehand (1975) conducted a study of the comparative effectiveness of time-out procedures with 24 5-year-olds. Time-out within the room and out-of-room-time-out was contrasted as to effectiveness in influencing compliance and oppositional behaviour. Mothers were instructed how to respond via a receiver placed in their ears. If within 5 seconds of a request the child did not comply, the mother would not interact for 2 minutes (within-room time-out). Out-of-room time-out involved the mother leaving with the toys for 2 minutes and then coming back. Strikingly, within-room time-out was as effective as out-of-room time-out — both significantly modified behaviour. Within-room time-out required more repetitions to affect behaviour. Mothers learned the procedures in a brief time.

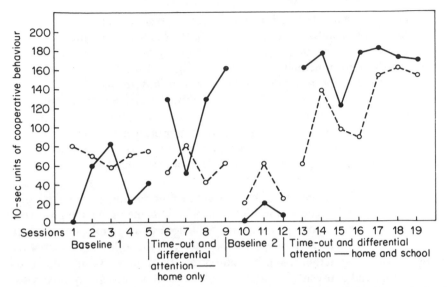

Figure 6 Cooperative behaviour in home and school setting during baseline periods of contingency management in the home alone or in both the home and school (o————o: *home behaviour; o- - - -o: school behaviour) (From Wahler, 1969b)*

COGNITIVE RESTRUCTURING

Masters (1970) made use of discussion and behavioural assignments to alter the extent to which a 17-year-old boy felt that he controlled his environment. He had a great deal of difficulty with any authority figures. He was quite jealous of his older brother's freedom (and his being the favourite of the parents). He frequently disobeyed his parents. Therapy focused on analysing the 'rules of the game' so that by 'playing the game' he could become, and feel, more in control. The boy realized that he could comply and be able to influence his parents' behaviour. By performing chores without being asked, he preempted their commands; furthermore his father felt obligated to him. By reinterpreting his family as neutral rather than negative, he engaged in fewer family arguments and offered fewer complaints of overcontrol. Masters feels that stimulus reinterpretation led to a change in perception, a change in behaviour (complaints), and a change in family interactions.

CONTROL GROUP STUDIES

Wiltz (1969) carried out a study — rare in the field of the conduct disorders — using as it did observational data to validate a behaviour modification technique through use of a treatment group and a control non-treated group. All of the participating families had been referred for treatment in the Social Learning Project, Oregon Research Institute. Parents in treatment met once a week with a therapist who taught them how to control their conduct-disordered children through principles of social learning. The waiting-list control group parents and children received no therapy from any source.

Six boys and their parents in each of the two groups comprised the sample. Children were matched for age, sex, socioeconomic status, and both mean and variance for the dependent variable (viz. the proportion of observed deviant behaviour of the boy to his total social interaction during a session of baseline observation). The control group started from a somewhat higher mean rate per minute of deviant behaviour than the experimental group — as measured during the baseline period. The matching comparison was based on the proportion of deviant behaviour and comprised the mean of each group on the sums of three clusters of coded deviant behaviour in the home. The differences were not significant. Deviant behaviours included the following: disobedience, aggression, hyperactivity, temper-tantrums, theft, absconding, destructiveness, lying, and enuresis. The mean age for the treatment group boys was 9. 8 years (range 7 to 14 years). The intervention programmes were based on procedures described by Patterson et al. (1969) and Patterson, Ray, and Shaw (1968). The parents used a programmed text (Patterson and Gullion, 1968). Treatment group families were observed over a 2-week baseline and then again after 5 and 9 weeks of intervention. Control families were observed for a 2-week baseline and then again 5 weeks later. Pre(baseline–and post(intervention)–observations made in the home served as the criteria for evaluating treatment outcome.

Two hypotheses were tested: (1) that the experimental group of boys would show a decrease in deviant behaviour attributable to the behaviour modification training programme for the parents; (2) that the control group boys would not show a reduction in deviant behaviour. The criterion used to test the hypotheses was based upon a total score comprised of three clusters of out-of-control behaviour. The clusters included 'aggressiveness', 'commanding', and 'non-compliance'. The analysis of total score for these three clusters showed a significant effect of intervention for the experimental group. There was a mean decrease of nearly 50 per cent. in the proportion of deviant behaviour in the treatment group and a mean increase in proportion of about 30 per cent. for the control group. Patterson, Cobb, and Ray (1972) have reanalysed this data to show that:

(1) *In the treated group*, four out of the six subjects showed reduction in the rate of treated behaviour, while two showed no changed ($t = 2.08$, $p <$ 0.05 on a one-tailed test).
(2) *In the control group*, four of the six subjects increased in the rate of deviant behaviour, but to an extent that was not statistically significant.

Any conclusions which might be drawn from this study are weakened by the fact that although the treated and control subjects were matched for *proportion* of deviant behaviour, their actual *rates* of deviant behaviour were very different, the rates for the controls being almost twice those for the treated subjects, so that the groups were not equivalent before treatment.

Walter and Gilmore (1973) have essentially replicated Wiltz's study, by taking twelve consecutive cases of aggressive boys and assigning them randomly to treatment or to a placebo control condition consisting of 'a warm supportive interchange'. In the treatment group the treated deviant behaviour was reduced. In the placebo group there was no such change. The results of these two studies may indicate that the operation of a differential reinforcement programme by the parents of aggressive boys is followed by a reduction in this behaviour which does not occur in similar subjects on a waiting list or in a placebo condition.

ACTIVE INGREDIENTS

The study by Walter and Gilmore (1973) bears also upon the important matter of identifying the therapeutically active ingredients in the differential reinforcement treatment strategy. It suggests that the non-specific factors of a warm, supportive relationship or parental expectancies of therapeutic change are not sufficient to achieve such change (although they may, of course, be necessary or facilitative in achieving it). In particular, although the measured parental expectancies of therapeutic change were high throughout the study, the children's behaviour in the placebo group did not change. A final point on this matter is that both the Wiltz and Walter studies suggest that the pre-treatment assessment procedures were not sufficient to produce the observed therapeutic change.

Eyberg and Johnson (1974) note that the adequate demonstration of successful treatment effects requires an analysis of successive cases assessed by multiple outcome criteria. Sadly, the majority of studies of behaviour modification of childhood problems using parents as mediators is characterized by single-assessment criteria.

CASE STUDY

The present author and a colleague (Roscoe, 1976; Herbert, 1976b) treated a case of severe non-compliant behaviour. Tommy M., aged 3½ years, was referred by his family doctor to the CTRU as a serious management problem for his parents. His mother stated that Tommy was a problem to both parents but that *she* felt his tyrannical and impossible behaviour more keenly, having him at home all day and every day. She felt he was beyond her control and that it had come to the point where, in her words, 'it is either Tommy or me!' At times she feared she would 'beat him to a pulp'. Such feelings made her feel guilty and depressed.

The family, particularly the mother, were relatively isolated from social contacts within the neighbourhood. This meant that Tommy and his 16-month old sister seldom met outsiders and, in particular, no other children. The father, out all day, was more worried by his wife's state of mind than Tommy's behaviour, although he admitted he was a problem. The mother appeared to be a tired, harrassed, and depressed-looking woman, for whom any activity, however small, seemed a tremendous effort to accomplish. Often on the verge of tears, she communicated a sense of desperation at her impotence to cope with the difficulties she was experiencing with Tommy. She admitted that she had had to overcome her pride in accepting help, which seemed to her an admission of failure as a parent. It was precisely because both parents endeavoured to provide a warm, caring, and stimulating environment for their children that they were so confused and demoralized by the difficulties Tommy presented. Mrs. M had been a secondary school teacher until she became pregnant with Tommy. As she said with bewilderment: 'I could stand up to a large class of hulking sixth-formers, yet this child reduces me to a jelly.'

During the early observations and interviews, Tommy appeared to be always 'on the go' and his commanding and disruptive behaviour constantly compelled his mother's attention and intervention. When we conducted our interviews at his home he would physically block eye contact between ourselves and his mother by standing between us; or he would make hearing difficult by making a noise which his mother interpreted as deliberately disruptive. He sought proximity to his mother most of the time.

(1) Specification of the problem

Four main techniques were used to obtain the necessary information concerning Tommy's behaviour. First, a structured interview produced verbal descriptions by the mother and, later, the father, of Tommy's problematic behaviours — but descriptions of observable behaviours couched in very precise terms rather than vague global statements. Another strategy used was 'a typical day in the life of the child'. This technique often teases out a very comprehensive and yet detailed picture of the child within the context of his family's life. Again, the method is designed to elucidate sequences of behaviour — antecedent and consequent events — in the confrontations between child and family, in fine (indeed pedantic) detail. Third, we spent periods at Tommy's home devoted exclusively to recording our observations of the child in his environment. In this case, our observations matched Mrs. M's report. We asked Mrs. M. to keep a diary of events (ABC) leading up to and flowing from several carefully defined target behaviours based on a preliminary estimate of what they were. She also kept a chart recording the frequency of these problems. She was to record how many times each occurred in each hour over the day. (A slightly unusual procedure that we adopted was to ask her to chart her feelings through the day.) The combination of these techniques led to a final specification of six target behaviours which were problematical.

'Lunatic' moods Mrs. M. coined this generic term to describe Tommy's

hyperactive goal-less behaviour — rushing about, giggling, and being silly. She stated that it was as if Tommy was a clock winding himself up until the spring snapped — a good metaphor for what happened to her. This mood appeared to have an involuntary quality and, as it continued, it seemed that Tommy was looking for ways in which to reach breaking point. His mother tended to wait until her nerves were at breaking point; then her intervention took the form of an overreaction. At this point the mood culminated by Tommy lying on the floor, raging and screaming, both of which gradually tapered away. Afterwards Tommy became quiet and usually sought out his mother.

Aggression   This consisted of pushing/hitting/kicking doors and his little sister Claire. There were also verbal threats, usually aimed at his mother.

Temper-tantrums   This took the form of lying on the floor screaming and crying.

Non-compliance   This took the form of a refusal to do something or to stop doing something, when asked.

Whining   This involved talking to his mother in a babylike, petulant, and whiny manner.

Tormenting   This was directed at Claire, and consisted of teasing or poking her or taking away her toy of the moment.

The baseline record indicated that in order of frequency, non-compliance came first, then aggression, whining, tormenting, and finally temper-tantrums and 'lunatic moods' together. The last item was the one to which she attributed the greatest importance. The recording indicated that non-compliance took the highest priority in terms of frequency. The baseline record also showed that peaks of difficult behaviour were found at certain times during the day, e.g., 2.30 p.m. to 4.00 p.m. Similarly, the record also showed the times the mother could predict reasonably good behaviour from Tommy.

Mrs. M. was also asked to delineate Tommy's prosocial behaviours and behaviours that he could do well and/or enjoyed doing. (These were sought as behaviours that might be incompatible with his problematic actions and therefore increased, or built upon in a treatment programme if one was instituted). In fact Mrs. M. felt that there were very few occasions when Tommy did anything praiseworthy, but she could predict that at least he was quiet and more approachable on three different occasions, one of these being teatime, an informal affair in front of the television just after his father arrived home from work.

(2) Controlling factors

(a) Contemporary events

A search for stimulus conditions or discriminative stimuli in the emission of Tommy's non-compliant behaviour revealed two main settings: first, a request to do something or to stop doing something and, second, the incidence of another target behaviour, particularly a lunatic mood. Tommy's other behaviours seemed to be precipitated by an absence of something, such as having something interesting to do or experiencing a withdrawal of his mother's attention (e.g., when she was talking to someone). To a considerable extent, Tommy's behaviours, both acceptable and unacceptable, were associated with particular times of the day.

In terms of consequences, Tommy's behaviour resulted in attention, mainly from his mother. He managed to obtain:

The limelight   This always had to be focused on Tommy to the detriment of the needs of other members of the family. He always managed to upstage others in the room.

Verbal disputations   Tommy (a highly verbal child) involved his mother in endless verbal discussions and arguments. Sometimes these would be followed by a smack, but when mother did smack Tommy she felt she was losing her control. This frightened her and made her feel guilty.

Entertainment   Because his mother could often predict the times of difficulty with Tommy she tried to avoid a confrontation by providing activities that she knew would amuse him, e.g., taking him out to the park.

Nursing   Tommy had been worryingly ill off and on as an infant and during these periods the negative aspects of his behaviour would be particularly intense. Nursing him would be one of the ways of avoiding or overcoming such difficulties.

(b) Somatic (organismic) factors

Mrs. M. reported that Tommy would cling to her and pester her when he was sickening for something, or actually ill. She also felt that he sometimes 'acted ill'

(c) Previous learning experiences

A reinforcement history and more general case-history suggested three important themes.

(i)   From the time of Tommy's conception he had been a very 'precious' baby. His mother had been trying for a baby for 2 years before she fell pregnant with Tommy. She was required to rest completely for the first 3 months of pregnancy to prevent a miscarriage. The labour was of normal duration but a hard one; following the birth his mother was ill both with urinary infections and post-natal depression. Her capacity for coping with a new baby was understandably diminished. This was not made easier when Tommy proved to have a difficult temperament. He suffered from colic, and his frequent and prolonged screaming drove his mother to distraction. Picking Tommy up and nursing him were means by which the mother could hope to at least have some calming effect on her child and herself. This she had to do a great deal. For the first 3 years of Tommy's life he had many bouts of illness; his constant demands and Mrs. M.'s vulnerability kept her always close at hand so as to nurse him. (Mr. M. was equally sensitive to Tommy.) Both parents feared that they might 'lose' the child through illness. Tommy received inordinate amounts of attention (positive reinforcement) during his illnesses which generalized to other areas of his life. His demands for his mother's attention (even when she was in the toilet) seemed to her insatiable. She kept going on tranquillizers.

(ii) Another theme concerned the mother–son relationship. There was a symbiotic quality to their relationship; temperamentally, they were both extremely sensitive individuals who acted like barometers for each other's moods. Thus Tommy's worst days often coincided with the days when his mother felt particularly low. This reciprocal interaction was highlighted by the fact that many of the mother's nervous mannerisms and idiosyncracies were mirrored in Tommy.

(iii) A third theme involved the parents' child-rearing philosophy. Both parents wanted to treat Tommy as an individual in his own right, not being overly intrusive or dominating. Therefore they tended to give commands to Tommy as if he had a choice, although in reality there was often no choice — in the sense that he only knew how to act in an immature manner. The hesitant way in which their 'commands' were often issued made for ambiguous signals. For example, mother would say 'Tommy, would you mind clearing your toys up as I want to hoover now?' or 'Darling, won't you stop doing that?' A command in the form of a question is likely to invite the answer 'No!'

(3) Clinical formulation

In a very real sense Tommy's problems could be considered 'normal' for a 3-year-old. Negativism, temper-tantrums, and attention-seeking behaviours are not unusual in a child of this age (see Herbert, 1974). What made Tommy's behaviours serious enough to merit treatment was their frequency, intensity, persistence, and pervasiveness. This judgement was based on a crucial question: what are (and what could be in the longer term) the consequences — favourable or unfavourable — of the child's pattern of behaviour and style of coping with life? The dynamic of much of this child's behaviour seemed to be an insatiable search for attention. He was certainly getting a large amount, but much of it taking a negative form. It was precisely because of the endless round of disputations between parent and child that Tommy was precluded from many of the usual range of symbolic rewards or social reinforcers which belong to happy and meaningful family communications. Tommy gave the appearance of being an unhappy child. He rarely smiled. This situation would be unlikely to improve if he exhibited the target problems at nursery school (which he was soon to attend) or in peer-group situations. Tommy had learned that certain antisocial behaviours were guaranteed to gain attention from his parents. This lesson, applied in the school situation, could have aversive consequences for him and reduce his ability to learn. It was our opinion that they had affected his social development adversely — his manner was babyish and off-putting.

From the point of view of other members of the family, Tommy's monopolistic and immature behaviour was undoubtedly undermining their well-being. His sister was also beginning to imitate some of his behaviours. As his parents saw things, they had endeavoured to provide 'the best' for Tommy and yet they were faced with a situation in which they no longer enjoyed their child. These considerations, among others, contributed to the decision that intervention was necessary.

(4) Selection of goals for treatment

Treatment objectives were negotiated between the therapists and the parents. The first goal was to reduce the frequency of all six target behaviours specified during assessment. The second goal was to increase adaptive behaviours in certain specified situations, as identified by the parents, with the main aim of creating opportunities for Tommy to win positive reinforcement for socially appropriate behaviour. There were four specified situations, one of which was tidying up his toys.

(5) Treatment programme

With regard to the reduction of the six target behaviours, a programme was designed to change both the stimulus and consequential events associated with Tommy's problems, using mainly modelling and operant techniques.

(a) Stimulus events

Mrs. M. was instructed to alter her methods of issuing commands to Tommy. Rather than using repetitive, pleading, and question-like 'commands' put in a hesitant manner, she was asked to give a simple, firm command to Tommy in those situations that required compliance. These situations were discussed with Mrs. M.

Another alteration involved the timing of setting events during the day. Mrs. M.'s day had all the periodicity of a school teacher's timetable. The baseline recording indicated (as we saw earlier) that Tommy's target behaviours reached peaks at certain times of the day. His mother was advised to try and alter the pattern of the day in order to preempt the onset of target behaviours, particularly the lunatic moods.

(b) Consequent events

It was predicted after discussion with the parents that, for a variety of reasons, ignoring would not be feasible for use as an extinction procedure. So time-out was chosen. It was applied as a sanction after one warning given at the earliest onset of a target behaviour (e.g., at the first display of a defined category of disobedience). If Tommy failed to heed the warning, his mother made him go to an upstairs room for a 5-minute period. One of the therapists spent the first day of the programme with Mrs. M. helping her to initiate it (and when necessary cueing and modelling commands). This initiation process was somewhat 'painful' for the mother (see page 134). Tommy's initial response to the programme was dramatic. His environment had changed from an inconsistent to a predictable one; he knew that what his mother said as a threat would be carried out. Attention was valuable and therefore highly rewarding to Tommy. Time-out deprived him of this. His quick 'capitulation' belied the therapist's warning that Tommy's behaviour might deteriorate before it improved. It was, in fact, to do this later on.

With regard to the second goal, namely, increasing adaptive behaviours, four activities were chosen that spanned the whole day, (e.g., dressing/undressing, together with any other behaviours that parents judged to be praiseworthy). It was worked out that there should be a chart for tokens (pictures called 'happy faces'). Happy faces denoted good behaviour and were to be exchanged for rewards in the form of outings and/or Smarties at the end of the day. Verbal praise and physical hugs were also to be given.

The reasons for a programme of positive reinforcement were explained to the parents in terms of time-out teaching Tommy what he could not do, and positive reinforcement providing guidance and encouragement with regard to what he could do, what is approved of. This was particularly the case with Tommy, a child who was manifesting so many maladaptive behaviours that the opportunities to gain rewards were few and far between. Sometimes, precisely because of the high frequency of target behaviour, his parents unwittingly forgot to provide him with those positive reinforcements which are vital for the healthy development of self-esteem. Other factors have been listed on page 131). There seemed to be a need for a more systematically planned reward system, a matter to which Mrs. M. agreed, but with some reluctance.

What followed underlines the necessity for frequent direct checks on the implementation of a programme. Complacency led to a slippage in criteria for parental action. Tommy's ingenuity at manipulating his parents and his verbal skills were also underrated. Thus two difficult periods arrived which held up the progress of the programme, and both parents, the mother in particular, became very despondent about its effectiveness. The first came 8 days after the programme commenced. Tommy displayed a series of delaying strategies at the time that the parents tried to implement time-out, such as running away, endless arguments, refusals, dawdling on the way to his bedroom, appeals to go to the toilet, etc. The antecedent events to such 'subversive' tactics were situations where the parents felt some confusion about the application of the programme or disagreed about criteria. This transmitted itself as indecisiveness to Tommy. As a result of the child's delaying strategies — a variation of his non-compliance — Mrs. M. responded by repeating a request, calling his name in a warning voice after she had given the initial warning, following him to see if he had obeyed her command to go to the room, and generally hovering over him when he had to carry out a request. Mr. M. (if dealing with the situation) would repeat a request, followed by physical punishment used in conjunction with time-out. Tommy would then start screaming. Furthermore, Tommy's behaviour led to open disagreement between the parents in front of the child as to the application of the programme. This last consequence reflects a fundamental mistake that the therapists made, namely, the failure to include the father (who was not easily available) in the finer details of the working out of the programme. They left too much to Mrs. M. to communicate to her husband. Tommy, a subtle child, soon took advantage of this situation 'to divide and rule'. He managed to create ambiguous situations in which it was difficult for the parents to be sure if they were being manipulated as part of Tommy's more immature repertoire (e.g., a babylike request for help) or whether he was expressing a legitimate request for parental help.

To counter this, the parents and therapist spent much more time going over again the theoretical principles operating in the programme. They worked out precisely what *both* parents were going to say when they issued commands to Tommy. What came through very forcibly was that both parents wanted to avoid forcing themselves in an 'authoritarian' manner on their son. So there tended to be an internal debate when action was required. They would silently argue with themselves 'should I?' or 'shouldn't I?' before they gave Tommy a command. Precise cues were suggested to the mother so that she might avoid this agonizing dilemma and so she could act at the right time in a *decisive* manner. Authoritative commands, it was hoped, would nip Tommy's target behaviours in the bud and prevent their unpleasant repercussions. On the consequential side, it was suggested that when Tommy tried his delaying strategies, at the point of implementing time-out, he was to be picked up, with no eye contact and no verbal communication, and placed in his room, thus eliminating the attention he was gaining from his diversions. The response to this detailed plan was encouraging and the frequency of the target behaviours fell again to below baseline.

Another critical point came at the sixth/seventh week of the programme. Mrs. M. again became very despondent about the programme, feeling that Tommy's target behaviour of aggression was not responding to her efforts. But despite protestations, hostility, and resentment that she expressed to the therapists, she persevered. Reinforcement (in the form of encouragement and praise) are as important to the mediators of change in the child (his parents) as to the problem child himself. After all, they are being asked to change and are in a learning situation too. Perhaps the acid test of the programme came during the eighth/ninth week when Tommy fell ill. This crisis was weathered. Following these two weeks, the frequency of the target behaviours decreased even further than they had already until they were a rare occurrence.

The record showed that from baseline frequency, non-compliance had reduced by 54 per cent. Aggression had fallen by 68 per cent.; whining by 95 per cent.; interfering by 94 per cent.; and tantrums by 100 per cent. There was an *increase* of lunatic moods by 36 per cent. The reason(s) for this increase are speculative. Possibly the mother was still finding it hard to prevent the onset of the mood. However, by the end of the programme (eleventh week), there was an average occurrence for both non-compliance and aggression of less than one per day. There were no occurrences of the other target behaviours.

The introduction of the positive side of the programme (rewards) was not a smooth one. Mrs. M. tended to verbalize the programme, talking about Tommy's opportunity to earn a happy face. As a result there arose a series of disputations between mother or father and Tommy. It was evident that we had planned a reward system which contained several loopholes as far as a perceptive and resourceful entrepreneur like Tommy was concerned. As so often happens in behavioural programmes, we had to think again. A detailed plan was worked out with regard to the four behaviours that the parents wished to encourage. A more careful contract was designed, one which specified precisely how the parents were to respond to Tommy — determining (for example) a reasonable length of time to put toys away, deciding upon the parents' activities during this task, and determining when this task should take place. Happy faces were to be given to Tommy if he completed the task successfully without any prior cajoling or verbal warning of their delivery; the child himself was to be involved in sticking them on to the chart. As before the tokens would be exchanged for sweets and/or trips, and praise and physical hugs were to be given as before.

Mrs. M. objected, not to social reinforcement but to tangible rewards which she felt constituted a form of bribery and, what is more, developed a 'sweet tooth' in Tommy. The therapists were of the opinion that the token system acted as a reminder to the mother to praise and smile at Tommy for his acceptable behaviour, and, in retrospect, the use of tangible rewards (Smarties) were probably redundant. Tommy did in fact achieve all four tasks that his parents delineated for him. As Tommy's maladaptive behaviours decreased, there were more opportunities for the parents to 'enjoy' Tommy, which in themselves stimulated a high degree of mutual social reinforcement.

(6) Termination

This phase came at the end of 12 weeks of treatment. Mrs. M. faded out the token reinforcement programme but retained the use of positive social reinforcement (on an intermittent schedule consistent with real life) and the occasional use of time-out as a back-up to her now generally effective verbal control. The goals that were selected for treatment were achieved to the satisfaction of both parents. This expression of satisfaction which was confirmed by the monitoring of Tommy's behaviours constituted the main criteria for terminating the case. As a by-product of the programme, Tommy now gave the appearance of being a far happier child to the therapist (and more important) to his parents and their relatives. Mrs. M. no longer looked the harrassed woman of 12 weeks previously; she now had a lightness in the presentation of her personality.

(7) Follow-up

A series of checks by telephone and visits indicated that Tommy maintained his improvement for 12 months (our standard follow-up period). Mrs M. felt that she had successfully reintroduced the programme for short periods as and when it was necessary. Mrs. M. experienced a setback when, as she said, she let her criteria slip and began to take the line of least resistance. A booster programme was contemplated, by the present author, but within a week of going back to recording Mrs. M. found that she had the situation in hand, and the need for an intervention disappeared.

8

Hyperactivity (and Associated Difficulties)

It has aptly been said that when referring to brain-injured or hyperactive children we enter a 'semantic jungle'. The problem, variously called 'hyperactivity', 'hyperkinesis', or 'overactivity', has been defined (Werry et al., 1966) as a chronic, sustained, excessive level of motor activity which is the cause of significant and continued complaint both at home and at school. It is a highly subjective judgement as to when activity is excessive. And the other problems or 'symptoms' which supposedly constitute the 'hyperactivity syndrome' have yet to be objectively defined, although attempts are being made (see Barkley, 1982). There are no necessary and sufficient criteria for the diagnosis of hyperactivity. Neurological signs, when they exist, are 'equivocal'. Yet, like the other ambiguous concept 'psychopathy', the notion of a hyperactivity syndrome refuses to die. And perhaps it persists with justification. The hyperactive child is like the proverbial elephant: difficult to define, but, by golly, we know one when we see one. His frenetic and wilful approach to life is unmistakable. He can be so disruptive and uncontrolled (at times) that the victim is often brought to the attention of the doctor, paediatrician, or psychologist by his parents or teachers who perceive themselves to be the real victims. Hyperactivity is one of the primary reasons for referral to school psychologists (Heussey, 1967) and mental health clinics (Patterson, 1964) in the United States. Given the problem of definition mentioned earlier, epidemiological findings have to be treated with caution. The disorder is probably the most common of the childhood disorders, accounting for approximately 3 to 5 per cent. of the school-age population depending on the definition used and the source of opinion (see Rutter, 1977a).

This is a heavily researched topic; more than 2,000 articles have been published on the subject, not to mention the many books both for professional (e.g. Barkley, 1982) and lay audiences.

The majority of factor-analytic investigations have failed to isolate a specific *hyperactive* syndrome in the medical sense of a disease entity (see Werry, 1968). Rather, the 'symptoms' of hyperactivity emerge as part of a conduct disorder. There is evidence that the children reflect similar basic behavioural or personality dimensions. Indeed, the sole distinguishing criterion appears to be the amount of overactivity manifested by the child. Oppositional, antisocial, and learning problems are common in both.

It is this aspect — the *management* of behaviour problems in children who have been labelled/diagnosed as hyperactive — which has been of interest to the author. An assessment was made (Herbert, 1980b) of associated problems and background factors in a series of hyperactive children. What was impressive was the *large number* of behaviour problems they presented. Certain features kept recurring in our clinical and research data. There is a characteristic (though not invariable) profile of behavioural and interactional tendencies. Typically the child presents as a 'mobile disaster area'. With his short attention span, rapidly changing goals, and insatiable touching combined with a ham-fisted approach to the environment, he leaves in his wake broken toys, smashed ornaments, and upset grocery shelves (if his mother is foolhardy enough to take him into a supermarket). Other children, too, tend to get the rough edge of his tongue and sometimes his fist. His lack of fear (perhaps a function of his impulsiveness), his nomadic peregrinations ('he never sticks to anything for long'), and his gift for choosing to do things which compel his parents to intervene either to prevent injury to himself or others, means that they too can seldom settle to anything for long. He is attention-seeking and manipulative to a degree that is so all-embracing that his parents feel themselves to be on a 20-hours-a-day duty roster. Teachers find that not only does the hyperactive child fail to learn efficiently but he disrupts his classmates' concentration. These children are usually at their best in the one-to-one situation where they do not have to compete for attention.

The behaviour problem has the following elements: serious disobedience and failure to heed; defiance; 'excesses' of behaviour and predominance of negative mood (whiny petulance, excessive crying, screaming, tantrums); aggressiveness (fighting, destructiveness); low frustration tolerance (inability to delay gratification); extreme attention-seeking; commanding behaviour (pestering, nagging, demanding, clinging, etc.); lack of empathy (self-centred inability in the older children to see the other's point of view). From the parents' point of view the child seems out of control. They report that they very rarely 'enjoy' their children. The parents and child get involved in endless nagging sessions and tearful disputations which end up with smackings and only the briefest respite before the child is up to the same misdemeanour as before, or a new one.

For the purposes of the present discussion a 'hyperactive child' is simply a child with a variety of conduct problems among which overactivity features in a prominent fashion. The clinical task is not to find a diagnostic label which has no implications but to assess the child in such a way that a programme can be designed to modify inappropriate surplus behaviours or to produce appropriate responses where there are deficits. The all-round despair and misery generated in the homes of these children leaves little doubt that even by the tender ages of 3, 4, or 5 years, and at older ages (in the classroom, too), these children can have potentially serious behaviour problems. In the wake of such problems comes social isolation (for parents and child), learning difficulties at school, and much unhappiness (see Figure 7). The little evidence there is suggests a poor prognosis if nothing is done about the hyperactive child's behaviour problems (see Barcai and Rabkin, 1974).

What is one to make of the diverse problems shown by hyperactive children? Is there an underlying organic condition or some other unifying process? It is not clear whether some of the behaviours these children exhibit are primary or secondary to other problems. For example, hyperactivity, lack of attention, and distractibility could represent the random response pattern of an over-aroused individual who has not found the operant that terminates aversive stimulation. In the case of a child, the stress may be the social pressures to learn difficult academic and social skills. The reason for his failure to produce the appropriate behaviour might be an inability to perceive the relevant discriminative stimuli or an inability to make the responses in the manner demanded by the environment (see page 55). It could also be argued that lack of attention, distractibility, and hyperactivity themselves provide the reasons as to why the child is unable to attend to the discriminative stimuli, and therefore not learning. This possibility raises a further question: why, in the first place, is the child distractible and hyperactive?

ORGANIC FACTORS

Various aetiological theories have been offered for the disturbed motor and attentional behaviour, but the cause or, more probably, causes are unknown. Explanatory theories include brain damage, biochemical disorders, minor congenital physical anomalies, abnormally low central nervous system arousal, genetic disorders, food allergies or simply a biological variation made manifest by universal compulsory education. All these theories are rather speculative (see Barkley, 1982).

In the study of hyperactive children aged from 5 to 11 years by Stewart et al. (1966), 47 per cent. of the patients' mothers felt that their children began to behave abnormally before their first birthday. The hyperactive children had all developed the great majority of their problems by the time they started school. This might suggest some very early congenital pathology, and, indeed, a common anamnestic finding from the pregnancy and birth histories is of a difficult gestation and/or delivery. The ancient Chinese were well aware of the psychological sequelae of birth complications. Modern empirical studies bear out their aphorism: 'difficult birth, difficult child'. There is evidence (Shirley,

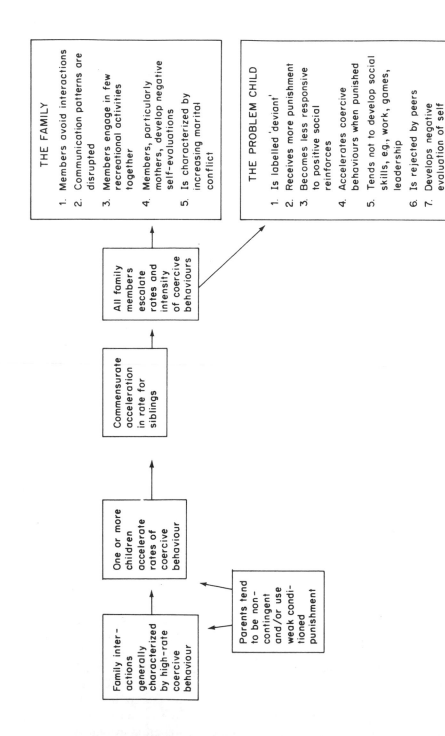

THE FAMILY

1. Members avoid interactions
2. Communication patterns are disrupted
3. Members engage in few recreational activities together
4. Members, particularly mothers, develop negative self-evaluations
5. Is characterized by increasing marital conflict

THE PROBLEM CHILD

1. Is labelled 'deviant'
2. Receives more punishment
3. Becomes less responsive to positive social reinforces
4. Accelerates coercive behaviours when punished
5. Tends not to develop social skills, eg, work, games, leadership
6. Is rejected by peers
7. Develops negative evaluation of self and others

All family members escalate rates and intensity of coercive behaviours

Commensurate acceleration in rate for siblings

One or more children accelerate rates of coercive behaviour

Family inter-actions generally characterized by high-rate coercive behaviour

Parents tend to be non-contingent and/or use weak condi-tioned punishment

Figure 7 Coercive family interactions (Patterson, 1982)

1939) that babies born precipitately after a short, sharp labour, or born after their mothers have endured difficult pregnancies (as in the case of full or partial placenta praevia) tend to be irritable, hyperactive, and difficult as babies and as older children. Drillien (1964) found that the most common behaviour problems associated with very severe prematurity (birth weight of 3 lb or less) were hyperactivity and restlessness. These problems, and distractibility, are probably the only types of behaviour disorder of childhood which can be associated (with any degree of confidence as to causality) with perinatal factors.

However, when Werry et al. (1972) carried out a neurological examination of 20 hyperactive, 20 neurotic, and 20 normal children, the finding that the hyperactive children could be distinguished from the others by an excess of minor neurological signs indicative of sensorimotor incoordination was not backed up by differences in the frequency of major signs, EEG abnormalities, or abnormal medical histories indicative of brain trauma. The researchers admit that the source and significance of this abnormality is unclear.

Stewart et al. (1966) report that only four of their hyperactive patients had a history which suggested probable brain injury, a proportion of 11 per cent. However, they conclude that the prevalence of delayed speech development, speech problems, poor coordination, and strabismus in their patients suggests that brain dysfunction rather than primary psychological factors is often the basis for the problem.

Doubtless in many cases of hyperactivity (e.g., those associated with epilepsy and cerebral palsy) there is strong suggestive evidence of some organic involvement in the high level of activity. However, hyperactivity can and does occur in children without any other independent indication of cerebral dysfunction (Werry et al., 1966). Kaspar et al. (1971) have demonstrated that while brain-damaged children are more active and distractible than normal controls in a structured-test situation, brain damage does not lead to hyperactivity and distractibility under any and all stimulus conditions 'but rather to certain forms of hyperactivity in certain children, certain forms of distractibility in others, and so on'. Yet the organic basis of all hyperactivity cases remains an article of faith for some researchers.

It is the global identification of the hyperkinetic syndrome with another vague diagnostic entity 'minimal cerebral dysfunction' or 'minimal brain damage' (m.b.d.) which seems unproductive. The concept of m.b.d. has few, if any, descriptive, aetiological, prognostic, or treatment implications (Herbert, 1964) and in any event is not a unitary dimension (Schulman, Kaspar, and Thorne, 1965; Werry, 1968). As it is, the hyperactive syndrome is only too susceptible to being used as a diagnostic wastebasket for children who are odd and who display puzzling symptoms including some above-average or disruptive level of activity.

PREVIOUS LEARNING EXPERIENCES

The histories (Herbert, 1974) of hyperactive children suggest that many are difficult from birth. Their parents often feel defeated by the combination of the intensity of the oppositional behaviour of the children and their own uncertainties about how to cope. This occurs, in many cases, long before their decision to seek professional help. For the mothers this is a desperately difficult time of their lives and many exist with the doubtful help of tranquillizers. From soon after birth their hyperactive babies have been too squirmy and restless to feed or nurse with ease. There are chronic feeding problems, colic (intermittent, prolonged, but unexpected crying), and severe bedtime and sleeping problems.

We know that the young child's activity level and ability to sustain attention can influence the expectations of its caretakers. Halverson and Waldrop (1970) observe that mothers of (presumably congenitally) more impulsive 30-month-old boys seem to be set for trouble when attempting to get their offspring to perform a series of experimental tasks. They suggest that this set probably stems from past experiences with their sons, since the same mothers seem less negative and controlling in the same situation with other, equally impulsive children. Bell and Ainsworth (1972) demonstrate that by the second half of the first year of life, infant crying seems to make their mothers reluctant to respond promptly. Because maternal delay is significantly associated with greater infant crying, it is suggested that for some mothers a tendency on the part of their babies towards prolonged crying could set up a vicious circle — maternal refractoriness leading to more infant crying, leading to increased maternal refractoriness, and so on. Persistent crying is a common finding in the early histories of hyperactive children. Cause and effect are difficult, if not impossible, to unravel in retrospective analyses. What parents often say is that they were reacting to a difficult and miserable child, and they point to his 'normal' sibling(s) by way of saying: 'You see we can't be blamed altogether; we didn't fail with this one. He was easier to rear.'

Negativism is a significant feature of the early behaviour of hyperactive children. An infant's negativism may arouse caregiver hostility (Yarrow, 1968).

Research into the behaviour problems of hyperactive children is incomplete, but it is possible to speak again about a strong but tentative conviction that a significant factor in the development of their problems is a temperamental or congenital factor (and in particular one to do with activity) which has powerfully modified the parents' expectations and the manner in which they have reared the child (Herbert, 1974). Early learning is shaped in a particular way. Patterson et al. (1965) state that empirical findings suggest an interesting hypothesis: that there is a curvilinear relationship between activity level of the child and the acquisition of socially acceptable behaviour. Up to moderately high levels of activity, the child's behaviour will call forth an increasing number of reactions from peers and adults. Assuming that these reactions are, by and large, positive, this probably means that the very active child will acquire social skills at a faster rate than the less active child. It is further assumed that *extremely high* rates of behaviour are aversive for other people; thus the reactions from society are more likely to be punitive. In this situation, the child functioning at high levels of activity is quite likely to be punished *even* when he is displaying socially acceptable behaviour, e.g., friendliness or cooperation. This higher ratio of punishment to reinforced behaviour for the hyperactive child may well result in his acquiring social behaviour at a slow pace.

Another potentially adverse influence in the life experiences of hyperactive children is the high prevalence of psychopathy, hysteria, and alcoholism in the mothers and fathers of hyperactive children (Cantwell, 1972; Morrison and Stewart, 1971). A substantial proportion of these parents were themselves hyperactive as children. Rutter (1966) has demonstrated a close association between psychiatric and physical illness in parents and psychological disorder in their offspring.

CONTEMPORARY INFLUENCES

The planning of a programme of treatment for a hyperactive child can only be discussed realistically with regard to individual circumstances. However, it is possible to make a few generalizations. The following considerations (most of which are current influences) are likely to enter into most assessments:

(1) The child's high level of arousal and excess motor activity.
(2) His poor performance (socialization) at home and his performance (scholastic attainment) at school.
(3) His distractibility and poor attention span.
(4) Concomitant behaviour problems such as non-compliant, attention-seeking, and commanding behaviour (surplus behaviours such as excessive crying, tantrums, and whining may also be a feature).
(5) In all likelihood there is a reinforcement history which is unusual in its ratio of punishments to rewards. The hyperactive child's behaviour is so below the norm in so many aspects that he has a remarkable experience of failure.
(6) He has a great need of attention and success. So great may be his need that he may actively seek any attention even if it looks to other people like punishment (e.g., naggings and smackings).
(7) The child often suffers from social isolation, being rejected by his peers. This may be a result of his oddity and aggression.
(8) His mother and father are likely to have lost confidence in their effectiveness as parents; they may feel that the child is beyond their control and is manipulating them. They are also likely to be exhausted (hyperactive children tend to have sleeping problems), despairing, and guilty about their feelings of rejection and violence towards the child.
(9) The child is unrewarding to his parents; they don't enjoy him (and, sometimes, the reverse must be true).

In designing a treatment strategy for the problems of hyperactive children, their hyperactive behaviours can be conceived of as operants. Grindee (1970) and Patterson (1965) have successfully employed operant techniques to reduce the high rates of behaviour associated with the syndrome. Of course, it is quite likely that hyperactive behaviours are a final common pathway for the expression of various disorders. Thus high levels of cortical arousal (due to brain dysfunction) may influence the probability of the maladaptive behaviours being emitted.

MEDICATION

Werry and Sprague (1970) make the point that excess motor activity is characteristic of inefficiently functioning organisms — e.g., developmentally immature organisms. Pharmacological agents have been used since the 1930s to control hyperactivity. Their use, of late, has been a matter of considerable public controversy in the United States (Schrag and Divoky, 1975; Weithorn, 1973), where the diagnosis of hyperactivity is somewhat popular.

Among the drugs in use are central stimulant or stimulant-like drugs (such as dextroamphetamine, methylphenidate, and pemoline); major tranquillizing phenothiazines (such as chlorpromazine and thioridazine) and butyrophenones (such as haloperidol); tricyclic antidepressants (such as imipramine and amitriptyline) and sedatives (such as barbiturates).

As a rule, pharmacotherapy will extend for several years. All these compounds carry their risks of side-effects. Perhaps the greatest risk is the psychological one for therapists — that they are so easy to prescribe in the context of a busy general, psychiatric, or paediatric practice. Their availability may short-circuit the necessary detailed technical and ethical analysis of the child's motor, attentional, and behavioural problems. In the absence of such care, drug therapy can degenerate into a facile and dangerous method of social control in the home and the classroom. A behavioural approach may make the use of drugs unnecessary or may, in combination with medication (see Christensen, 1975), make prolonged drug dependence and the abdication from personal parental responsibility less likely.

Another risk is also psychological in the sense that the patient is likely to attribute change to an outside agent (the drug or 'the pill') rather than to himself or herself. In any event, the responsivity rate to central stimulants is only between 50 and 70 per cent. (Wender, 1971), and recent long-term follow-up studies indicate a poor prognosis for the hyperactive child despite drug treatment (Heussey, Metoyer, and Townsend, 1973). The value of the various drugs and their side-effects are reviewed by Achenbach, 1982; Barkley, 1982; and Conners, 1974. In view of the side-effects, the ineffectiveness of medication with many hyperactive children, and the reluctance of many parents to use medication, physicians may in many cases require an alternative treatment.

Unfortunately, there are few well-controlled studies of the effects of behaviour therapy on hyperactive behaviour and no study which systematically compares behaviour therapy and drug therapy with hyperactive children.

Among the most useful treatments available are the stimulants caffeine, dextroamphetamine and methylphenidate. Researchers (Conners, 1972; Wender, 1971) report that stimulant drugs are beneficial in one-half to two-thirds of cases. Sadly, there is no way to predict the effectiveness of such drugs in the individual child. These are the less toxic of the compounds mentioned above. Nevertheless, high doses of methylphenidate carry the risk of weight loss, anorexia, and the suppression of growth (Safer and Allen, 1975).

Weiss et al. (1968) in a double-blind uncrossed study of the effects of individualized dosage of dextroamphetamine and placebo on a group of 38 hyperactive children of normal intelligence showed that dextroamphetamine is superior to placebo in reducing hyperactivity and distractibility. Chlorpromazine was also highly effective in reducing hyperactivity but had no demonstrable effect on distractibility. The therapeutic effect of dextroamphetamine was more variable than that of chlorpromazine, more often resulting in dramatic improvement or in no appreciable change.

The therapeutic effects — the suppression of overactivity and impulsivity and lengthening of attention span — are sometimes described as 'paradoxical' because when stimulants are given to adult patients their activity is increased rather than calmed. This notion is criticized by some theorists; all that is known is that the pharmacological effect in many adults *and* children is heightened efficiency. Dosage is a very individual matter from child to child, but with any drug a thorough trial should be undertaken.

Werry et al. (1966) in a double-blind study of 39 out-patient chronically hyperactive children of normal intelligence (mean age 8.5 years) demonstrated that chlorpromazine was significantly superior to placebo, its maximum therapeutic effect being manifest in the area of hyperactivity. Other symptoms seemed less amenable to the influence of this drug, though more subtle refinements of measurement may subsequently reveal smaller and still hidden therapeutic effects. The effect of chlorpromazine did not seem to be influenced by other variables such as a positive history of brain damage, an abnormal EEG, a poor family environment, or added psychopathology. The severity of the hyperactivity tends to diminish any therapeutic effect slightly. Placebo effects were conspicuous, over half the placebo group showing improvement. Changes in intellectual functioning were minimal.

The available evidence about sedatives such as barbiturates is that they are not helpful and, indeed, may exacerbate the hyperactive child's behaviour problems.

BASELINE DATA

Attempts (see Barkley, 1982) have been made to quantify and objectify the activity dimension. Bell, Waldrop, and Weller (1972) developed six rating scales for hyperactivity* and three for withdrawal from a series of studies on

* Items, 4, 10, 14, 15, 20, 25.

202 early pre-school-age children. The scales were tested for factor composition and it was found that they formed one bipolar hyperactivity-withdrawal factor for males and separate hyperactivity and withdrawal factors for females. The authors have produced a scoring system that can be applied by teachers on a periodic basis to keep a running account of hyperactive and withdrawn behaviour. The scales are useful for assessing the results of treatment programmes for hyperactive and withdrawn children.

Similar attempts have been made to measure objectively the second major dimension in the hyperactivity syndrome: the problem involving a disorder of attention (see Sykes et al., 1971). It is worth noting — in the light of the absence of an agreed definition of hyperactivity — that the attentional problem may be primary. The supposed overactivity of 'hyperactive' children may be a reflection of the short attention span and rapidly changing goal directions of such children.

The Connors' teacher rating scale (Sprague and Sleator, 1973) has been widely used as a standardized measure of change with hyperactive children. Indeed, it is probably of only limited value to concentrate on highly elaborate quantitative measurements of activity level. What is required is information about specific problem behaviours (motor, attentional, and others), the situations in which they occur, antecedent events (i.e. controlling stimuli) and response-reinforcement contingencies (i.e., environmental consequences).

Werry (1968) recognizes that the essential issue confronting the behaviour therapist is what situation is likely to facilitate substantial and lasting behaviour change. He conceptualizes the hyperactivity problem as follows: each of the child's days consists of an infinite number of successive learning trials in which hyperactivity is being strengthened or weakened. Thus, it follows that a successful behaviour modification programme for hyperactivity should utilize at least a majority of these learning trials. Werry maintains that this can be achieved only by a substantial and significant alteration of the eliciting stimuli and response-reinforcement contingencies — by restructuring the child's environment where these problem behaviours are displayed and by involving those persons who ordinarily dispense rewards and punishments and who have control over eliciting stimuli.

As in the case of all problems, an ongoing record is kept of the frequency of the targeted behaviour problems. Baseline data provide an objective evaluation of the severity of the problem and a yardstick against which to measure change (see Appendix A) during therapy. It sometimes has a 'placebo' effect. Sulzbacher (1975) reports that some 15 to 20 per cent. of hyperactive children improve by simply having the parent or teacher gather baseline data.

ANTECEDENT CONTROL

A major characteristic of the hyperactive child is his distractibility. He finds it difficult to cope by means of selective perception, ignoring irrelevant, inessential stimulation. O'Malley and Eisenberg (1973) suggest decreasing the amount of extraneous stimulation, decreasing the choices and alternatives, and encouraging patterns of behaviour which earn the child approval. There are several down-to-earth suggestions which can be made: avoiding potential 'disaster areas' such as supermarkets, restaurants, cinemas, the front seat of the car, and so on, when in company of the child. Making special provisions can be helpful, like arranging a play space separate from the main living room or (when this is not possible) 'baby-proofing' the room by removing precious and delicate objects. Having a separate bedroom from siblings, making mealtimes and other 'confrontation' situations carefully structured in terms of rules and routines, avoiding long and futile arguments about getting ready for school by being firm and decisive — all these ideas for pre-empting tiring clashes of will can be worked out in advance, subject to the constraints upon the family. Whatever the limitations, the principles can be translated into practical suggestions for parents and written into a parent–child contract. They have to be specific and detailed, and the parents may require help in putting them into practice. The classroom setting and its unsuitability for the idiosyncracies of the hyperactive child is another aspect of the environment that will need close attention. It is in planning for home management and education that target assessment is particularly helpful. First, it is vital for the therapist to find a level of social or academic performance at which the child has already experienced success. This provides a realistic basis on which to begin whatever therapeutic or educational programme is planned. Second, the programme for a given child must directly reflect the problems which the child is presenting. Third, the programme is presented to the child within a learning situation and time span which permits conditioning to take place — a critical point given his learning difficulties. Finally, the therapeutic or educational programme is highly structured environmentally and methodologically for the child.

Meichenbaum and Goodman (1971) suggest that the therapist can instruct the hyperactive, impulsive child in the concept of talking to himself and gain the child's attention by using his natural medium of play. For example, while playing with one hyperactive child, the therapist said, 'I have to land my airplane, now slowly, carefully, into the hanger.' The therapist then encouraged the child to have the control tower tell the pilot to go slowly, etc. In this way he is able to help the child to build up a repertoire of self-statements to be used on a variety of tasks. Training begins on a set of tasks (games) in which the child is somewhat proficient and for which he does *not* have a history of failures and frustrations. The therapist employs tasks that lend themselves to a self-instructional approach and which will encourage the use of cognitive strategies. The method of self-instructional training is flexible and usually follows the principle of successive approximations. Initially, the therapist models and has the child rehearse simple self-statements such as 'Stop! Think before I answer.' Gradually the therapist models (and the child rehearses) more complex sets of self-statements.

The procedure can be supplemented with the manipulation of imagery, especially in treating young children. The impulsive child is trained to imagine and to subsequently instruct himself as follows: 'I will not go faster than a slow turtle, slow turtle.' Schneider (1973) has used such a turtle imagery procedure to foster self-control in hyperactive, disruptive school children. Schneider incorporates the turtle image into a story which is read to the class. Following the story the students imitate the turtle who withdrew into his shell when he felt he was about to lose control. This was followed by relaxation, self-instructional and problem-solving exercises to teach self-control. In the Schneider study the teacher spent 15 minutes each day for approximately 3 weeks in training and achieved reduced aggressive behaviour and fewer frustration responses. The therapist could use a variety of different stories and cognitive techniques to teach self-control behaviours. It is possible to train children to control their own behaviours by saying sentences to themselves such as 'Stop, look, and listen' or 'Count to ten'. Self-instruction is still a relatively neglected area but one that is worthy of exploration for anyone interested in teaching self-control to children.

OUTCOME CONTROL

According to Cruickshank (1968) the basic need of hyperactive children is for *success* — success in something in which adults and adult society genuinely believe. All children have this need, but unlike most children hyperactive youngsters seldom enjoy a reasonable share of success. Unfortunately, hyperactive children are likely to have experienced a sort of 'built-in' failure. As Cruickshank explains, their unacceptable behaviour increasingly excludes them from the circle of acceptance in the family, the neighbourhood, the school, and in the community at large. They tend to be strangers to the usual range of symbolic rewards or social reinforcers which regulate appropriate behaviour.

Defective attention is a primary factor in the hyperactive child's lack of success. During the last decade research on academic achievement has demonstrated that attention is a basic skill, underlying or preceding learning effectiveness, and thus one of the main variables differentiating high and low achievers. A positive relationship between attention and school learning has been demonstrated with kindergarten subjects and with sixth-grade students (Ladhaderne, 1968). Other authors have described attention as a basic skill, underlying or preceding other learning (Gagne, 1965).

Alabiso (1975) defines attention as a multibehavioural process involving the length of time that the subject can spend at a given task (concentration span), his ability to respond correctly (focus), and his ability to make two-stage stimulus discriminations (selectivity). The hyperactive child falls short in all of these aspects. Attending behaviour obviously becomes a crucial and desirable alternative to hyperactivity.

PROMOTING PROSOCIAL BEHAVIOUR IN CLASSROOM SETTINGS

Therapists have utilized principles of operant conditioning to supplant inattentive (and disruptive motor) behaviours by strengthening incompatible but socially acceptable alternatives. It is assumed (see Patterson et al., 1965) that both environmental and internal stimuli have become discriminative for the emission of such behaviours as pinching, squirming, looking around, tapping, and walking about the room. Theoretically, it should be possible to condition a set of responses to these same stimulus configurations that would interfere with the occurrence of these hyperactive behaviours.

In the classroom setting, *differential reinforcement* has been used to strengthen 'attending' responses. These might include looking at a book, looking at the arithmetic problem, or listening to the teacher. Because of the relatively high strength of the hyperactive behaviours, it is necessary to arrange for potent reinforcing stimuli to be contingent upon the occurrence of these desirable responses; furthermore, the latency between their emission and the occurrence of the reinforcing stimulus must be very short — a practical desideratum which is not easy to achieve in a busy classroom of several pupils.

Patterson et al. (1965) describe a method for conditioning attending behaviour in hyperactive children. Attention in the classroom implies keeping relatively still and is incompatible with behaviours such as shuffling chairs, looking out of the window, fiddling with objects, wiggling one's feet, and so on. These are easily recorded. It is not easy to observe something as vague as 'paying attention' in a direct and objective manner. Patterson and his colleagues suggest that in order to focus on observable behaviour the formulation of a double negative is necessary in designing a treatment programme: reinforcement is made contingent on the 'non-occurrence of non-attendance behaviour'. The researchers illustrate their procedure in the case of Raymond, a brain-injured hyperactive boy aged 10 years referred to the Oregon University Clinic. Observations of his behaviour (and that of another hyperactive brain-injured child, Ricky, also aged 10, acting as a control) were made in the classroom setting. The observations were made from an observation booth adjoining the classroom and provided data on the frequency of occurrence of seven categories of non-attending behaviour including the following high rate responses: walking, talking, distraction, and 'wiggling'. Each child was observed for a minimum of 10 minutes a day, 4 days a week. Following several weeks of baseline observation, the conditioning procedure was begun with the experimental subject. Using a radio transmitter device, a signal was sent for each 10-second interval in which none of the non-attending responses occurred. This fixed-interval schedule was maintained for the first four conditioning trials and sweets were used for rewards. The first conditioning trial lasted 7 minutes, and the trials were increased one by one for 3 minutes each day until 20-minute trials were reached. After the fifth trial, a variable-interval schedule was used. The total number of reinforcers for a given trial ranged from 15 to 70. There was a significant reduction in Raymond's non-attending behaviour. This improvement was maintained over a 4-week extinction period. Ricky showed no significant change over the 3-month period.

In work of this nature, it is customary and desirable to have some form of contract which makes clear the reinforcement contingencies to the child. Patterson, in his treatment of 9-year-old Earl, did just this (Patterson, 1965).

Earl was a hyperactive child who was almost always misbehaving in the classroom: talking, pushing, hitting, pinching, looking about the room and out of the window, leaving his desk, tapping, squirming, and fiddling with objects. In addition, he was aggressive, pinched other children, and threw himself into groups of children, disrupting their work or play. He occasionally engaged in shoving his desk around the classroom, pushing aside all the children and desks in his way. As an aggressive 9-year-old in a classroom of 7-year-olds. Earl was not surprisingly socially isolated; the other children consciously avoided him. Isolated children are prepared, often, to accept attention (and self-esteem) in any way they can get it — and sometimes this involves being a buffoon. Earl's disruptive behaviour was reinforced by laughter from the class and other signs taken by him to be 'approval'. So, in planning a treatment strategy. Patterson announced not only to Earl but also the entire class what would happen. A small box containing a light bulb and a counter was placed on Earl's desk. He was told that at the end of each 10-second interval, if he had paid attention to his work for the entire time, the light would flash and the counter would add a count. Each time this happened he had earned one sweet or one penny and these would be given to him at the end of each lesson. The daily lessons lasted from 5 to 30 minutes. The students were told that some of the pennies and sweets which Earl earned for working hard and paying attention to his lessons would be shared with all of them and that they could help Earl earn more if they did not distract him when he was working. The decision to include the other pupils in the rewards provided the additional bonus of social reinforcement. At the end of each conditioning session when the score was announced, the children applauded Earl. They also frequently walked by his desk to check the counter and to see how many reinforcements he had earned and spoke approvingly to him, thereby giving him the added encouragement which encouraged him to work even harder.

During the baseline period. Earl spent 25 per cent. of his time making disruptive or inattentive responses. By the end of the 10 days of treatment, he misbehaved less than 5 per cent. of the time. Near the end of the therapeutic experiment. Earl was observed for a 2-hour period. He now presented as a well-behaved child in the classroom and was also less hyperactive and destructive in the playground. He played with the other children rather than hurling himself at them. Four months later, he was still much quieter in the classroom and, for the first time, other children were coming to his home to play. In addition, he was making progress in a remedial reading programme.

Doubros and Daniels (1966) are critical of Patterson's method of announcing the contingencies to the child and his classmates. They are of the opinion that this introduces uncontrolled social reinforcement and awareness, factors they attempted to control in their own work. Of course, it is on issues like this that the basically 'research' and 'clinical service' orientated psychologists differ. Not that there is any necessary dichotomy between being a good clinician and a diligent and critical researcher. However, the priorities and therefore the emphasis given to a treatment design may vary between the two. As long as it is necessary to test the effectiveness of a specific therapeutic procedure, a verbal statement of the contingencies announced to the patient (as in this example) would confound the experiment. Where a therapeutic programme has advanced beyond the experimental stage, or where the problem is particularly disturbing, anything that enhances the treatment process — be it a placebo effect, parent counselling, or verbal instructions — is legitimately brought to bear in helping the child.*

Doubros and Daniels (1966) controlled for social reinforcement and awareness in their own work on the reduction of hyperactivity in six mentally retarded boys. The results of their experiment suggest that differential reinforcement of other behaviour (DRO) can be an effective method for reducing hyperactivity and increasing constructive play. They worked with six hyperactive, mentally retarded children aged from 8 to 13 years. The subjects were first observed individually for a period of 8 days in the playroom in order to obtain a baseline performance on a specially constructed checklist of hyperactive behaviour. Following this, the conditioning phase began under a fixed schedule of reinforcement with tokens as the reinforcing agents (later to be exchanged for sweets). A fading-out phase was instituted after a 30-day conditioning period in order to maintain resistance to extinction at a higher level. Postconditioning observations were then made. It was demonstrated that the disturbed, hyperactive behaviour came under stimulus control with 'grasshopper' play decreasing substantially during the latter part of the conditioning and extinction periods. It is not known whether the responses the children learned in the playroom generalized to other settings.

Allen et al. (1967) conducted a study to ascertain whether social reinforcement procedures would alter the attention span aspect of the hyperactivity of James, a 4-year old, who tended to flit from activity to activity. Records kept over five school mornings showed that the average duration of James' activities was less than I minute. The authors were able to control the child's behaviour by providing social reinforcements only if James persisted in a single activity for a period exceeding 1 minute. The hyperactive behaviour was reduced by 50 per cent. in this way.

* This issue is raised by the ABAB design. See Appendix A. Where complex behaviour patterns must be modified a combination of treatment methods may be required (and not all necessarily from the behavioural field), thus confounding precise treatment-effect evaluation. Another shortcoming, if such it is, is that the elaborate equipment, electronic devices, independent judges, and observers are not always available in clinical practice as they seem to be in research centres.

Woolfolk and Woolfolk (1974) compared three conditions in the management of inattentiveness: one experimental and two control conditions. These were (1) participation in small-group lessons incorporating a token reinforcement programme (E); (2) participation in the same lessons without the token programme (C1); or (3) participation in the regular classroom activities during the entire investigations (C2). Within each condition were children whose classroom teachers had received in-service training in reinforcement principles and others whose classroom teachers had received no such training. The subjects were 54 first-, second-, and third-grade students from a public school in Austin, Texas. Three classes from each grade and six children from each classroom were involved in the project. Subjects were selected on the basis of their scores on an observational measure of attention (attention rating instrument), the least attentive children in each classroom being chosen. The authors tested the following hypotheses:

(1) A contingency management strategy involving a vigilance task and token reinforcement would be associated with increased task attention during treatment lessons.
(2) These increases in attention would generalize to the ordinary classroom.
(3) Generalization of gains in attention to the ordinary classroom would be greater for those pupils whose teachers received in-service training in the theory and practice of social reinforcement.

The children were observed and scores assigned on the attention rating instrument during the treatment lessons (treatment attention score) and during the ordinary classroom activities (in-class attention score). A second index of student attention was the child's vigilance score, earned during the special treatment lesson. This score represented the number of correct responses made by the subject to a signal instruction given by the teacher.

Subjects assigned to the experimental (E) group left their ordinary classrooms for 30 minutes each school day for 4 weeks. During this time the students from each grade level met together in small groups of six with a specially trained teacher. The content of these lessons included stories, songs, sound effects, and other listening activities. At ten randomly preselected times during each session, seemingly as a part of the lesson, directions were given to the subjects to make some motor response. Examples of these directions included 'Touch your nose', 'Open your mouth', 'Raise your hand', and 'Close your eyes'. The entire lesson, including these directions, was scripted so that content would be the same for both the E and C1 groups. After the signal was given, the teacher recorded one point for each child who responded appropriately within 2 seconds.

A special scoreboard was designed to record the points earned by each child. Each child's name was followed by a row of ten moveable wooden beads on a wire. One bead was moved from the left side of the board to the right each time a child earned a point. This gave him immediate feedback, provided a visual representation of his progress, and avoided the frequent interruptions of the lesson necessitated by the dispensing of tokens.

During the second week of the investigation, after the children became familiar with the individual point-earning system, a group contingency was added. At five randomly preselected times during the lesson the teacher assessed group attention. If all members of the group were attending, as defined by the behavioural criteria established for the attention rating instrument, a group bonus point was awarded by moving a large gold bead from the left to the right side of the scoreboard. This automatically added one point to each child's score for the day. Throughout the point-tallying procedure, a child's name was used only when he earned a point, and teacher praise was systematically paired with the awarding of points.

At the end of each day the children's points were recorded on individual tally cards and on a group chart. Initially, points were exchanged for sweets at the end of each lesson, and then after two lessons. After the first week points were saved to be exchanged for the opportunity to play with an assortment of toys at the end of a two-lesson period. When each child had earned a specified number of points, the entire group was allowed to play. Points earned by individual subjects in excess of the quota were saved toward the 'purchase' of a toy at the end of the treatment period. Quotas were established in such a way that points had to be saved for increasingly longer periods of time before a reward period could be earned.

Subjects assigned to the control condition 1(C1) participated simultaneously in the same lessons as the E condition subjects, meeting in small groups with another special teacher. The same vigilance signals were given, but points were not awarded contingent upon appropriate response. On days when the E condition subjects were given sweets or allowed to play with toys, the C1 subjects received identical non-contingent privileges. Subjects assigned to the control group 2 (C2) remained in their regular classrooms during the study and continued their usual activities.

The results (with regard to hypothesis 1) indicated that the treatment techniques *were* effective in eliciting and maintaining the attention of the subjects during the special lessons. Although the children were selected on the basis of their low rates of attention in their regular classrooms, they were immediately able to produce high levels of attention in the special lesson. Furthermore, these high rates of attending behaviour were maintained during the entire 4-week treatment period. Children taking part in the same lessons, but not receiving the experimental treatment techniques, initially exhibited lower levels of attention. The attention levels of these youngsters fell sharply over the 4-week period. The observations of the special teachers were in keeping with the experimental findings. They reported that, while the E group subjects were enthusiastic and task oriented, the C1 condition subjects frequently exhibited disruptive behaviours, were very erratic in their participation in the lessons, and were not eager to come to the lessons. With regard to hypothesis (2), the increments in attention did not generalize to the ordinary

154

classroom, in spite of the fact that differences between E and C1 subjects were immediately exhibited and highly significant. The authors note that the thesis (that simple practice in exhibiting attending behaviours should lead to increased attention in other situations) was not confirmed by the results. In connection with hypothesis (3), teachers were observed (in a separate study) and their behaviour assessed. No overall differences were identified between the trained and untrained groups in the dispensing of reinforcement for attentive or inattentive behaviours. Before, during, and after the treatment period, in-class attention scores of children whose teachers had received in-service training were compared with the scores of those whose teachers had received no training. No significant differences were found. Increases in classroom teacher's recognition and praise of attention were not associated with increased student attending behaviours in the ordinary classroom. These changes in teacher behaviour were not sufficient to maintain the attending behaviours that had been established by the more powerful and systematic token reinforcement programme.

Alabiso (1975) also attempted to confirm the hypothesis that attending behaviours can be brought under operant control and their frequency increased to the point of inhibiting hyperactive behaviour. The subjects were eight institutionalized, hyperactive retardates, ranging in age from 8 years 3 months to 12 years 4 months (mean IQ 44). They were selected on the basis of their level of attention span, focus of attention ability, selective attention ability, and degree of hyperactivity. All the children were receiving drug therapy and were rated by their teachers as being the most active children in their special education classes. Measures of span, focus, and selective attention consisted of the length of time that a subject could remain seated, the frequency of correct responses to an eye–hand coordination task, and the number of correct responses to a two-stage stimulus discrimination task. The tasks themselves were chosen on the basis of the teacher's requests. Teachers targeted out-of-seat behaviours, poor motor coordination, and deficits in concept formation as the learning disabilities that they would most like to see changed. During the baseline period, measures of attention span were obtained in terms of the sitting and out-of-seat behaviours (OSB) response rates of all subjects. These were recorded for six 10-minute intervals at various times over a 10-day period. An eye–hand coordination task was also used; this requires subjects to resist distraction and to focus their attention in order to copy digits and symbols. Finally, all subjects were required to discriminate between the test stimulus and an array of other stimuli on the basis of dimension (form) and cue(size). The baseline data for focus of attention and selective attention were collected by the classroom teachers.

Span training

Token and social reinforcements were made contingent upon being able to sit according to the increased fixed interval (IFI) schedule. If the child remained seated for a specified interval, a red light came on and the subject received token and social reinforcements. After ten training sessions of 30 minutes each a 30-minute extinction period was initiated.

Focus training

After a warm-up period of ten reinforced responses, the children were trained in focusing attention. The training task consisted of copying digits and symbols in correct order. After the child had earned 50 continuous reinforcements (CRF), fixed ratio 3 (FR 3) and fixed ratio 5 (FR5) reinforcement schedules were introduced over the next hundred trials. In addition, children received concurrent variable interval 5-minute (VI5) reinforcement for sitting behaviour. Finally, performance was recorded during 50 extinction trials.

Selective attention training

Selective attention training required the children to make stimulus discriminations. The stimulus dimension and the stimulus cue were varied at each trial. After ten successful one-stage stimulus discrimination trials, the subjects received CRF during a 50-trial period followed by successive, 50-trial FR3 and FR5 periods. Concurrent VI5 reinforcement of span for sitting behaviour was also in effect. Finally, responses during a 50-trial extinction session were recorded.

These reinforcement training procedures were remarkably effective in improving attending behaviour, as reflected in the rapid acceleration of correct responses associated with span, focus, and selective attention training. Correct responses increased directly with increases in the response–reinforcement ratio. The results certainly support the hypothesis that attention is a learned behaviour and that span, focus, and selective attention behaviours can be brought under operant control. Post-training classroom baselines of span, focus, and selective attention behaviours were made by classroom teachers to measure generalization. Laboratory training did generalize to the classroom, a number of generalization trials having been built into the treatment programme.

Rosenbaum, O'Leary, and Jacob (1975) assessed the effectiveness of group and individual reward programmes with hyperactive children. An ABAB design was employed in order to assess maintenance effects. The relative popularity of group and individual reward programmes among teachers was also evaluated. The experimenters discussed with teachers of grades three to five the general type of treatment programme offered. They described the hyperactive, poor school performance, and distractibility. Children taking medication were excluded from the study. Ten boys (mean age of 10.3 years) were selected. All subjects had scores on the abbreciated Conners' teacher rating scale (TRS) greater than 1.5 (mean 2.18. SD = 0.34) (Sprague and Sleator, 1973). The TRS has been widely used as a standardized measure of change with hyperkinetic children.

The subjects were first divided into two matched treatment groups. Following the collection of pre-treatment data, each teacher received a written instruction manual outlining the rules of the programme and providing suggestions for presenting the programme to the target child and the class, a set of reward cards consisting of index cards with a smiling face mimeographed on the front, and a supply of back-up reinforcers consisting of a selection of penny sweets.

Target behaviours were selected individually for each child. One experimenter met with each teacher in order to determine the most appropriate target behaviours for each subject. An attempt was made to avoid targets which involved vague or ambiguous feelings about the child's general behaviour pattern. Sample target behaviours included complete assigned work, stay in seat, no fighting, stay in room, and work on one task at a time.

It was stressed to the teachers that the individual reward (group I) programme involved a private contract between the teacher and child. The teacher was asked to explain the programme, contingencies, and target behaviours to the child on a private basis. The following sample explanation is given:

> Johnny, you know that you have trouble sitting still and concentrating on your work. You are lucky to have been chosen for a special programme designed to help you do better. There are certain rules you must follow. These are . . . (list targets) . . . At the end of each hour I will come over to your desk and give you a reward card (show card) if you have been following the rules. After school, you will be allowed to trade in each card for a sweet from this box (show selection of sweets). No one else in the class has to know about it . . . it will be our secret deal.

In the group reward programme (group G), class involvement was emphasized. Teachers were instructed to present the programme to the entire class, including the target child, using some variations of the following presentation based on Patterson (1965):

> Class, we all know that Johnny has trouble sitting still and completing his work. He has been lucky enough to have been chosen for a special programme designed to help him work better. There are certain rules Johnny must follow (list target behaviours). At the end of each hour I will evaluate Johnny on how well he has followed the rules, and if he has been good, I will give him a reward card (show card). If he has not been good, I will not give him a reward card (show card). If he has not been following the rules, he does not get a card. At the end of the day, everyone in the class will get a sweet for each card he has earned. You may get from zero to four sweets each, depending on how well Johnny has followed the rules. You can all help Johnny earn sweets by ignoring him when he is acting bad and by telling him when he is behaving or working well.

The teacher had to repeat the rules at the start of each day to the class in the group reward programme or to the child in the individual programme. At the end of each hour of the 4-hour day, the teacher was required to rate the subject on his behaviour for the previous hour and give the child a reward card, when appropriate. When giving the rating, teachers were supposed to enumerate those behaviours which were or were not displayed and the reason either for the reward or its absence. Even if the child had not earned a reward card for that rating period, teachers were instructed to emphasize any positive behaviours that occurred and to stress that the subject could still earn reward cards for future rating periods. Group G teachers were asked to draw a chart on the blackboard and to record each reward card earned so that the class could keep track of the number of sweets it had coming.

Teachers were asked to rely on their subjective opinions of the child's behaviour in determining the criteria for reward. They were advised to consider progress, effort, and relative improvement, rather than some absolute performance criteria. They were instructed to begin with criteria which were relatively easy to reach, but to change them gradually so as to require more effort from the child. All exchanges of cards for sweets were made at the end of the day. The token phase lasted for 4 weeks, followed by 4 weeks of withdrawal. At the beginning of the withdrawal phase, the children were told that they had been doing very well and that although the supply of sweets was depleted and they would no longer receive cards, the teachers still expected them to behave well.

The two primary dependent measures were the Connors' teacher rating scale (TRS) which the teachers completed four times during the course of the study (pre-treatment I, in January; pre-treatment II, in April; post-treatment, in May; and post-withdrawal, in June) and the problem behaviour report (PBR) which was completed at the end of each week. The TRS scores provided a repeated measure of hyperactivity across the study. The PBR provided a weekly subjective measure of the severity of each target behaviour. A third measure was a questionnaire (the post-token summary) designed to assess teacher satisfaction with the programme. Teacher satisfaction was assessed with regard to a child's improvement, positive and negative peer pressure, and practical concerns regarding programme implementation. These were filled out at the conclusion of the token phase and were scored by two uninformed raters for the number of positive, negative, and neutral statements.

The results as measured by the standardized teacher ratings of hyperactivity *and* the ratings of problem behaviour indicate a highly significant treatment effect. Differences between groups, although failing to reach an acceptable level of significance, were in the expected direction (i.e. favouring group reward) on both the rating scale and the PBR. On the post-token summary, group G teachers made more positive and fewer negative statements than group I teachers; programme utilizing a group reward were significantly more popular with the teachers than were programmes employing an individual reward. The authors made the point that the importance of the teacher satisfaction measure lies in the fact that a programme which is popular with teachers not only has a great probability of being used but, once used, has a higher probability of success and of being maintained. Given that more time was required to dispense reinforcers in the group reward condition than in the individual reward condition, the teachers' preference for the group reward condition seems especially interesting.

The results of the post-token summary were corroborated by other dependent measures. The results of the present study indicate that decreases in hyperactive behaviour were maintained 4 weeks after the discontinuation of reinforcement.

There have been several other studies of the effective use of behavioural techniques on hyperactive behaviour, especially with regard to increasing attention and reducing disruptive behaviour in classroom settings (e.g., Ayllon, Layman, and Kandel, 1975). Among the procedures used are overcorrection — positive practice (Azrin and Powers, 1975), time-out (Carlson et al., 1968; Kubany, Weiss, and Sloggett, 1971; Wahler, 1969a), group contingencies (Barrish, Saunders, and Wolf, 1969), response-cost (Wolf et al., 1970), and aversive stimulation (Hall et al., 1971). We have dealt, so far, with the difficulties of concentration of hyperactive children and the disruptive behaviours that flow from them. Much of the work that has to be done with these youngsters is concerned with other behaviour problems that they present, ones which are dealt with in other chapters, e.g., oppositional behaviour (Herbert and Iwaniec, 1981) and aggression (Hawkins et al., 1966).

There are times when it is inappropriate to engage in a therapeutic programme — as was the case of a child in residential care. Henry aged 10 years was referred to the Centre by his housemother with the following complaints: he taunted other children, was abusive to staff, and ate noisily. In addition, he was so uncontrolled when out of the Home that the guide who escorted him to the school bus had been obliged to use a restrainer to stop Henry running off and across busy roads. Henry was also reported to have severe temper-tantrums about three times a week and he was said to be highly disruptive, often upsetting the whole household by banging on the floor and by shouting obscenities at some members of staff.

The comprehensive assessment of this child helped to identify several possible factors that seemed to indicate real obstacles to any possible approaches to treatment. As regards biological deficits, it was clear that Henry was very considerably handicapped by intellectual retardation. Bearing this in mind and the related poor social development, it seemed that some of the specific complaints suggested that perhaps staff were setting too high expectations for Henry's capacity (e.g., his unpredictability in traffic). He was also found to have a genetically determined clinical syndrome which made more understandable his reported clumsiness and hyperactivity, as well as deficient social and intellectual development. As regards the antisocial behaviour problems, the initial assessment identified several factors which were of relevance. It was clear that such problems occurred only with some staff members. His houseparents were able to control Henry. It seemed that three members of staff had real difficulties in dealing with him, and it appeared that they helped to reinforce the bad behaviour by the very considerable attention they paid to it. His housemother noted that by ignoring his swearing, and so on, she very rarely found that it caused her any problem.

It was also apparent that any hyperactive behaviour and difficulties arising out of the child's poor social skills were exacerbated by the rather restrictive regime. For example, when the unit therapist had tea at the Home as part of assessment, it emerged that the children were not usually allowed to talk at the table. Second, all children were ready, washed, and in nightclothes by 6 p.m. each evening, and, as the tables were set for the next day's breakfast, the children had little space in which to play. Finally, it was apparent from the comments of staff that no one was able to think of positive characteristics in the child; the emphasis was almost wholly on his bad points.

Rather than attempt to set up any specific treatment plan, the unit therapist emphasized the child's very real handicaps, arising out of his intellectual, physical, and social retardation. Second, a considerable correspondence ensued which stressed the advantages of planned social casework designed to facilitate the child's rehabilitation with relatives who lived some considerable distance away from the Midlands.

COMBINED BEHAVIOURAL AND DRUG TREATMENT IN THE HOME AND SCHOOL SETTING

O'Leary et al. (1976) successfully treated eight out of nine children (average age 10 years) by means of a home-based reward programme. Daily classroom goals were specified for each child. At the end of each day the child's behaviour was evaluated and the parents received a report card to take home. The parent rewarded the child according to progress. Only one subject in an untreated control group showed an improvement comparable to the eight members of the treatment group.

There are limitations to all the methods described above. The improvements recorded are not always maintained when treatment is terminated and they do not transfer readily to other situations than the one in which the intervention takes place (Kazdin and Bootzin, 1972; O'Leary and Kent, 1973). Then again, some procedures have simply failed to affect significantly the behaviour of a proportion of the children treated (Kazdin, 1973; Madsen, Becker, and Thomas, 1968).

MODELLING

Goodwin and Mahoney (1975) have successfully modified aggression in three hyperactive impulsive boys by modelling a young boy who copes with verbal aggression by means of covert self-instruction. This cognitive modelling is worth detailing. One week after the baseline session, subjects viewed a 3-minute videotape of a young boy participating in the verbal taunting game. The tape showed a 9-year old being taunted by five other children. In addition to remaining ostensibly calm, looking at his taunters and remaining in the centre of the circle, the model was portrayed as coping with verbal assaults through a series of covert self-instructions. These thoughts, which were dubbed in on the tape, consisted of statements such as 'I'm not going to let them bug me' and 'I won't get mad'. Immediately after viewing the tape, subjects participated in another taunting session.

One week later, subjects again viewed the videotape of the coping model. However, this time the dubbed-in thoughts and overt actions of the model were pointed out, discussed, and verbally emphasized by the experimenter. Each coping self-statement was repeated by the experimenter and labelled as an effective way to handle verbal aggression. After viewing the tape, each subject was asked to verbalize as many of these coping responses as he could recall. A third taunting session was then conducted (see Goodwin and Mahoney, 1975, p. 201).

This study was carefully designed to isolate treatment effects and the results are very promising. It should be added that the children received coaching and practice in the coping skills that were modelled.

SELF AND BODY CONTROL

At the Centre for Behavioural Work with Families we employ training exercises which have the purpose (1) of helping the child to develop better self-control, thus reducing the frequency of outbursts of overexcitement, aggression, and impulsive acts, (2) of teaching the child to exercise better control over his body movements, and (3) of developing body awareness with a view to increasing his consciousness of his body movements and activity level, e.g., fidgeting, running, shuffling, arm flapping, and so on. Further aims are (4) to give the parents some means of controlling their child during 'crisis' periods of excessive activity and excitement, (5) to help the child with coordination problems such as those associated with the description 'cross-lateral' which applies to many hyperactive children and (6) to improve attention through breathing control (see Simpson and Nelson, 1974).

The exercises are divided into three types, each concentrating on a different problem area. Within each group are several exercises, any number of which may be used depending on the individual child's needs and capabilities. The types are as follows:

(1) body control and awareness
(2) self-control
(3) coordination
(4) stop, look and listen

All the exercises are based on learning principles and make use of behaviour modification techniques. Both response increment and response decrement procedures are used in order to ensure the child's cooperation and effort, such as positive and negative reinforcement (including self-monitoring and reinforcement), star charts, shaping, and response-cost.

In group (1) the child is required to do the following exercises for progressively longer periods, and which are themselves progressively more difficult:

(a) Keep parts of the body and then the *whole* body still.
(b) Move parts of the body in turn, keeping all others still.
(c) Move very slowly on the spot, copying the therapist's arm and leg movements, etc., and at the same time 'talking through' the exercise. For this, the three stages in verbal control of the inhibition of voluntary motor behaviour described by Luria (1961) are utilized.
(d) The 'talking through' procedure is also used in the final stage of this group of exercises, where the child is required to carry out various instructions including gross movement actions, such as making a cup of coffee, fetching objects, etc. The procedure used here is similar to that described by Schneider (1973) who used 'turtle imagery' to foster self-control in hyperactive children. The main imagery used in these exercises is perhaps more topical for the children, i.e., that of a character currently popular on TV. The procedure is very similar to that used by Meichenbaum and Goodman (1971) who evolved a treatment paradigm for training verbally mediated self-control in children.

In group (2) (self-control) exercises, a procedure similar to thought-stopping is used. Whenever the child feels the first sign of a reaction within him, such as an aggressive outburst or a mounting overexcitement possibly leading to a loss of self-control, he is instructed to stop on the spot and to count slowly to ten, at first aloud and later to himself. The child monitors and reinforces his own behaviour. The other type of exercise in this group, which is at present being developed and investigated, is role-playing, where the subject may be instructed, for example, to take the role of a quiet, submissive child.

Group (3) consists of various coordination exercises, e.g., simple finger exercises for a child with fine motor control problems.

Group (4) makes use of methods designed to encourage reflective actions (see Kendall, 1977) in impulsive children. The child is trained to consider (verbally) alternative courses of action and to focus on essentials prior to taking action. The slogan is 'stop, look and listen!'

PROGNOSIS

What can be said about the 'natural history' of the overactive pattern of behaviour without therapeutic intervention?

What evidence there is suggests that hyperactive children, in many cases, lose their hyperactivity by adolescence but remain underachievers with conduct disorders (see Wender, 1971). But this is an oblique inference and there are certainly no grounds for a 'he'll grow out of it' complacency. There is very little direct evidence about the prognosis for hyperactive children considered as a specific group. Follow-up studies (Riddle and Rapoport, 1976; Weiss et al., 1971b) suggest that hyperactive children may become less active, excitable, and impulsive by adolescence but that restlessness and aggressiveness tend to persist. A substantial minority manifest antisocial behaviour (Mendelson, Johnson, and Stewart, 1971) and academic difficulties (Anderson and Playmate, 1962). Hyperactivity may show its ill-effects beyond adolescence into adulthood (Menkes, Rowe, and Menkes, 1967).

Weiss et al. (1971b) reported a 5-year follow-up study of 64 hyperactive children who met the following criteria: (1) they had suffered long-term and sustained hyperactivity; (2) they were 6 to 13 years of age; (3) their IQ was greater than 84, as measured by the Wechsler intelligence scale for children; (4) they were not psychotic; (5) they had no major brain damage or dysfunction such as epilepsy or cerebral palsy; and (6) they were dwelling at home with at least one parent. Sixty were boys with a mean age of 8 years 7 months at referral; they were 13 years 3 months at the time of follow-up. Whereas hyperactivity had been the chief complaint on referral, it was no longer so 5 years later. However, 30 per cent. of the 64 mothers reported that restlessness was still present, though not severe. Rating scales and classroom observation of hyperactivity suggested that these children did 'not necessarily or entirely outgrow their restlessness, but rather expressed it in less gross or disturbing ways'. Distractibility, aggression, and emotional immaturity (reported by 70 per cent. of mothers) remained prominent. Eighty per cent. of these children were performing at a poor academic level. Only 20 per cent. of the children had not repeated at least one grade as compared to 85 per cent. of the control group. Ten per cent. had been in special classrooms, 5 per cent. expelled, and only 5 per cent. were doing above-average work.

Weiss and his colleagues conclude that hyperactivity diminishes but that other major handicaps remain, namely disorders of attention and concentration. Associated with this is chronic underachievement in school despite normal intelligence. In keeping with the gloomy findings of Robins (1972) these children seem to have a poor prognosis because of a significant tendency toward psychopathology with emotional immaturity, inability to attain goals, poor self-image, and feelings of hopelessness. They are differentiated from their peers by greater restlessness, aggression, and more antisocial behaviour at the time of reassessment.

There is undoubtedly a crying need for the wider application of preventive and management programmes with regard to this major problem of childhood. Iwaniec, Herbert, and McNeish (1985) have shown how fear and exhaustion are perennial enemies of parents, sapping their energy, confidence, and ingenuity. Good advice about increasing the sleep (see Schmidt, 1975) of overactive infants would be a boon. An understanding of the benefits of structure in the child's environment (predictability and firmness over rules and routines) and of principles of behaviour management, are just two items that would represent a promising starting point in an educational agenda for the parents of hyperactive children.

CASE STUDY 1:

Holmes and Roscoe (1976) have reported the successful treatment of a 3-year-old hyperactive child, Clive. On referral he showed several hyperative behaviours: he was on the go all the time, manifested an endless supply of energy, and was very clumsy. He had an extremely short attention span and was easily distracted. He also displayed many attention-seeking behaviours, especially clinging and pestering, and he performed many acts which necessitated intervention by his mother. He was very disobedient and would often have a temper-tantrum when his mother tried to force him to comply.

Clive had caused his mother difficulty since his premature birth. As a baby he was difficult to feed and nurse, and had been very active since he had started to crawl. His speech development had been very slow. On psychometric assessment he obtained an IQ of 88 on the Merrill Palmer scale of mental tests, and he presented during testing as a very active, distractible, destructive, and defiant child.

Clive's mother, Mrs. W. aged 21, married Mr. W. in 1974, before which she and Clive had lived in a hostel. Mrs. W. had to work during the day from shortly after Clive's birth. He was cared for by a baby-minder from 9.00 a.m. to 4.00 p.m. In the time Mrs. W. did spend with Clive she felt that she could not cope with him at all, and he frequently reduced her to tears. Mrs. W. was referred to the Centre after appealing to her GP for help, as she saw herself to blame for Clive's behaviour. The situation was not helped in her mind by the fact that Clive behaved very well for Mr. W. She felt that he rejected her mothering. As she had suffered rejection as an illegitimate child herself and had had to live in institution after institution, this 'repudiation' in the child who she had always hoped would be her 'very own loving baby' was a cruel blow.

BEHAVIOURAL ANALYSIS

(1) Specification of the problem

Two target behaviours were identified and recorded over a baseline period of 14 days.

Defiance　This was defined by Clive not obeying a request to do or stop doing something when the request had been repeated once.

Tantrums　These were defined by Clive shouting, crying, and throwing himself on the floor.

(2) Controlling factors

As the tantrums followed from his mother trying to force Clive to obey her, the main emphasis was on defiance.

Antecedent events   Mrs. W. would make a request for Clive to do something or ask him to stop an ongoing activity.

Behaviour

Clive would defy his mother's request in a high ratio of refusals to requests. He also engaged in coercive behaviours (tantrums) if she tried to insist. Over the baseline of 14 days, he displayed relatively few instances of defiance. Mrs W. felt that Clive was being somewhat better than usual during this period.

Consequences   Mrs. W. gave Clive a great deal of attention whenever he was defiant, ranging from talk to shouting and smacking him. She would get very upset at times and ended up in tears. She gave in to most of Clive's demands.

Decision   Although the rate of defiance was relatively low during baseline observations and did not reflect the usual state of affairs according to Mr. W. — an impressive and reliable informant — it was decided to intervene. The episodes were very intense and disruptive. Mrs. W. had no verbal control over Clive and this was affecting their relationship adversely. In addition, the graph on the last few days of observation showed an upward turn. As Mrs. W. was about to have Clive at home all day (she had changed to evening work) it was felt that a time-out (TO) and positive reinforcement programme would be helpful.

(3) Treatment programme

Mrs. W. was instructed in the use of time-out and giving praise, and was asked to start using the programme the next day. The need for keeping calm and using the TO immediately was carefully explained, and the contingent use of tangible rewards and praise when Clive did behave in defined ways was also emphasized (he was given a sweet for compliance).

In the first week Mrs. W. stated that she could cope with the programme, but after 3 full days at home with Clive, the following week she felt she could not manage on her own. A 4-hour visit was arranged for the next morning. The long stay was made to model and instruct Mrs. W. in her use of TO and to give moral support. After this Mrs. W. became more confident and used the TOs as needed. A further 4-hour visit confirmed that Mrs. W. was using the programme correctly.

Over the following 4 weeks Mrs. W. continued to record occurrences of defiance, the frequencies of which gradually diminished. When Clive had only two occurrences of defiance in each of two 10-day periods (12–21 and 21–31 October) the programme was discontinued, Mrs. W. felt that Clive was now much better.

CASE STUDY 2: CLASSROOM-BASED

Bornstein and Quevillon (1976) investigated the effects of a self-instructional package on three overactive 4-year-old pre-school boys. Scott was described as a 'disciplinary problem because he is unable to follow directions for any extended length of time'. He could not complete ordinary tasks within the pre-school classroom setting and often manifested violent outbursts of temper for no apparent reason. He was also considered to be non-compliant and uncooperative. Rod was described by teachers as 'being out of control in the classroom'. He displayed several problems and behavioural deficits, including short attention span, aggressiveness in response to other children, and a general overactivity. Tim was reported to be highly distractible both at home and in pre-school. Most of his classroom time was spent walking around the room, staring off into space, and/or not attending to a task or instruction.

After an 8-day baseline period of observations, the children were seen individually for a massed self-instruction session lasting 2 hours. Each child worked with the therapist for about 50 minutes, was given a 20-minute break, and then resumed work for another 50 minutes. The self-instructional training was similar to that described by Meichenbaum and Goodman (1971): (1) the therapist modelled the task while talking aloud to himself, (2) the child performed the task while the therapist instructed aloud, (3) the child then performed the task talking aloud to himself while the therapist whispered softly, (4) the child performed the task whispering softly while the therapist made lip movements but no sound, (5) the child performed the task making lip movements without sound while the therapist self-instructed covertly, and (6) the child performed the task with covert self-instruction.

The verbalizations modelled were of four types: (1) questions about the task (e.g., 'What does the teacher want me to do?'), (2) answers to questions in the form of cognitive rehearsal (e.g., 'Oh, that's right, I'm supposed to copy that picture'). (3) self-instructions that guide through the task (e.g., 'OK, first I draw a line here . . .'), and (4) self-reinforcement (e.g., 'How about that; I really did that one well').

The entire training session was presented in a story format. In each situation, the subject was told that the teacher (not the therapist) had asked him to complete the task in question. When using self-instructions the child would make a response as if he were in the classroom (e.g., 'Mrs. B. wants me to draw that picture over there. OK, how can I do that?'). The self-instructional protocol consisted of the therapist initially instructing the child: '. . . (child's name), watch what I do and listen to what I say.' Immediately, on gaining his attention, a sweet was placed in the child's mouth. When the first trial was completed, and if the child's attention had not shifted away from the ex-

166

perimental task, he was again given a sweet reinforcer. The experimenter then said to the child: '. . . (child's name), this time *you* do it while I say the words.' Contingent on correct performance, the experimenter dispensed a sweet to the child, paired with self-praise at the conclusion of this second trial. The provision of sweet reinforcers was then reduced quite rapidly and given only at the close of a trial. No more than ten reinforcers were given to any one child during a training session. Later in the training sequence, when the child was asked to verbalize on his own, acceptable responses were those that included correct performance and the four elements outlined above (i.e., questions about the task, answers, self-instructions, and self-reinforcement). If the child did not produce an acceptable response, the therapist again modelled the task while talking aloud to himself. Following such demonstrations, the child was then returned to that part of the sequence where his error had been committed. If the child refused to comply, the therapist merely repeated his instructions and again modelled an appropriate response.

The dependent variable in this study was on-task behaviour, and was defined as those subject behaviours directed towards the assigned tasks. During teacher instruction it was expected that the child would be attentive and silent. When asked to participate during a work period (e.g., figure-drawing exercises, story reading, etc.), on-task behaviours included performing the prescribed and accepted classroom activity. Off-task behaviours included engaging in unassigned activity, such as movement about the room, playing with toys, shouting, fighting, kicking, and leaving the classroom without permission.

The authors used a multiple-baseline design across subjects. Behavioural observations of the three target subjects indicated transfer of training effects from the experimental tasks to the classroom. On-task behaviours increased dramatically, concomitant with the introduction of the self-instructional package (see Figure 8). The therapeutic gains were maintained 22.5 weeks after baseline was initiated. Since observers had no knowledge as to the timing of treatment effects, results cannot be attributed to expectation biases in the observational process.

CASE STUDY 3: GROUP-BASED

Bardill (1972) applied group therapy incorporating behaviour contracting techniques during sessions with 9–13-year-old boys at a residential treatment centre. Characteristically, the boys were impulsive, acted out their aggressive feelings, and lacked skills necessary for engaging in cooperative interpersonal transactions. The contracting in this study involved a point system in which each boy was awarded points for certain specified behaviours during the therapy sessions. Each boy could earn a maximum of fifteen points for appropriate conduct and up to ten points for 'therapeutic responses'. The therapist and co-therapist met at the end of each session to agree on the total

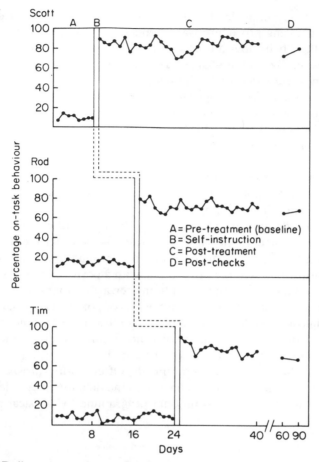

Figure 8   Daily percentage on-task behaviours for Scott, Rod, and Tim across experimental conditions (From Bornstein and Quevillon, 1976)

points for each child. Conduct points were earned for (1) arriving for therapy at the scheduled time, (2) not taking items from the office, (3) not physically hurting or abusing anyone, and (4) obeying the institutional rules regarding such behaviours as cursing and smoking. Therapy points were earned by (1) listening to others, (2) making verbal comments designed to be helpful to others, and (3) talking about one's own concerns. Specific explanations and examples of each of these guidelines were given to each boy. The goal of the therapy points was a traditional one — to get the boys to talk out rather than act out their negative feelings, as well as to learn more positive ways of relating to others.

Each boy could earn an extra two points by correctly guessing, within two points, the number of points awarded to him for each session. The therapists met with each boy individually after each treatment session to discuss his points. This guessing procedure was intended to encourage a more realistic appraisal of their behaviour during therapy. Moreover, a sponsor system was established whereby each boy acted as a sponsor for two other boys in the group. Whenever a sponsored child earned top conduct and therapy points (twenty-five) for a session, his sponsor earned three extra points. It was hoped that the sponsor or buddy system would instil in the boys a sense of responsibility for the behaviour of others and for the formation of common goals. A listing of the points earned by each boy was posted on the office bulletin board every week.

On earning fifty or more points during the calendar month a boy became eligible to convert the points into money at the rate of 1 cent per point. He also qualified for a monthly off-campus trip to spend his money. The off-campus trips were considered part of the group therapy and a boy's behaviour off-campus was subject to the same point rules as the other therapy sessions.

Throughout the 8 months of this group programme the therapists made a conscious effort to present the programme with a positive orientation, that is, to show the boys a way of earning points and rewards rather than to emphasize the misbehaviours that would result in the loss of points. The programme was successful almost immediately in eliminating physical fights among the boys, destruction of furniture, and thefts of office items. The boys did 'test' the programme with minor breaches of conduct but this testing became less noticeable as the programme continued. Often more prosocial leaders emerged in the therapy groups, in contrast to the delinquent-type leaders who often reigned in the larger institutional programme by physical power and threats.

9

Disruptive Behaviour

Emotionally disturbed children frequently behave in a disruptive manner in the classroom. They interrupt, shout, tease, talk at the wrong time, get out of their seats, pester, disobey, and fight. The rationale for treating this problem in a section separate from the chapter on aggression (or for that matter the one on oppositional behaviour) is its group connotation. An individual can, of course, disrupt another's peace of mind, concentration, play, or some other ongoing activity, by doing any of a number of aversive things. However, in the behaviour modification literature, disruptive behaviour is usually a term applied to the interference with, or shattering of, some endeavour in which several individuals are involved as part of an organized group (e.g., a classroom of pupils). This chapter, therefore, focuses particularly on management of acting-out disruptive youngsters in school and residential settings.

Schools are in a powerful position to exert influence on their students — children and adolescents — because, in essence, they have a 'captive audience' for some 15,000 hours. This is the average amount of time spent by British children at school. They enter an environment providing work and play for nearly a dozen years during a formative period of development. Children spend almost as much of their waking life at school as at home. And it is not only an influence in terms of the transmission of academic and technical skills and cultural interests. The school introduces boys and girls to social and working relationships and to various forms of authority which they would not experience in the family. The areas of particular influence — academic success, social behaviour, moral values, and occupational choice — represent major themes in the socialization of young people.

Here then is another force shaping the youngster's growing independence from the family. There is no doubt that it does matter which school he goes to;

certain features of school curriculum and social ethos are of vital importance to its young consumers. Many parents will not be surprised to hear that research confirms the assumptions they make in trying desperately to get their offspring into a 'good' school. Adolescents are more likely to show socially acceptable behaviour and good scholastic attainment if they attend certain schools rather than others.

Differences in the ways that schools 'perform' are not related to the age of buildings, the space available, the size of the school, or its organization.

In other words, they are not due to physical factors, even when seemingly unpromising. Rather, they owe their favourable or unfavourable outcomes to their attributes as social institutions:

(a) teacher actions in lessons,
(b) the availability of incentives and rewards,
(c) good conditions for pupils,
(d) opportunities for pupils to take on responsibility, and
(e) an emphasis on academic work

The cumulative effect of various social factors (according to Rutter et al., 1979) is greater than the effect of any of the individual influences taken alone. Rutter believes that the implication is that the individual actions, approaches, or measures combine to create a special ethos, or set of values, attitudes, and behaviours which could be said to be characteristic of the school as a whole. The qualities of the school as a social institution really matter.

The school ethos

The researchers found outcomes for pupils to be better when both the curriculum and approaches to discipline were agreed and supported by the staff acting together. Thus, attendance was better and delinquency less frequent in schools where courses were planned jointly. Group planning provided opportunities for teachers to encourage and support one another. In addition continuity of teaching was facilitated. Much the same was found with regard to standards of discipline. Examination successes were more frequent and delinquency less common in schools where discipline was based on general expectations set by the school (or house or department), rather than left to individual teachers to work out for themselves. School values and norms appear to be more effective if it is clear to all that they have widespread support.

CONTINGENCY MANAGEMENT

The chief characteristic of behaviour modification procedures suitable for classroom management is the systematic application and/or withdrawal of reinforcement, the aim being to increase desirable behaviour, such as academic performance, and reduce, disruptive activities. There is evidence (Patterson,

1975) that many boys who are assessed as conduct problems perform disruptive behaviours at higher rates than their normal counterparts. The data suggest that the conduct-disordered boy manipulates his immediate social environment in a style characteristic of a 3- or 4-year-old child. He is without doubt a severe trial to his teacher.

Perhaps the most obvious and natural reinforcement available to the classroom teacher is the attention she can give to her pupils, in the form of a smile, word of encouragement, or even mere proximity. Adult attention is a powerful secondary reinforcer for the child acquired over the years by an association between adult attention and the provision of primary reinforcers, such as food, comfort, security, and so on. The giving of attention by the teacher will tend to increase those behaviours which attracted it in the first place. Thus, if a teacher pays attention to a child who is working well she will tend to increase this behaviour. However, if she pays attention to bad behaviour, that behaviour will also tend to increase.

Madsen and his colleagues (1968) demonstrated how reprimands can inadvertently reinforce the very troublesome behaviours they are intended to diminish. When teachers admonished pupils for disruptive activities, the number of transgressors promptly increased. In subsequent phases of the study the numbers declined when teachers reduced their reprimands and rose again when they resumed their admonishments. This chronic problem was solved by ignoring annoying actions and praising instances where pupils were engrossed in learning activities.

It can be appreciated how many interventions intended as punishments actually serve as positive reinforcers that maintain troublesome behaviour. Self-defeating practices usually go unnoticed by those who use them because they only see the immediate results, but rarely assess the full or long-term effects their behaviour may have on others. These interactions are unwittingly set in motion and maintained because ineffective control techniques are reinforced in the users by their 'success'. This success is more apparent than real; there is only a *temporary* suppression of deviant behaviour. The teachers have rewarded annoying conduct in students who, in turn, have rewarded the teacher's shouting by their momentary compliance; the net effect is that both kinds of performance are mutually escalated. To give one example of the potency of attention in influencing disruptive behaviour, Thomas, Becker, and Armstrong (1968) were able (by systematically varying teacher attention) to change an initially well-behaved class with an average rate of disruptiveness of only 8.7 per cent. to one in which disruptiveness reached a level (on average) of 25.5 per cent. This was achieved by seeing that approval was not given to attending behaviour. It went down to 12.0 per cent. on reversal to baseline, increased again to 19.4 per cent. on return to the non-approval condition and rose higher to 31 per cent. when frequent disapproval was given to disruptive behaviours. Disruptiveness went to 25.9 per cent. in the third no-approval condition and fell to 13.2 per cent. on the final return to baseline conditions.

CONTINGENCY MANAGEMENT USING TOKEN REINFORCEMENT

O'Leary and Becker (1967) and O'Leary et al. (1969) utilized a token reinforcement programme to reduce the disruptive classroom behaviours of elementary school children. Their aim in the former study was to evaluate the effectiveness of the token economy system in a situation involving a class of eight disruptive children and a single teacher. In addition they wished to investigate whether a transfer from the token system to more 'natural' reinforcers such as teacher attention, praise, and grades could be effected gradually without a return to the previous levels of disruptive behaviour. Unfortunately, the secondary aim could not be carried out for organizational reasons. To keep the system manageable, it was put into effect only from 12.30 to 2.00 p.m. each day. Ten-cent spiral notebooks were taped to each desk. These cue words were written on the blackboard: 'in seat', 'face front', 'raise hand', 'working', 'paying attention', and 'desk clear'. The children were told they could earn from 1 to 10 points each 15 minutes for following the rules or showing improvement. The points could be exchanged for prizes of differing values which were shown to the children. The prizes were grouped in boxes labelled 10, 25, and 50 points. The teacher arranged instructional units so she could stop each 15 minutes and take 2 minutes to write the points earned on the notebooks and tell the children what they had done to earn them. While she was handing out points, the class could earn a group point towards a Friday popsicle party for good behaviour. After a few days, the time period was changed to 30 minutes rather than 15, and then, progressively over several weeks, the children were required to save points for 2 days, 3 days, and 4 days. Also, the number of points required for various prizes was increased. The children had to work harder and longer for a smaller reward. This was to have been the means by which the token system was to have been faded out, leaving praise and attention for appropriate behaviour and ignoring of inappropriate behaviour as the sole reinforcement contingencies. With the introduction of the token reinforcement programme, an abrupt reduction in deviant behaviour occurred. The percentage of off-task behaviour for the eight children on days 11 and 12 (the first 2 days of the token reinforcement programme) was less than 5 per cent. The children showed a few bad days as more points were required and delayed pay-offs introduced, but over the rest of the term the teacher could begin to teach and the children could begin to learn.

The token system (as measured by observer ratings) was effective in reducing deviant behaviour from means during the baseline period ranging from 66 to 91 per cent. to means ranging from 3 to 32 per cent. The programme was equally successful for all children observed, and anecdotal evidence suggests that the children's appropriate behaviour generalized to other school situations. Delay of reinforcement did not lead to an increase in deviant behaviour.

In their later study, O'Leary and his colleagues (1969) tried a variety of techniques for modifying disruptive behaviour. They found that classroom rules written on the blackboard were ineffective. So was structuring the day into 30-minute sessions, or even praising appropriate behaviour and ignoring inappropriate or disruptive behaviour. When all these techniques were combined, the disruptive behaviour of one child appeared to be controlled, but not the others. A token system was also tried. Tokens were dispensed according to how well the children followed the rules on the blackboard. This proved effective in controlling the disruptive behaviour of six out of the seven children involved in the study. Tokens also reflected, wherever possible, the quality of a child's classroom discussion and the accuracy of his schoolwork. Even though the tokens were not contingent solely upon the absence of disruptive behaviour, behaviour was clearly controlled.

Several investigators have arranged token reinforcement contingencies for appropriate classroom behaviour (e.g., Birnbrauer et al., 1965; Walker, Hops, and Fiegenbaum, 1976). These have proved to be effective. However, these token reinforcers have been dependent upon back-up reinforcers such as sweets and money — rewards that are unnatural in the ordinary classroom. Also these studies are usually designed to demonstrate the feasibility of using behavioural procedures in *special* educational settings. The target behaviours — academic achievement and social disruptiveness — are also issues which directly concern the classroom teacher in the normal school. The reinforcement procedures were not so esoteric as to exclude applications in the ordinary or 'normal' classroom. As we saw earlier, praise, attention, and the ignoring of inappropriate behaviours are methods which can be used more systematically by teachers. Although the token systems are not found in the typical school, the possibilities of the method (perhaps with alternative incentives) are worth exploring.

In a psychiatric hospital, 'emotionally disturbed' children participated in a classroom project in the hospital (Santogrossi et al., 1973). The effects of teacher-determined versus self-determined points were evaluated on disruptive student behaviour. The points each child received were exchangeable for snacks, fruits and prizes. When the teacher administered points, disruptive classroom behaviour decreased. However, when the students were given the opportunity to reward themselves, they did so *non-contingently* and disruptive behaviour increased. Thus, self-reinforcement led to administration of rewards for undesirable behaviour.

A very significant prototype for work in normal school classrooms was provided by the study of Becker et al. (1967). It drew attention to problems arising in 'natural environment' work which are not present in laboratory and other more controlled special settings. The authors state that the conduct of their research was guided to some extent by the necessity of establishing good relationships within the school system. They had to convince the teachers of the classes into which they were going that the interruption of normal routine would be outweighed by positive advantages. In order to achieve this, seminars were conducted prior to the commencement of the experiment, even though it was realized that this might influence teacher behaviour during the baseline period. There was a further constraint upon the experimental design. This was the feeling that employment of the classic reversal design might alienate the teachers who might not tolerate a return to the pre-treatment levels of disruptive behaviour. The therapists therefore used only an AB design. In justifying this weaker experimental design they point out that the value of the experimental processes involved had already been demonstrated many times elsewhere, and that since they were working with ten different children in five classes, the possibility that an interfering variable would affect them all equally, and therefore be undetected, could be discounted. They argued, also, that by not using a reversal design the period of controlled reinforcement could be extended and longer-term effects demonstrated.

Becker and his associates were concerned with the use of teacher attention as a reinforcer in the control of disruptive behaviour manifested in the junior school classroom, and also in the training of teachers to be more effective in the use of a behavioural approach to problems of behaviour management. Teachers were given instructions for the experimental period regarding making classroom rules explicit to the pupils, ignoring inappropriate behaviour where possible, and giving praise and attention to behaviours which facilitate learning. In order to ensure that these instructions were carried out, teacher behaviour was observed, coded in categories, and teachers were given daily feedback concerning their own behaviour. It was thought that a procedure involving signals by lights or hand signals when the appropriate times for praise and ignoring occurred would be too disruptive in a full classroom. Difficulty was found by some teachers in implementing the regime, as some had previously relied heavily on reprimand as a method of control. This early study checked on observer reliability, which was measured by getting observers to work initially in pairs. Observation intervals were 20 seconds each followed by a 10-second period for recording and were carried out within a 20-minute daily session. Coded categories for behaviours incompatible with learning were devised: e.g., X symbolized gross motor behaviours such as getting out of the seat, standing up, running, hopping, etc., and N symbolized disruptive noise with objects, such as tapping pencil, clapping, tapping, etc. The categories were established on the basis that they reflected undesirable disruptive behaviours which were defined in a mutually exclusive way and in a way which involved minimal inference from actual observation. Agreement rarely fell below 80 per cent. Praising behaviours incompatible with undesirable responses took the form of remarks such as 'That's the way I like to see you work' and 'I'm calling on you because you raised your hand'. The experimenters found that ignoring behaviours which interfered with learning or teaching was somewhat difficult for teachers to implement since it was their habit to draw critical attention to inappropriate behaviour of problem children rather than ignore it. Nevertheless, the differential reinforcement procedures — the combination of explicit rules, praise for on-task behaviour, and ignoring — was effective in reducing disruptive behaviour from an average for the ten children during the baseline period of 62 per cent. to 29 per cent. during the experimental period. The regime was, however, not very effective with two of the children and with these a token system was instituted and was somewhat more successful. The effectiveness of praising a child who was behaving appropriately while ignoring a nearby deviant was noted.

This study by Becker and his colleagues provided guidelines for many of the classroom studies which followed it. Among the major contributions it made was the definition it provided for observable behaviours, clear reporting of procedures, and recognition of practical problems in the natural setting. The researchers themselves comment on the limitations of their study in terms of experimental design and in terms of the confounding of independent variables (rules, ignoring, and praise). These were introduced in combination rather than one at a time, a method which would have allowed an assessment of the comparative strength of rules, praise, and ignoring. The study lacked other controls. The teachers were in a seminar on behaviour theory and practice during baseline conditions. Some target children improved during baseline, apparently because some teachers were beginning to apply what they were learning even though they had been requested not to do so. A reversal of teacher behaviour was not attempted. Such a reversal would more conclusively show the importance of a teacher's behaviour in producing the obtained changes.

Evaluation of these strategies has been the subject of a number of studies. Several investigators have utilized teacher attention (Hall et al., 1968; Madsen, Becker, and Thomas, 1968; Zimmerman and Zimmerman, 1962) to improve behaviour in the classroom. The most effective procedure seems to be a combination of approval for constructive behaviours and ignoring for disruptive conduct (Hall et al., 1971; Hall, Lund, and Jackson, 1968; McAllister et al., 1969; White, Nielsen, and Johnson, 1972).

Not all investigations have been an unqualified success. A study of behaviour modification in a British primary classroom was carried out by Barcroft (1970). He found his results inconclusive; although on-task behaviour increased from 25 to 53 per cent. when the attend-on-task/ignore-off-task strategy was adopted with a highly disruptive pupil, a significant increase in on-task behaviour was observed in one of the control pupils. Ward (1971), in another United Kingdom study, found that one of his three teachers acting as a mediator of change was unable to adopt the praise or ignore strategy successfully. There was no reduction in the target disruptive behaviour. There were, however, significant improvements in the other two classrooms.

Many of the studies concerning the contingent application of teacher attention have considered it primarily as a secondary reinforcer, whereas it could be argued that in many of these applications it has also served, when verbally expressed, as a re-specification of rules. Praise or reprimand can have a directive quality.

Madsen, Becker, and Thomas (1968) followed up their 1967 study (see page 171) with a design which introduced rules, ignoring and approval, one at a time, in order to determine their individual contributions. Two disruptive children in each of two classrooms were observed under the following experimental conditions: baseline; rules; rules plus ignoring deviant behaviour; rules plus ignoring plus praise for appropriate behaviour; baseline; rules plus ignoring plus praise. During the rules condition the teacher specified explicit classroom rules, posted a notice, and verbally reminded the class an average of over five times per day. Previously developed behavioural categories (Becker et al., 1967) were modified for use with these particular children and baseline recordings were made to determine the frequency of problem behaviours. At the end of the baseline period the teachers entered a workshop on applications of behavioural principles in the classroom, which provided them with the rationale and principles behind the procedures being introduced in their classes. Various experimental procedures were then introduced, one at a time, and the effects on the target children's behaviours observed. The experiments were begun in late November and continued to the end of the school year. The main conclusions were that: (1) rules alone exerted little effect on classroom behaviour, (2) ignoring inappropriate behaviour and showing approval for appropriate behaviour (in combination) were very effective in achieving better classroom behaviour, and (3) showing approval for appropriate behaviours is probably the key to effective classroom management.

O'Leary et al. (1969) made a study of the disruptive behaviour of seven children in a primary class and they, too, found that rules without reinforcement did not influence the behaviour of these subjects. The data are not available to assess precisely the importance in the classroom of using a combination of rules and reinforcement, but O'Leary points out that the clear specification of rules can serve to prompt the children to rehearse the rules themselves (symbolic modelling) and act as a discriminatory cue when moving from one classroom situation to another. Some behaviours are appropriate to particular activities, e.g., children are expected to behave differently in maths, PE, and art lessons. O'Leary and his colleagues (1969) examined the differential effects of rules, lesson structure, praise and ignore, and token reinforcement conditions in the study of seven primary-school children mentioned earlier. The conditions were introduced successively but disruptive behaviour did not decrease consistently until the token reinforcement programme was introduced (see Figure 9).

Follow-up showed that the teacher was about to transfer control from the token and back-up reinforcers to the reinforcers existing within the educational setting, such as stars and the occasional sweets. Back-up reinforcers used in the study included toys, sweets, and comics. The usefulness (as opposed to effectiveness) of the token economy system is that it allows immediate secondary reinforcement and delayed gratification when the tokens are redeemed, at a time most convenient for the teacher. Tangible reinforcements such as the one so far mentioned may not be considered suitable for the typical classroom on the grounds of expense and the difficulty of transfer to more natural reinforcers. However, the token economy may equally well be used with a 'reinforcement menu', offering activities or privileges readily available in the classroom, such as outings, free time for painting, reduced homework, etc.

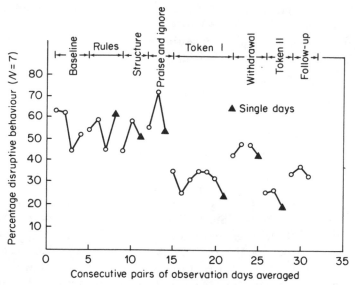

Figure 9 Average percentage of combined disruptive behaviour of seven children during the afternoon over the eight conditions: base, rules, educational structure, praise and ignore, token I, withdrawal, token II, follow-up (O'Leary et al., 1969)

PUNISHMENT

Not uncommonly, teachers will say that although they can accept intellectually the advantages (on the one-to-one basis) of ignoring a child's disruptive behaviour, to do so in practice is very difficult. They cannot refrain from expressing disapproval despite its 'paradoxical' reinforcing potentialities. The question arises as to the possibility of using *only* positive reinforcement for the child's positive actions. In studies that have attempted this total exclusion of expressions of disapproval, the teachers were observed nonetheless to use disapproval frequently (Thomas, Becker, and Armstrong, 1968). Similarly, in the token economy procedure which was designed to emphasize positive reinforcement, token fines were still required for some disruptive behaviours such as aggression (Ayllon and Azrin, 1968). Consequently, many studies that have attempted to reduce classroom disruptions have used both procedures.

Disapproval for disruptive conduct has been exemplified by reprimanding the child (Hall et al., 1968; O'Leary et al., 1970; Sajwaj et al., 1972) by positive practice (overcorrection) (Azrin and Powers, 1975; Madsen, Becker, and Thomas, 1968), by time-out procedures such as isolation, loss of recess time, or detention after school (Hall et al., 1971); McAllister et al., 1969; O'Leary and Becker, 1967; Zeilberger, Sampen, and Sloane, 1968), or by response-cost procedures. These may be loss of privileges as by subtraction of tokens (Hall et al., 1971) or by presentation of minus points which must be earned-off to avoid some other form of aversive event (Broden et al., 1970). The use of time-out usually involves moving the child out of the classroom situation to a setting which is ideally less reinforcing to the child whenever he engages in the disruptive behaviours. This latter setting might be a barren room, the principal's office, the hallway, or a chair in the back of the classroom itself.

REPRIMANDS

O'Leary et al. (1970) found that teacher attention did not increase the disruptive behaviour of the majority of target children in the study if it was in the form of a soft reprimand. Only the child concerned heard the reprimand and therefore did not receive contingent peer attention at the same time, as might be the case with a loud reprimand. A loud reprimand might represent contingent teacher and peer attention, whereas a soft reprimand might represent teacher attention only. Since in the latter condition disruptive behaviour decreased, it could be suggested that peer attention was largely maintaining disruptive behaviour and that teacher attention had comparatively little effect. The question cannot be resolved from this study since there was no baseline period when no reprimands were given; loud reprimands were baseline (usual) teacher behaviour. Two children of the nine in this study increased their disruptive behaviour during the soft reprimand period. O'Leary suggested that this might have been because their teacher's proximity was particularly reinforcing for these two children: 'a child might realise that he could draw the teacher to his side each time he misbehaved during the soft reprimand period.' It might also have been due to the teacher's loud reprimand acting as a more aversive stimulus than her soft ones.

OVERCORRECTION

We mentioned in Chapter 5 (page 96) the use of the positive practice method as a way of eliminating disruptions in the classroom (Azrin and Powers, 1975). We return to this study shortly. In applying the positive practice rationale to classroom misbehaviour, Madsen et al. (1968) characterize the behaviours in terms of the child speaking or shouting aloud or leaving his seat to misbehave. In order to apply the positive practice rationale to the problem of a disruptive child constantly leaving his seat to engage in mischief, it is necessary to ask what would have been the correct form of conduct. Leaving the seat may not be misconduct as such, but the child should have asked for permission first. The same answer applies to the problem of a child speaking up in class. With the positive practice rationale the teacher requires practice in asking for permission from a child whenever he has spoken out of turn.

TIME-OUT

Clark et al. (1973) studied the effects of four intermittent schedules of TO on disruptive behaviour of a retarded girl. Their results suggested an inverse, non-linear relationship between the percentage of responses punished and the frequency of the response. However, since the responses in question had already been reduced to a low frequency by the use of a continuous schedule, their conclusions apply to the maintenance of previously established response suppression.

There seems little doubt that behaviour modification provides a formidable technology for classroom management of disruptive behaviour and encouragement of constructive activity. Where the evidence is meagre is with regard to the crucial questions of whether the changes in behaviour generalize from one class to another, and the degree of this generalization. It is a subject we take up in more detail in Chapter 13. However, two studies which have examined generalization yielded somewhat contradictory results. Schwarz and Hawkins (1970), in a study of a sixth-grade child, were able to point to a high degree of generalization in the effects of delayed reinforcement from one class to another. Wahler (1969b), on the other hand, reported little generalization between home and school in the elimination of similar disruptive behaviours through the use of operant techniques.

Blanchard and Johnson (1973) conducted an experiment to examine the degree of generalization of several commonly used operant classroom procedures. A second concern of the study was the relative efficacy of these operant classroom control procedures for achieving significant improvement in a short period of time. This was done by applying each procedure for only one week. The third interest of the study (given the predominant attention in the literature to work with primary schoolchildren) was to extend the age range of applicability of current operant classroom control technology by systematically applying it to five 'behaviour problem' children in each of two seventh grades.

Three categories of student behaviour were recorded: (1) *appropriate study* or *attention* behaviour, (2) *inappropriate non-disruptive* behaviour, and (3) *disruptive* behaviour. Each time a student's behaviour was recorded, the teacher's behaviour was also scored in three categories: (1) *praise* or any other form of *positive attention* and approval, (2) *neutral attention*, defined as the teacher performing her routine instructional duties, such as answering a question or delivering a lecture, and (3) *censure*, defined as the teacher using any disapproval technique such as scolding, threats, sarcasm, etc. It was also noted whether the teacher's behaviour was to the class as a whole or to an individual. When the teacher was silent, teacher categories were left blank.

Throughout the 12 weeks of the experiment proper, baseline conditions were alternated with experimental conditions on a weekly basis. During the baseline periods the two teachers conducted their experimental classes in their own typical manner. Generalization effects were measured on the target students in the non-experimental, or generalization, classroom under the second teacher. The teachers were instructed to control these latter classrooms in their own typical manner throughout the experiment.

The first experimental procedure was that of ignoring inappropriate behaviour; the second was giving frequent verbal approval and positive attention for appropriate behaviour; in the third procedure the teachers were instructed to indicate disapproval of inappropriate behaviour through verbal reprimands, sarcasm, threats, and/or frowns immediately after the transgression; the next procedure combined the first two procedures by praising appropriate behaviour while ignoring inappropriate. There was also a condition involving tangible individual rewards and punishments (T-G).

The results of the study were as follows:

(1) There was a change in student behaviour (an increase in appropriate classroom behaviour and decrease in disruptive behaviour) within 1 week of the application of operant conditioning methods. Although the use of contingent rewards was effective for the older children, the nature of effective reinforcement was somewhat different for this age group. Whereas teacher attention and praise are very effective reinforcers for younger children, with the older children tangible rewards and punishments were more effective rewards, regardless of the teacher applying them. The reinforcing value of teacher attention was specific to the individual teacher in this study.

(2) The experimental effects generalized to some extent, but in an inconsistent manner. In the case of the students for whom teacher attention was effective there was no generalization of the improvement to a situation where they were taught by a second teacher. When tangible rewards were effective there was a significant improvement in all categories of behaviour for both classes. There was a concurrent generalized improvement in behaviour for class 7A in the situation where teacher Y was conducting the class in his normal manner.

RESPONSE-COST PROCEDURES

Researchers have found that a RC system used to withdraw reinforcement for the occurrence of disruptive classroom behaviour may also be an effective method for reducing these behaviours. Iwata and Bailey (1974) compared token withdrawal (for rule violations) with token presentation (for following rules) in a special education class. Both systems were effective in reducing the transgression of rules. Also, academic output doubled under both systems. In this case an individual contingency was used for determining the loss of reinforcement. The consequences for each individual depended solely on his own behaviour. By way of contrast, a study of retarded children has involved a group contingency RC system. Here the consequences for each student depend not only on his own behaviour but also on the behaviour of other group members. Greene and Pratt (1972) utilized a RC group contingency to reduce rudeness, obscenity, insults, and disruptions in eleven special education classes. Each incidence of a targeted behaviour resulted in a 1-minute loss of a 30-minute free-time period for the whole class. The procedure resulted in a reduction in misbehaviour in ten of the eleven classes. The mean daily incidence of misbehaviour per student decreased from approximately 1.4 during baseline to 0.4 during treatment.

GROUP CONTINGENCIES

Consideration has been given to the effects on the other children if one child is singled out for teacher praise or token and back-up reinforcement. Christy (1975) found that if other children were given social reinforcement for desirable behaviour and if their requests for other rewards were ignored, the overall effect on the class could be beneficial, both for the childdren concerned in the programme and their classmates. It may seem invidious to some teachers to single out a particular child. A group contingency system can be used as an alternative.

Schmidt and Ulrich (1969) describe a method in which class points were lost if there was excessive noise. They could be regained if the class remained quiet (as measured in decibels) for 10 consecutive minutes. Hall et al. (1968) successfully applied a 'response-cost' procedure involving loss of token points. The tokens could be used to gain extra breaktime or time for playing games. The system was operated effectively by newly qualified teachers.

Other methods have worked in reducing inappopriate classroom behaviour by the specification of group behaviours as targets. Reinforcement was given to a group of children when they did not exceed pre-arranged levels of disruption. Barrish, Saunders, and Wolf (1969) describe how a class containing a number of disruptive children was divided into two groups, and any instance of disruptive behaviour during a maths period was marked on the blackboard. In this 'good behaviour game', as it became known, the team with the fewest points (or both teams if they had less than five marks) would be awarded badges and privileges, such as early lunch and free time. The researchers report that the game significantly and reliably modified the disruptive out-of-seat and talking-out behaviour of the pupils. One pupil caused problems and would not cooperate so he was dropped from the game, there having been numerous complaints that he spoiled his team's chances. It is possible to see how some disruptive children might use a system such as this to draw attention to themselves by misbehaving.

Group rewards have been made contingent upon the appropriate behaviour of individuals. Peers are encouraged to exert a desirable influence on the behaviour of the target child rather than support undesirable behaviour. Carlson et al. (1968) reported a reduction in the frequency of tantrum behaviour in a primary schoolgirl. She was awarded points for desirable behaviour and these could be exchanged for a class party (immediate individual token reinforcement and delayed group tangible and social reinforcement). The researchers also gave sweets to peers who ignored the tantrum behaviour (immediate tangible individual reinforcement).

Herman and Tramontana (1971) and Drabman and Spitalnik (1973) compared the application of group and individual reinforcement contingencies for modifying disruptive group behaviour and found both systems equally effective. Tsoi (1974) used a token system in a London primary school with free time as back-up reinforcement. Group reinforcement contingent on group behaviour was compared with group reinforcement contingent on individual behaviour. Results indicated that both systems were effective in reducing disruptive behaviour, but individual variations in response to the programme and the extent to which behaviour was maintained were observed.

The studies described suggest that the combination of rules, praising desirable behaviour, and ignoring undesirable behaviour can be effective with many children in increasing academic performance and decreasing disruptive behaviour. Success depends on the teacher's ability to apply the contingencies systematically and on the value of the individual teacher's attention on the individual child. It has been found in some studies that some teachers have had difficulty in remembering to praise disruptive pupils when they are behaving appropriately and even more difficulty in refraining from attending to their disruptive behaviour. For various reasons, some children may not find teacher attention rewarding and may be more subject to peer attention, which reinforces their disruptive behaviour. The teacher may therefore look for other forms of reinforcement which may be applied systematically. Symbolic rewards such as team points and grades and privileges such as free time, extra break, or special outings are commonly used in many typical school situations, and can be employed effectively in behaviour modification programmes.

A great deal of research (as we have seen) has focused upon the elimination of classroom behaviour which is labelled 'disruptive' because it competes with participation in study activities. The procedures researched have, for the most part, involved consequences which were administered within the classroom setting. Common to all is the use of classroom (or school)-related incentives. This tactic has always been considered basic to the implementation of behavioural efforts to reduce misbehaviour. However, reinforcers for the chronically disruptive student may not always be available in the classroom. There have been attempts made to explore the efficacy of alternative methods in reducing discipline problems in the classroom. The management of classroom behaviours through the use of delayed consequences administered in home settings has been researched by Bailey, Wolf, and Phillips (1970), Clark (1972), and McKenzie et al. (1968), and has been shown to be successful.

Bailey, Wolf, and Phillips (1970) have provided one of the few attempts to investigate the effectiveness of other alternatives. They studied a system that combined the objectives of school with rewards in a residential setting for predelinquent boys. In this investigation, evaluations from the classroom teacher resulted in each boy earning privileges for good conduct and for studying, and losing them for failure to meet these criteria. These evaluations were sent to the residential setting where privileges were available the same day. The authors found this system to be both practical and effective in the control of classroom behaviour. The boys lived as a group in a highly structured residential environment under the management of a trained team of husband and wife.

Kent and O'Leary (1976) make the point that the context of most behavioural treatment studies may have contributed substantially to the positive outcomes reported, especially as so many behavioural intervention procedures have been assessed on a research basis. The special advantages likely to accrue in such a context are particularly clear in the classroom literature. The authors note that teachers involved in classroom projects have received college-course credits or stipends in return for their participation. In addition, the teacher's implementation of experimental procedures has frequently been monitored by research personnel, and such monitoring provides immediate feedback when the experimental procedures are not adequately executed. They provide correctives to misunderstanding or lack of motivation. Advantages such as these, unavailable to the clinician, may have contributed to an overestimation of the effectiveness of child behaviour modification in out-patient settings. Kent and O'Leary comment on the growth of studies conducted under circumstances similar to those of the clinician in private practice or at a community clinic and characterized by treatment of *actual* clinical referrals, reasonable limits on therapist time and resources, and the use of multiple-treatment procedures, rather than single techniques.

The authors set out to provide a comprehensive evaluation of child behaviour modification for school problems under typical out-patient clinical circumstances. The design features of their study included (1) objective measures of change from independent evaluators as well as ratings by clients, (2) multiple measures of academic as well as behavioural change, (3) random assignment of referred children to treatment and a no-contact control condition, (4) a 9-month follow-up evaluation, (5) a highly structured therapy programme that specified each of the intervention procedures and when they were to be implemented in a 55-page manual, and (6) a homogeneous population of children in grades 2 to 4 referred for the combination of conduct problems and academic difficulties. The study provided data on 32 children and teachers in their respective classrooms in six schools and on treatment by four therapists. With the exception of intermittent data collections, the present investigation simulated out-patient behavioural treatment of children with conduct problems and academic difficulties. Consultation with teachers at the schools and with parents and children in the clinic was limited to a total of 20 hours of direct contact per case. All children were treated in the context of normal classrooms with 30 to 32 children. None of the participants (parent, teacher, or child) received any incentives for participating. There were no drop-outs during the 3 to 4-month course of treatment.

Subjects were randomly assigned to treatment ($n = 16$) and a 'no-contact' control group ($n = 16$). A standardized 20-hour treatment programme involving the child, his parents, and his teacher was provided by Ph.D. clinical psychologists. A significantly greater behavioural improvement was demonstrated for treated than for control children. Both observational recordings and teacher ratings of social and academic behaviour showed this. However, at a 9-month follow-up, the control group had improved sufficiently that these differences in social behaviour were no longer significant. Although no differences existed between treated and untreated children in achievement test performance or grades at termination, follow-up revealed that the treated subjects had significantly better achievement scores and grades 9 months after termination. Ratings of therapists by teachers and parents were uniformly positive.

ILLUSTRATION OF CLASSROOM: GROUP MANAGEMENT

Azrin and Powers (1975) used the overcorrection method during a special Summer class to manage disruptive classroom behaviour. The procedure was compared with other methods of coping with such problems. These were (a) a clear statement at the start of each class of the rules regarding deviant acts, (b) a reminder/reprimand to the child, whenever he misbehaved, that he should not do so again, and (c) the loss of a forthcoming recess period whenever he misbehaved. The study took place in a special education class for children. The pupils were six boys, aged 7 to 11 years. Each child had been identified by his teacher, principal, and school psychologist as severely deficient in academic skills and extremely disruptive in the classroom; he was also characterized as hyperactive and aggressive. The high rate disruptive behaviours involved the child talking out or being out of his seat, always without permission.

There were several phases to the experiment:

(1) Warnings, reminders, and reinforcement

Before each class, the teacher reminded the children that no one was allowed to talk or leave his seat without permission and that permission could be obtained by the student raising his hand and waiting for the teacher to call on him. If the child either talked out or left his seat without permission, the teacher called the child by name and reminded him of the rules and told him, 'Do not talk unless called upon' or 'Do not get out of your seat without permission'.

(2) Loss of recess

As above, the teacher announced the rules beforehand and on each occasion that the child broke the rule. In addition, those pupils who transgressed were prohibited from going outside the class during the 10-minute recess period that followed each class period. They remained in the classroom during the recess and were to refrain from talking, but were given no constructive activities to perform during that time.

(3) Positive practice procedure (delayed)

As above, the teacher announced the rules at the start of each session. As in the loss of recess procedure, an infraction of the rules resulted in the culprit having to remain quietly in the classroom during the 10-minute break period. During recess, they were required to engage in the following positive practice procedures: (a) The teacher first asked the student what the correct procedure was for talking in class or leaving one's seat; (b) the student recited the correct procedure to the teacher; (c) the student was required to raise his hand, wait until the teacher acknowledged him by name, and (d) then he asked the teacher for permission; (e) the teacher acknowledged that he had practised correctly and then told him 'Let's practise again'; and (f) the child repeated the entire procedure for several trials.

(4) Positive practice (immediate)

During this procedure, the positive practice was the same as in the previous condition except that the student began it immediately and completed it later when it was more convenient for the teacher. When a student broke a rule, the teacher required him to state the correct procedure for the disruptive behaviour and then engage in the procedure for asking permission, but had him do so for one trial only. When the next recess was scheduled, the student practised asking for permission for 5 minutes during the recess period.

During the positive practice (immediate) condition, the duration of positive practice was gradually reduced (faded) in successive classes, until the student was required only to recite the rule. Similarly, during the recess period, the duration of positive practice was decreased by half each day if the number of disruptions the previous day was two or less. For example, if a student was disruptive only once during the previous day, the amount of time he spent in positive practice would be 2.5 minutes. If he again had only one disruption the following day, the duration would be 1.25 minutes. If the number of disruptions exceeded two on a given day, then the duration of positive practice was increased to 5 minutes.

Results

The researchers found that the positive practice procedure was more effective than the warnings, reminders, or the loss-of-recess penalty in reducing the disruptive conduct. Reinforcement for constructive classroom activity did not discourage the disruptions since the teacher was continually engaging in praising the students for their study efforts as she systematically walked from one student to the next. During the positive practice procedure the disruptive incidents were a rarity.

By comparison, disruptive actions were at a high level during a reminder and disapproval procedure and the disruptions were reduced by only 60 per cent. by a loss-of-recess penalty procedure. The principal advantage of the positive practice procedure over the alternative methods was its re-educative value as well as its greater effectiveness. The positive practice procedure reduced the disruptions immediately to about two per day, a reduction of about 95 per cent. Under the immediate positive practice procedure, the disruptions averaged about 0.4 per day, a reduction of about 98 per cent. Unfortunately, a statistical comparison between the delayed and immediate positive practice conditions were not meaningful because of the small number of students attending the final classes.

After the Summer session, the children returned to their ordinary classrooms. The special Summer class teacher instructed the teacher of each child how to use positive practice and phoned them several times during the school year regarding the child's behaviour. In the case of each child, his teacher consistently reported that he was no longer a problem and was behaving well.

ILLUSTRATION OF CLASSROOM: INDIVIDUAL MANAGEMENT

An investigation by Calhoun and Matherne (1974) was designed to examine the effects of intermittent schedules on the original suppression of disruptive aggressive behaviour. If schedules other than a continuous one can be shown to be highly effective, the practical advantages to parents and teachers are obvious. Three schedules of TO were compared for suppressing aggressive behaviour in a 7-year-old retarded girl. The child was attending a day-care and training school 5 days a week. She was considered an extreme behaviour problem by the Centre directors and teachers. Her behaviour included hitting, kicking, spitting on the teachers and the other children, cursing, leaving the classroom, taking toys and food away from the other children, repeatedly leaving her seat during organized instruction time, and throwing temper-tantrums when disciplined. She often refused to obey her teachers, calling them names, and threatening to tell her parents if they did not leave her alone. She constantly demanded attention and would ask the same questions over and over again or call the teacher's name repeatedly until she received a response. Ignoring her brought about pleas of 'Look at me', 'Talk to me', and eventual aggression if her pleading failed. The class was composed of eight to ten moderately retarded children between the ages of 5 and 8 years, supervised by one teacher and one assistant.

The target behaviours selected were the subject's disruptive behaviour, defined as destructive or injurious behaviour towards other people or objects, specifically hitting, kicking, spitting, or throwing.

The TO room was a four-sided plywood structure located in a storage room adjoining the subject's classroom. Baseline observations were made and TO administered by the experimenter between 9 a.m. and 12 noon. The treatment conditions were three different schedules of TO: in treatment I the subject was placed in TO after every fifth aggressive behaviour (FR5), in treatment II a 2:1

ratio schedule was used (FR2), and in treatment III each aggressive behaviour was followed by TO (CRF). During treatment periods, the subject's teachers continued to discipline her in their accustomed manner for all offences except aggressive behaviour. The experimenter was given complete responsibility for dealing with these.

Treatments I and II lasted a total of twelve 1-hour sessions each. Treatment III required twenty 1-hour sessions to obtain a stable rate of responding. All treatment conditions were exactly alike except for the schedule of TO used. During treatment periods the experimenter sat in a corner of the classroom and recorded aggressive behaviours. Immediately following the critical response for that treatment condition, the experimenter led the subject out of the room, saying 'When you hit (kick, spit, throw) you go in the TO room.' As the subject was put in the TO room, the experimenter said, 'You can come out only when you have been perfectly quiet for 2 minutes and not before.' After 2 minutes of continuous silence the experimenter unlocked the door of the TO room and said, 'You have been quiet, so you may come out now.' During TO the subject occasionally removed her clothing or urinated on the floor. An additional 2 minutes of TO were imposed for these offences.

The FR5 schedule had no effect on the child's disruptive behaviour. The FR2 schedule resulted in a significant decrease in aggressive behaviour, as did, to an even greater extent, the CRF schedule.

During the twelfth session of treatment III, there occurred a burst of aggressive responses which consisted mainly of the subject's hitting some inanimate object (a chair, the door, the wall) as she left the TO room. This happened ten times, resulting in the subject spending a total of 32 minutes almost consecutively in TO. In order to determine the nature of this unexpected behaviour, treatment III was continued for an additional eight sessions. The excessive, above-baseline rate of aggression did not recur.

10

Aggression

Concern about aggression and violence, especially among young people, has reached such a pitch that a note of despair, and sometimes hysteria, can be detected in the commentaries appearing in the news media. News items about acts of sadistic bullying, attacks on teachers, vandalism, arson, and even rape and murder, among school children, seem to abound. Causes are postulated and panaceas prescribed, yet still the statistics pour in, suggesting ever-increasing rates of juvenile criminal violence. The statistics have been challenged. However, in this feverish atmosphere it is easy to believe that we are sliding down a slippery slope into some sort of nightmarish scenario in which hordes of 'feral' children rise up to plague the parents who failed to socialize them properly.

Whatever the basis in fact for the pervasive public anxiety, aggression is certainly seen as a problem at the mundane child-rearing level. Geoffrey Gorer (1955) in his survey of the English character found that the undesirable behaviours which overwhelmingly preoccupied parents, and which they felt it was their duty to uproot, eradicate, or control, were ones concerned with aggression.

THE NATURE OF AGGRESSION

There are many definitions of aggression in the literature. The trouble with omnibus constructs like 'aggression' is that they can cover so many different activities. According to some theorists aggression is an instinct — an atavistic but autonomous impulse — to be tamed, channelized or sublimated in children as soon as possible. Problematical aggression is explained in terms of the vicissitudes of innate or inborn tendencies and the control systems which evolve to cope with them. Yet others conclude that aggression is a drive which is aroused by frustrating circumstances. Other theorists maintain that the important lesson to be derived from studies of the immense variations in the expression or inhibition of aggression in individuals and societies (e.g., the Hopi) is that the constructs of instinctive impulses to violence or aggressive drives are redundant. Learning theorists point to the fact that as progress is made up the evolutionary scale, living creatures depend less and less on reflex or instinctual patterns of behaviour and more and more on experience and learning; hence the fascinating variety of possibilities in man's patterns of behaviour. 'Feelings' of anger and hostile 'thoughts' may well be aroused in conjunction with involuntary physiological processes, but man is not stereotyped in his behavioural responses to the emotional state. Aggressiveness, in their view, is a learned habit or appetite. The belief here is that social (and learned) contingencies more than biological (and innate) characteristics determine the hostile acts and belligerence of individuals. According to this view, it is possible theoretically, at least, to lessen the likelihood of aggressive conflict between people by decreasing the occurrence of severe frustrations and by minimizing the gains to be won through aggression. In the words of Francois Rabelais: 'The appetite grows by eating.'

This is not the place to get bogged down in the debates about the nature of aggression. There are excellent critical reviews available (Bandura, 1973; Tedeschi, Smith, and Brown, 1970). They force one to conclude that 'aggression' is a generic term for complex and many-sided phenomena which still evade precise definition or specification. The term may be applied to aggressive actions (behaviour), to 'states of mind' such as rage, anger, or hostility (subjective feelings), to aggressive drives, inclinations, thoughts and intentions (motivations), and to conditions under which aggressive behaviours are likely to occur (environmental stimulation).

There is a tendency to reify aggression as though it resides in the child as a form of trait which manifests itself in a generalized way across a variety of situations and relationships, or as an instinctual force or energy, or as a physiological drive. The intercorrelations between different ratings of aggressiveness in the same child are in fact very low. Yarrow, Campbell, and Burton (1968) assessed aggression by means of questionnaires and interviews with mothers and by teachers' ratings — conducted with regard to the same nursery-school children. The correlation between mothers'–questionnaire and mothers'–interview responses only amounted to 0.29. The correlation between independent ratings of a child's aggression by two teachers was 0.65. This compares with a correlation of 0.33 obtained by an analysis of overall measures of the child's aggressiveness derived from two independent sources, namely parent and teacher. Sears, Rau, and Alpert (1965) compared reports and observations of direct and indirect aggression at home and at school in nursery-school children. The correlations ranged from −0.20 to +0.36. With such low correlations there is little evidence for the reality of a powerful general trait of aggression.

SOCIAL LEARNING APPROACH

For our practical purposes, aggressive behaviour refers to socially unacceptable ways of behaving which may result in physical or psychological injury to another person or in damage to property. Bandura (1973) delineates the social learning approach (the one adopted here) as follows: it treats aggression as a complex event which requires an explanation of behaviour that produces *injurious and destructive effects* as well as *social labelling* processes (i.e. the social judgements that decide which acts are labelled 'aggressive').

Jehu (1974, p.1) provides the following catalogue of various forms of aggressive response:

A child is said to be destructive when he destroys, damages or attempts to damage an object. Disruptive behaviour involves interference with another person so that he is prevented from doing something or caused displeasure. Physical attack is defined as an actual or attempted assault on another person of sufficient intensity to potentially inflict pain. Verbal abuse occurs either when a child screams or talks loudly enough for this to be unpleasant to another person if carried on for a sufficient time, or when the content of his speech is abusive.

Although biological factors do influence aggressive behaviour, children are not born with the ability to perform these specific acts; this ability must be acquired through learning, either by direct experience or by observing the behaviour of other people (Bandura, 1973).

Although new forms of aggressive behaviour (according to the social learning model) can be shaped by selective reinforcement of successive approximations to it, learning would be extremely slow and tortuous if it relied solely on this process. Most complex behaviour is acquired by watching the behaviour of exemplary models. These may be people the child observes in his everyday life or they may be symbolic models that he reads about or observes on television or in films. A distinction is made between the direct and vicarious learning experiences that contribute to the acquisition of aggressive behaviour and those contemporary influences (see page 77) which determine whether the child will perform the behaviour he has acquired (Bandura, 1973). Aggressive behaviour which has been acquired may not be performed, either because appropriate instigating conditions do not occur or because the consequences of aggression are likely to be unrewarding or unpleasant. The contribution of exemplary models to the acquisition of aggressive behaviour was considered above, and such models also influence the performance of previously learned aggressive responses. In the first place, models who behave aggressively may be emulated by children. Conversely, aggression can be reduced in observers by exposure to models who behave in a non-aggressive fashion in the face of provocation.

In the case of the maintenance of aggressive behaviour, this is largely dependent on its consequences. Aggressive actions that are rewarded tend to be repeated, whereas those that are unrewarded or punished are generally discarded. The reinforcement which strengthens aggressive behaviour may take the form of direct external reinforcement, vicarious or observed reinforcement, or self-reinforcement. Direct external reinforcement may be of a positive kind involving the presentation of rewards such as tangible resources, attention, approval, or social status.

The major effect of direct experience is to select and shape aggressive behaviour through its rewarding or punishing consequences. Aggressive responses which are followed by reward tend to be retained and strengthened, while those that are unrewarded or punished tend to be discarded.

There is convincing evidence (see Bandura, 1973) of the importance of reinforcement in shaping up and maintaining aggressive behaviour. Several theorists (Tedeschi, Smith, and Brown, 1970; Patterson, 1975) have looked at aggression in terms of the concept of coercive power. There is fairly good agreement in the clinical literature (see Feshbach, 1970) that there are two major types of aggressive response: (1) *hostile* or *angry aggression*, in which the only objective of the angry individual is to harm another person by inflicting some injury; and (2) *instrumental aggression*, in which the occurrence of harm or injury to another person is only incidental to the individual's goal of achieving some other goal. Bandura (1973) points out that hostile aggression is also instrumental, except that the actions are used to produce injurious outcomes rather than to gain status, power, resources, or some other goal. In either case the 'aggressor' exercises *coercive power* against another person. Coercive power involves the use of aversive stimuli, threats, and punishments to gain compliance, and can be used offensively to take something away from another person. It can also be used defensively to avoid doing something.

Patterson (1975) lists the following possibilities for the child's failure to substitute more adaptive, more mature behaviours for his primitive coercive repertoire: (1); the parents might neglect to condition prosocial skills (e.g., they seldom reinforce the use of language or other self-help skills); (2) they might provide rich schedules of positive reinforcement for coercive behaviours; (3) they might allow siblings to increase the frequency of aversive stimuli which are terminated when the target child uses coercive behaviours; (4) they may use punishment inconsistently for coercive behaviours; and/or (5) they may use weak conditioned punishers as consequences for coercion. He believes that the average 3-year-old, in American society has learned all of the 14 noxious behaviours described below, this early acquisition being facilitated by the ubiquitous presence of coercive models in the home, nursery school, and on television. The moxious behaviours are coded by the Oregon team as: command negative, cry, disapproval, dependency, destructive, high rate, humiliate, ignore, non-comply, negativism, physical negative, tease, whine, and yell. Observations in the homes of normal families showed that coercive behaviours occurred from a range of 0.02 to 0.50 responses per minute. These represent minimal estimates.

Outside the home, children, especially younger ones, frequently lash out if they cannot get their own way. It may be the teacher who is making demands and thus thwarting the child's wishes, and she becomes the object of the child's rage. Or it may be that young John wants the attractive toy that Jimmy is playing with. 'Hit and grab' gets him what he wants. Jimmy retaliates in the face of this offence by hitting out with his fists. Young children often act as if they invented the maxim 'attack is the best means of defence'.

Patterson and his colleagues (Patterson and Reid, 1970; Patterson and Cobb, 1971) refer to a fairly typical sequence of behaviour as 'the coercion process':

(1) John annoys Jimmy by grabbing his toy.
(2) Jimmy reacts by hitting John.
(3) John then stops annoying Jimmy, thus negatively reinforcing Jimmy's hitting response.

Jimmy has coerced John into terminating his annoying behaviour, A vicious circle is quite likely to be set in motion, an escalation of attack and counter-attack. To continue the sequence:

(4) John may, of course, react to Jimmy's hitting not by desisting from his grabbing at Jimmy's toy, but by hitting back in an attempt to terminate Jimmy's aggression.
(5) Jimmy now responds to John's aggression with more intense counter-aggression.

This exchange would continue until it is interrupted by an adult or until one of the antagonists is negatively reinforced by the cessation of warfare on the part of the other child. We can see how it carries within it the seeds for a perpetuation of aggressive behaviour in the child's repertoire.

Aggression may be positively reinforced if the aggressor gets away with his hitting and grabbing when he wants something from the victim. We also saw another pattern of negative reinforcement at work in the coercion process. Several researchers have shown how rewards heighten the likelihood of future violence. Walters and Brown (1963) gave 7-year-old boys intermittent rewards for punching a Bobo doll. When the boys competed against their peers several days later they proved to be more aggressive than boys in a control group. The occasional reinforcement had achieved more than strengthen the playful punching; they had also strengthened a broad spectrum of aggressive actions. Onlookers, if they approve of the child's hostility, can be a source of reinforcement for aggression. Hostile children who wish and expect to attack another child are often gratified to learn that their intended victim has been hurt. If they think the individual they wanted to injure has been hurt, whether by themselves or someone else, they are likely to experience a pleasant reduction of tension and even a lessened desire to attack the victim further. But there are later consequences, too. The information that an opponent or enemy has been hurt by hostile actions is rewarding. It acts in the long term to strengthen the angry person's aggressive habits. Patterson, Littman, and Bricker (1967) found that children who see their victim's defeat and submission are more likely to act aggressively again, not less so.

DEVELOPMENT OF AGGRESSIVE BEHAVIOUR

The younger the child, the stronger are its demands for the immediate gratification of all its wants. It is impossible to determine precisely how early these aggressive feelings appear in the child. However, the infant lashes out very early at the source of events that frustrate, restrict, or irritate him. The child uses any means at his command to eliminate unpleasant and undesirable stimuli. As the child gets older, the random, undirected, or unfocused displays of emotional excitement (crying or screaming) get more rare, and aggression that is retaliatory more frequent. It is not easy for young children to learn to 'wait patiently', 'ask nicely', and to be generous, considerate, and self-sacrificing. They try to get their way by fighting for it. The social interaction of young children is marked by aggressive, conflict-ridden behaviour. Anger, hostility, quarrelling, and combativeness are observable frequently in children's relations with each other. Dawe (1934) carried out an investigation of the quarrels of pre-school children as they arose in a relatively uncontrolled social environment — the morning free-play period at nursery school. Forty boys and girls (25 to 60 months of age) were observed using the behaviour sampling method. A total of 200 quarrels were analysed. Dawe summarizes her findings as follows:

(1)   The average duration of the quarrels, 23 seconds, is surprisingly short. Quarrels of the older children last longer than those of the younger.
(2)   Boys quarrel more frequently and are more aggressive during quarrels than girls.
(3)   Quarrelsomeness tends to decrease with age, at least quarrels of the type studied do.
(4)   The youngest children start the most quarrels but take the less aggressive role during the quarrel. As children grow older aggressiveness and retaliation increase.
(5)   A very slight negative correlation is found between IQ and frequency of quarrelling.
(6)   Children quarrel most often with those of the same sex, who are, however, either older or younger than themselves. The latter difference seems influenced by opportunity.
(7)   The majority of quarrels are started by a struggle for possessions. The number of quarrels of this type decreases with age but still holds the lead over other types for all ages.
(8)   Pushing, striking, and pulling are the most common motor activities. The older children indulge in the more violent forms more often. In only three quarrels was there no motor activity.

(9)　Crying, forbidding, and commanding are the most common forms of vocal activity, although silence is a more frequent reaction than any single activity. Talking during a quarrel increases with age but reciprocal conversation is rare. There is some indication that quarrels of the argumentative-type increase with age.

(10)　The average number of quarrels per hour is three to four, although this is probably an underestimation of the total quarrelling of this group. There seem to be more quarrels indoors when the children are crowded together.

(11)　The children settle the majority of the quarrels themselves, most frequently by one child's forcing another to yield. Most often the younger child is forced to yield to the older, and most often it is the older who yields voluntarily to the younger.

(12)　The great majority of the children recover after a quarrel very quickly and show no evidence of resentment.

Goodenough (1931) analysed records of angry episodes by 45 children from 1 to 7 years of age. Their mothers kept daily diaries of any angry incidents, recording the time, place, and duration of outbursts, their causes, and the kinds of behaviour manifested. A total of 1,878 angry outbursts were recorded over 4 months. Goodenough listed the following forms of expression of anger: kicking, stamping, jumping up and down, throwing oneself on the floor, holding one's breath, pulling, struggling, pouting, frowning, throwing objects, grabbing, biting, striking, crying, and screaming. Each child had his own particular repertoire with a preference for some but not for others. With time he would change the repertoire of behaviours used in expressing anger. The author found that there was a rapid decrease in outbursts as the child gets older after the peak age of 1½ years. Boys consistently show more anger outbursts than girls.

As the children increased in age from 2 to 5 years, there was a steady diminution in random directionless discharges of expressions of anger, and an increase in retaliatory behaviour aimed at someone or something. As the child gets older his motor resistance decreases as his verbal resistance increases. Fewer than one-third of the outbursts lasted for as long as 5 minutes. The immediate causes of anger could be divided into the following categories, which accounted for 70 per cent. of all incidents reported:

30%— Problems of social relationship (e.g., being denied attention, incomprehension of child's desires, etc.)

20% — Conflicts over routine physical habits (e.g., going to bed or the toilet, etc.)

20% — Conflicts with authority (response to punishment, prohibitions, etc.)

Goodenough found that problems of social adjustment constituted the most frequent single source of anger outbursts among children.

Krebs (1976) has investigated the existence of dominance hierarchies (pecking orders) based on aggression in nursery-school children. She found a linear dominance hierarchy for the sixteen children studied. This was stable over a 3-month period. The most common form of dominance was based on verbal aggression (commanding) and a quarter of dominance encounters on physical aggression. The only one of fourteen attributes which was significantly related to dominance rank was the amount of time a child had spent at the nursery. In other words, a child is more likely to win a dominance encounter if he is more familiar (by longer stay) with the school, irrespective of his size, IQ, etc.

Interference with the satisfaction of needs is one of the many sources of frustration leading to aggression. Another common source is in the conflict of motives. Observations of children demonstrate that one of the most frequent causes of fighting is the dispute over the possession of desired objects. Self-control obviously enters the picture as the child gets older. Hostility in older children is frequently inhibited from open expression (MacFarlane, Allen, and Honzik, 1954). Inner controls are learned. More effective and more socially acceptable ways of solving conflicts are developed, and rules governing the rights of persons and property become incorporated in the child's aware-ness. However, at every age there are wide disparities among individuals in the amount of aggressive behaviour displayed; in some children an aggressive component pervades to a marked extent their behavioural repertoire. Children differ, too, in the extent to which they will manifest aggressive behaviour in situations where retaliation may or may not occur.

From as early as the second year of life boys are, on average, more aggressive than girls, and there are differences in the way the sexes express their hostility. With girls, the aggression is more likely to consist of a verbal attack. Boys, by and large, express their aggression, especially to other boys, in physical assault.

A longitudinal study of the behavioural problems of 'normal' children (McFarlane, Allen and Honzik, 1954) showed differences in the aggressive outbursts of boys and girls. After peaking at 3 years of age, the more aggressive forms of behaviour such as temper-tantrums begin to be less frequent, in both boys and girls. However, at 9 years, more than 50 per cent. of the boys, but only 30 per cent. of the girls, were having quite frequent explosions of temper.

Robins (1966) suggests that by ages 7 or 8 the child with *extreme* antisocial aggressive patterns of behaviour is at quite considerable risk of continuing on into adolescence and indeed adulthood with serious deviancy of one kind or another. Lefkowitz et al. (1977) followed a group of New York children from age 8 to age 19 years; the study has a particular focus on the persistence of aggression. Aggression was much less common in girls than in boys but, in both sexes, children who were highly aggressive at age 8 years tended also to be unduly aggressive at 19 years (correlations of 0.38 for boys and 0.47 for girls). In West and Farrington's study of London boys substantial continuity was again shown (Farrington, 1978). Of the youths rated most aggressive at 8 to 10 years, 59 per cent. were in the most aggressive group at 12 to 14 years (compared with 29 per cent. of the remaining boys) and 40 per cent. were so at 16 to 18 years (compared with 27 per cent. of the remainder). The boys who were severely aggressive at 8 to 10 years were especially likely to become violent delinquents (14 per cent. versus 4.5 per cent).

The same study demonstrated the very considerable extent to which troublesome, difficult, and aggressive behaviour in young boys was associated with later juvenile delinquency. Both the measure at age 8 to 10 years of 'combined conduct disorder', which was based on combined ratings of teachers and social workers, and that of 'troublesomeness' at the same age, which was a combined rating of peers and teachers, proved to be powerful predictors of delinquency. This was especially so with respect to severe and persistent delinquency going on into adult life. Some half of such individuals showed deviant ratings on these measures compared with only one in six of non-delinquent boys.

Kagan and Moss (1962) in their longitudinal study from childhood to adulthood reported greater long-term stability of aggressive conduct in males than females. Some of the differences in aggressiveness between boys and girls may be due to the fact that parents tend to disapprove more of aggression in girls; in our culture females are supposed to fulfil the role of submissive, gentle, and nurturant creatures. Boys are expected to be assertive go-getters, so parents tend to approve aggression in their male offspring as 'manly'. Much of the time parents are quite unconscious of their 'reinforcing' behaviour. However, it is difficult to believe that environment is wholly responsible for producing the differences which are already apparent at the age of 2 years.

ORGANIC FACTORS

Upbringing *is* vital, of course, but there do seem to be inbuilt (hormonal and chromosomal) differences, leading to average differences in temperament. Boys show higher energy levels and greater activity than girls, and the restrictions placed upon them as they grow up — at home and in the classroom — may place greater strains on them, creating more irksome frustrations. Among nursery-school children, Walker (1962) obtained significant correlations between mesomorphic type and clusters of behavioural traits labelled 'energetic–active' and 'aggressive–assertive'. He concluded that variations in physical energy in bodily effectiveness for assertive or dominating behaviour, and in bodily sensitivity appear as important mediating links between physique structure and general behaviour (p.79). The recent (but disputed) claim that there is an extra male chromosome in the genetic make-up of certain aggressive impulsive criminals suggests, though it does not prove, that possibly the male chromosome is linked with impulsive and aggressive behaviour (see page 57).

There is no denying the importance of factors such as brain mechanisms mediating the aggressive behaviour of animals and humans (Avis, 1974). In experiments with animals and clinical observations of humans whose brains have been damaged by disease or in accidents it has been possible to locate centres in the brain (in particular neural mechanisms in the limbic system) which are involved in the production of rage and aggressive behaviour. These are activated and bring about the adaptive bodily changes which occur during the 'emergency emotions' of rage, fear, and excitement. In man, rage and anger are regulated by the highly developed cerebral cortex which both inhibits or gives release to hostile behaviour.

PREVIOUS LEARNING EXPERIENCES

Given the doubtful reality of a general trait of aggression it would seem rather ingenuous to hope for the formulation of reliable cause–effect equations linking child — rearing variables and aggressive behaviour. Nevertheless, there is a somewhat surprising consensus — and a confidently expressed one — that aggressive behaviour in children can be related to long-term attitudes and child-rearing practices. To summarize the findings (see Becker, 1964), parental *permissiveness of aggression* is said to increase the child's tendency to behave aggressively. More precisely, a combination of lax discipline combined with hostile attitudes in the parents produces very aggressive and poorly controlled behaviour in the offspring. The lax parent is one who gives in to the child, acceding to his demands, indulging him, allowing him a great deal of freedom, being submissive and inconsistent, and, in extreme cases, neglecting and deserting him. The parent with hostile attitudes is mainly unaccepting and disapproving of the child; she fails to give affection, understanding, or explanations to the child, and tends to use a lot of physical punishment but not give reasons when she does exert her authority — something she does erratically and unpredictably. Over a long period of time this combination produces rebellious, irresponsible, and aggressive children; they tend to be disorderly in the classroom, lacking in sustained concentration and irregular in their working habits.

The evidence (Bandura, 1965) suggests that children *model* their behaviour on that of their parents. Bandura and Walters (1959) compared families of adolescents who exhibited repetitive antisocial behaviour with those of boys who were neither markedly aggressive nor passive. It was found that the families differed in the extent to which they trained their sons to be aggressive through precept and example. Parents of the non-aggressive boys did not condone aggression to settle disputes, whereas the parents of the aggressive boys repeatedly modelled and reinforced combative attitudes and behaviour.

CONTEMPORARY INFLUENCES

Given that all children are subjected to aggressive acts, why do some children choose to manifest them more than others, in different ways and with different intensity. As Bandura (1973) explains, people rarely show aggression in blind, indiscriminate ways. Rather, aggressive actions tend to occur at certain times, in certain settings, towards certain objects or individuals, and in response to certain forms of provocation. People become aggressive at certain times because of current conditions and influences. There are two categories of contemporary influence to consider in planning treatment: contemporary circumstances which (1) instigate aggression (viz. physical or verbal attacks, deprivation, frustration, conflict, and exposure to aggressive models) or (2) maintain aggression (viz. direct, vicarious and self-reinforcement).

The interactions between parents and child go a long way (as we have seen) toward shaping aggressive behaviour because of the rewarding and reinforcing consequences inherent in their behaviour. The child is likely to generalize what he learns about the utility and benefits of aggression to other situations. In these circumstances he has to put to the test the consequences of being aggressive. For example, he may try being aggressive (because it produced results with his siblings) with his peer group in the playground at school. The example is given of one family member presenting an aversive stimulus to the child, say teasing. Over a series of trials the older brother learns that if he hits his younger sister, she will usually terminate the teasing; thus his hitting behaviour is strengthened. Teasing produces hitting a certain proportion of the time. In effect, pain produces pain — a functional relation which has been noted by several researchers (see Ulrich, 1966; Ulrich and Azrin, 1962). It is also hypothesized that some exchanges become extended and that when this occurs there is likely to be an escalation in the intensity of the painful stimuli (see page 192). It is assumed that family systems which permit behaviour control by the use of pain are quite likely to produce children who exhibit high rates of noxious responses. Patterson (1975) observes that negative reinforcement is most likely to operate in certain closed social systems where the child must learn to cope with aversive stimuli. In such a family the boy's aggressive behaviour will be supported by *both* positive and negative reinforcement. His hitting terminates much of the aversive stimulation. In addition, as many as a fourth to a third of his coercive behaviours are likely to receive positive reinforcement for deviant behaviour as well (Johnson et al., 1973; Patterson, Ray, and Shaw, 1968).

The wider environment in which the child lives can also act as a powerful reinforcer of aggressive behaviour. The child may reside in a neighbourhood where aggressiveness is regarded as a highly valued attribute. In such an environment he is valued through being known as a pugnacious and successful fighter. Successful aggressors are the prestigious models upon whom the other children in the area model their behaviour. The combination of aggressive modelling plus potent reinforcements for being known as a 'tough guy' makes aggressiveness a high probability response in the child's repertoire. Even in highly aggressive subcultures there are children who are not aggressive. The opposite also applies in the case of children who grow up in non-aggressive subcultures or who do not come in direct contact with aggressive models. Some children, of course, do not have the physical equipment to employ aggressive behaviour in a successful manner. Beyond that, modelling theory is not sufficiently accommodating to explain all aggressive children's adoption of these strategies, especially when exemplars or instructors in assaultive actions are lacking in both home and the immediate environment. Some people would argue that the mass media have greatly expanded the range of models of aggression for the child (see page 241).

Bandura (1973) states that aggressive instigators are often established through symbolic experiences. Because of prior learning individuals tend to pair stimuli together like names and words which can evoke negative feelings in the person — hence the symbolic transference in functioning as triggers to aggression. According to Das and Nanda (1963) evaluative responses established through symbolic means tend to generalize along previously established networks of association. In this way effects are produced that extend beyond the specific experience. People also regulate their behaviour according to what they think the consequence of their actions is likely to be (see page 89).

ANTECEDENT CONTROL

There are several methods for reducing aggression based on a modification of the antecedent side of the ABC 'equation'. These procedures include:

(1) Reducing discriminative stimuli for aggression

The absence of, say, the mother in the playroom may be a cue for the eldest child that threatening or hitting his younger brother is likely to gain him certain advantages, e.g., the best toys. In other words, certain stimulus conditions provide signals to the child that aggressive behaviour is likely to have rewarding consequences for him. Several treatment programmes could be planned to reduce discriminative stimuli for such aggression; one way would be to provide parental supervision of play until such time that it is no longer necessary.

(2) Providing models for non-aggressive behaviour

Acceptable alternatives to aggression may be enhanced by exposing youngsters to prestigious or influential individuals who manifest such alternative behaviours, especially when they are instrumental in obtaining rewards for these models. Davids (1972) reports a study in which institutionalized boys with behavioural disorders observed male and female adults playing with toys in either an aggressive or non-aggressive manner. A comparison of the boys' play activities before and after viewing these models showed that the male aggressive model had the greater influence in producing an increment in the boys' aggressive behaviour. The female non-aggressive model had the greater influence when it came to increasing their non-aggressive behaviour. The male model of aggressive behaviour tended to have the effect of reducing the boys' verbalizations, both aggressive and non-aggressive.

However, the most significant changes with regard to verbalization consisted of an increase in verbalizations of a non-aggressive kind after viewing the non-aggressive female model and a reduction of verbalizations of a non-aggressive kind after viewing the female aggressive model.

(3) Reducing the exposure to aggressive models

We have already seen that there is evidence that exposure to other people behaving aggressively may facilitate the imitation of such behaviour by the observer. An attempt to reduce the exposure of a child to such aggressive models is likely to decrease the likelihood of him behaving similarly.

(4) Reducing aversive stimuli

Violent reactions may be instigated by a large variety of aversive stimuli: by conflict, by physical assaults, by words of a threatening or humiliating nature, and by deprivation of the child's proper care, rights, and opportunities. It is reasonable to expect that a reduction of such aversive stimuli might be accompanied by a decrease in aggression. One technique is to resolve conflicts before they flare up into violence (Kifer et al., 1974).

(5) Increasing social skills

Social skills training has been of particular interest to therapists working with disruptive and aggressive children and adolescents (Patterson, 1974). Social skills training has been used to eliminate aggressive behaviour in nursery-school children (Brown and Elliott, 1965) as well as to reduce various confrontational problems between special education students and their teachers (Graubard et al., 1971). A typical example of a social skills training programme for educational settings would be a programme of instruction, modelling, role playing and feedback (see Beck and Forehand, 1984; Herbert, 1986) (also typically) to change the behaviour of aggressive, uncooperative, underachieving pupils in the direction of positive changes in school work (following directions and rules), showing courtesy and consideration, etc.

DESENSITIZATION

The defusing of aversive stimuli by diminishing their power to arouse anger in the child can be achieved by using densensitization procedures (Rimm et al., 1971).

O'Donnell and Worell (1973) provide an example of the effectiveness of three procedures to reduce anger. They generated anger experimentally by exposing young white males to provocative black racial stimuli. The angry response aroused by this experience (considered to be an appropriate reaction for these white males) was assumed to be the result of long exposure to a racially conscious subculture. It might therefore be more resistant to modification than most other emotional responses, such as anxiety about snakes. The therapeutic procedures were: desensitization, desensitization with cognitive relaxation, and desensitization in the absence of relaxation training. The desensitization group reported decreases in anxiety and disgust relative to a control group which received no treatment. Ratings by therapists showed reductions in anger for subjects in both the desensitization with and without cognitive relaxation groups. In the latter group there were reductions in anger concurrently with increases in diastolic and systolic blood pressure. The subjects for whom desensitization was most effective reported less anger after the anger-arousing procedure carried out before treatment, greater depth of relaxation during treatment, and were liked more by their therapists. These subjects also reported a greater reduction in ethnocentrism and a trend toward lower overt hostility following treatment.

Kifer et al. (1974) observe that one of the factors contributing to the delinquency of many youths is their inability to cope with conflict situations with authority figures. Conflict situations are defined by the authors as interpersonal situations in which the youth and authority figure (e.g., a parent or teacher) have opposing desires. The youth may want to buy a motor bike, but his mother wants him to purchase an old car because she thinks bikes are dangerous and will get him into bad company. Youngsters often make inappropriate responses to conflict situations (such as fighting, withdrawing, tantrums, or destructive behaviour); an escalation of the conflict may bring them into contact with clinics, courts, and other agencies. Negotiation could sometimes defuse these situations and produce more acceptable consequences for both parties. There are two broad approaches to conflict resolution: (1) arbitration or mediation of specific conflicts and (2) modification of communication processes (see Carter and Thomas, 1973). Behavioural contracting is the most common example of the arbitration approach. This procedure has been described in detail elsewhere (see page 72), it involves the therapist in the role of a mediator or arbitrator who facilitates mutual agreements between opposing parties about reciprocal exchanges of specific behaviours and reinforcers (Stuart, 1971a).

Verbal instructions, practice, and feedback are the major techniques used to modify communication processes. Kifer et al. (1974) describe attempts to modify communication processes. Their emphasis was entirely on learning new adaptive behaviours, rather than eliminating problem behaviours, and the techniques were primarily educational rather than therapeutic. The training was designed to teach one specific skill. Two mother–daughter pairs and one father–son pair acted as subjects. The youths (aged 13, 16, and 17 years) had at least one contact with the County Juvenile Court. The boy and one girl were in Achievement Place Homes, and the other girl was a candidate for Achievement Place. Only one parent was involved in each case because two of the youths were living with only that parent and the father of one of the girls declined to participate.

The procedures involved analysing the negotiation process into component behaviours and using instructions, practice, and feedback to train these behaviours. Trainers visited subjects' homes and asked them to identify 'the three most troublesome problem situations between the two of you at this time'. Any conflict situations identified by both parent and youth were discussed. In case different situations were identified, at least one selected by the parent and one by the child were discussed. Subjects were instructed to discuss each situation for 5 minutes without help from the trainers, and were told to 'try to reach a solution acceptable to both of you'. At the end of the first discussion, the trainers gave brief general praise for discussing the situation, restated the next conflict situation, and repeated the instructions. Each parent-child pair attended their own weekly session. The same three-step format was used in all sessions: (1) pre-session simulation, (2) discussion and practice simulations, and (3) post-session simulation. Results indicated that the procedures were successful in training youths and their parents in negotiation behaviours that produced agreements to conflict situations, and that these behaviours generalized to actual conflict situations in the subjects' homes.

COGNITIVE CHANGE (WITH REGARD TO ANTECENDENT EVENTS)

The performance of aggressive behaviour and its alternatives may be determined by the child's thought processes as well as his external environment. For example, the instigation of aggression may be influenced by antecedent cognitive events such as aversive thoughts (e.g., remembering a past grudge), being aware of the probable consequences of aggressive actions, or being capable of solving problems mentally instead of 'lashing out' reflexly. The patient's search for various possible courses of action in the face of provocation and frustration can be made more flexible by attention to the thinking processes that precede, accompany, and follow violent actions. A skill that hostile children sometimes lack is the ability to identify the precursors to an aggressive outburst, so that they can bring into play more adaptive solutions to their problems. Modifying a child's cognitions concerning an unpleasant experience might reduce its probability of triggering violent behaviour. To take an example, if the incident of another child knocking over the potential aggressor is redefined as an accident rather than an attack, there may be less risk of a pugnacious reaction. The influence of pleasant or aversive consequences on a child's actions are enhanced by his awareness of these consequences. Thus, increasing a child's consciousness of the penalties contingent upon aggressive behaviour may reduce its performance. On the other hand, a word of approval before reinforcing an alternative form of behaviour to aggression will tend to make such approval into a signal for reinforcing consequences and thus increasing the probability of the prosocial action.

There is evidence that the performance of aggressive acts is influenced by cognitive problem-solving process. D'Zurrilla and Goldfried (1971) identify the processes which often precede and guide subsequent overt behaviour as follows: (1) being able to recognize problematic situations when they occur; (2) making an attempt to resist the temptation to act impulsively or to do nothing to deal with the situation; (3) defining the situation in concrete or operational terms and then formulating the major issues to be coped with; (4) generating a number of possible responses which might be pursued in this situation; (5) deciding on the course(s) of action most likely to result in positive consequences; and (6) finally, acting upon the final decision and verifying the effectiveness of the behaviour in resolving the problematic situation.

To facilitate the problem-solving process in children, they require help in identifying their aggressive behaviour and recognizing the conditions which provoke and maintain it. The problem situation is analysed, broken down into its component parts, and (hopefully) represented in a manner most likely to lead to a solution. A number of procedures are available for this purpose (Thoresen and Mahoney, 1974). They include self-recording by the child of his hostile activities, together with his observations of the circumstances in which they occurred and their consequences. This information is used to show the child the relationships between his behaviour and its controlling conditions.

COVERT SELF-INSTRUCTION

An example of how aggressive conduct problems have been successfully modified by methods incorporating self-control training is given by Goodwin and Mahoney (1975). They reduced aggressive behaviour in three hyperactive, impulsive boys by modelling a young boy who copes with the provocation of verbal aggression by means of covert self-instruction. One week after the baseline (taunting) session, subjects viewed a 3-minute videotape of a 9-year-old boy being taunted by five other children. In addition to remaining ostensibly calm, looking at his taunters and remaining in the centre of the circle, the model was portrayed as coping with verbal assaults through a series of covert self-instructions. These thoughts, which were dubbed on the tape, consisted of such statements as 'I'm not going to let them bug me' and 'I won't get mad'. Immediately after viewing the tape, subjects participated in a further taunting session. One week later, subjects again viewed the videotape of the coping model. However, this time the dubbed thoughts and the overt actions of the model were pointed out, discussed, and verbally emphasized by the experimenter. Each coping self-statement was repeated by the experimenter and labelled as an effective way to deal with verbal aggression. After viewing the tape, each subject was asked to verbalize as many of these coping responses as he could recall. A third taunting session was then conducted. The study was carefully designed to isolate treatment effects; the resultant ability of the children to control their outbursts seems very promising. It should be added that the children received coaching and practice in the coping skills that were modelled.

Theoretically, the discontinuation of the reinforcing consequences of aggression (if they have been identified correctly) could result in a temporary persistence (or increase) in the unwanted behaviour before it finally extinguishes. Obviously, it is crucial for the clinician operating an extinction programme to take account of this phenomenon, which may for various reasons be unacceptable. Pinkston et al. (1973) attempted to deal with the kind of aggression which cannot simply be ignored, by using a modified type of extinction programme. This involved ignoring the aggressor while sheltering the victim from further assault. (This is not always viable in open-ended situations such as the bully trapping his victim on the way back from school.) Another problem in treating the aggressive child arises when the extinguished aggression (in the absence of any intervening reinforcement) reappears — as it may — after an interval of time. This 'setback' (spontaneous recovery) is a transitory phenomenon and the frequency of the recovered response is usually limited. Again, the therapist needs to be on the lookout for this possibility and the parent or teacher forewarned.

There is a constructive way to mitigate the troublesome initial period of treatment. Several researchers (Bernal et al., 1968; Johnson and Brown, 1969; O'Leary, Repp and Dietz, 1974, O'Leary and Becker, 1967; Sloane, Johnston and Bijou, 1967; Zeilberger, Sampen, and Sloane, 1968) have demonstrated the success of methods combining non-reinforcement of aggressive behaviour with positive reinforcement of considerate behaviour. Essentially they concentrate on 'reprogramming' the social environment using one or other variations on a *differential reinforcement* theme.

OUTCOME CONTROL

There is sound evidence (to be reviewed) that procedures based on selective reinforcement can reduce aggressive behaviour. In some studies aggressive behaviour is consistently ignored; in others it is ignored while a competing pattern of prosocial conduct is rewarded. In other cases prosocial behaviour is positively reinforced, but aggression is punished by removing the child from the scene (time-out).

EXTINCTION OF AGGRESSIVE BEHAVIOUR

It should be possible to extinguish aggressive behaviour by discontinuing its reinforcing consequences if they can be identified. Brown and Elliott (1965) note that while there are many theories which try to explain aggression in children, perhaps the simplest is the best. One formulation is that many fights, etc., occur because they bring with them a great deal of fuss and attention from some adult. Brown and Elliott demonstrated with twenty-seven 3-to-4-year-old boys that by systematically ignoring their aggressive behaviour and attending to their cooperative behaviour they succeeded in reducing the aggressive behaviour. However, there is no information about follow-up; nor was information provided about how well trained the parents were to maintain the behaviour changes on their own or to deal with new problems arising in the future.

TIME-OUT AND RESPONSE-COST

Time-out and response-cost programmes have been designed to provide stimulus conditions which signal to the child that his aggressive behaviour will not only fail to have rewarding consequences but, indeed, will result in punitive consequences. The provision of such discriminative stimuli may bring aggression under control while more acceptable alternative behaviour is being acquired. Burchard and Tyler (1965), for example, report how a very difficult boy named Donny (aged 13 years) responded to such a procedure. This youngster had been in an institution for delinquents since he was 9 years of age. The problems that had brought him there included behaviours that were criminal, disruptive, destructive, and cruel. Donny was diagnosed as psychopathic and even schizophrenic. After commitment to the institution, it had been recommended that the child be given regressive therapy: '. . . that he should be regressed to the point of taking a bottle from his therapist . . . and that if he could be brought to smearing faeces, it would surely be good for him' (p. 247). After 2 years of unsuccessful regressive therapy, contingency management procedures were instituted. Donny was so uncontrollable that, in the year before treatment was initiated, he had spent 200 days off and on in an isolation room. His intractible behaviour tended to attract considerable staff attention. When Donny first began to 'act up', staff members would try to ignore his behaviour for as long as possible. During this time, peer approval and attention tended to reinforce the behaviour. As the behaviour continued and increased in magnitude, attendants attempted to use supportive persuasion to get him to desist. When this (reinforcement) was unsuccessful, the staff became angry and only at that point was punishment finally introduced. Staff members now felt guilty and visited the boy in isolation, where they would also give him snacks. The other boys tended to reinforce Donny's misbehaviour with attention, praise, and sympathy. In contrast, good behaviour brought little attention or praise because the overextended staff had to focus their efforts on the troublesome boys. With the contingencies operating in this fashion, it is not unexpected that Donny's unacceptable behaviour increased over time. Staff and peer attention occurred immediately after the response, while the punishment was delayed and ambivalently administered.

A new treatment programme was instituted, in which any unacceptable behaviour requiring punishment was followed immediately by placement in isolation (time-out) for 3 hours, during which communication with staff and peers was reduced to bare essentials. The staff was instructed to approach this intervention in a matter-of-fact way and at the onset of carefully specified target behaviour, i.e. before they themselves had become emotionally aroused by the behaviour. It was also stressed that isolation had to be on an all-or-none basis and that it should never be used as a threat. On the positive side, contingencies were established to promote acceptable behaviour. For each hour during the day that the child was *not* in isolation he received a token, and if he stayed out over night he was given three tokens upon waking up. These tokens could be exchanged for cigarettes, soda pop, trips to town, movies, etc. The opportunity to exchange tokens was given daily. The system evolved with improving behaviour. After a while (2 months), the child was required to stay out of isolation for 2 hours, not just 1, in order to gain a token, and there was a bonus of 7 tokens for each 24-hour period completed without isolation. Finally, the time-out period was shortened to 2 hours, thus allowing the child greater time with the staff and other inmates.

Isolation was used relatively rarely, eighteen times in the first month of treatment and only twelve times in the last. Still, there was a clear effect upon the child's behaviour. In addition to the slight (33 per cent.) decline in the use of isolation, the offences for which it was invoked became much less serious. During the first month of treatment these included glue sniffing (twice), stealing while on a field trip, stealing from the staff, fighting, and sniffing from a stolen bottle of bleach. During the fifth month the offences included running in the dormitory, disrupting the classroom at school, and insolence to staff.

Brown and Tyler (1968) succeeded in 'dethroning' (as the authors put it) a tough delinquent who exercised powerful bullying control over his peers. They excluded him whenever he or his gang intimidated the weaker members and forced subservience from them. His tyrannical control now proved too costly and he ceased to exercise it. Since he was held accountable for any trouble that might develop in the cottage, he not only ceased promoting disruptive behaviour but tried to dissuade others from it. There is always a problem in modifying such powerful delinquent systems. While punishment may usurp the throne from a domineering leader there is likely to be a pretender awaiting the succession. It therefore becomes necessary to restructure the peer reinforcement system to a significant degree — and this is no easy task.

We have claimed that treatment in home settings seems to promise well (see page 106). The evidence suggests that this is true of problems of aggression. The limited time available for treatment by the clinician makes it more efficient to involve the parents by encouraging them to follow procedures offered by him. It is obviously crucial to observe the parents interacting with their children before such training commences. There may be significant anomalies in the parent–child interactions and relationship. One method of training is for the therapist herself to model appropriate interaction with the child. This can be observed by the parents through a one-way screen. Mothers are trained in this way to modify their own behaviour in relation to their children. Hanf (1968) worked with nineteen mothers and trained them in about 6 weeks through modelling and direct training in mother–child rearing. Placing a telemetric instrument in the mother's ear helped advise her immediately on differential reinforcement and how she could enhance certain behaviour and eliminate other types.

This type of instruction was particularly useful in dealing with aggressive children. Bernal et al. (1968) studied two children manifesting the so-called 'brat syndrome'. One was an 8-year-old boy with frequent temper-tantrums, rocking, social isolation, and peculiar verbal behaviour, as well as stereotyped motor responses. He frequently attacked parents and teachers as well as peers with physical violence. The second was a 5-year-old who presented as being disobedient, defiant, hyperactive, destructive, and physically authoritative to his younger brother. Bernal analysed the parent–child interaction and had the parents observe the child at home. In the clinic videotaping was also done. Mothers were then shown how they interacted with their own children through replay on the television screen. Mothers were trained not merely to concern themselves with discrete behaviour but also with an interaction system of behaviour and the maintenance of new desirable behaviour in children. The first case reported cessation of 'brat' behaviour after 15 weeks of training and a 2-year follow-up showed that the improvements were maintained. In the second case, improvement was noted by observers in the home, and by parents' and teacher's reports. After termination, follow-up contacts over several months indicated maintenance of the improvement in behaviour and in the parent–child relationship.

Patterson and Brodsky (1966) report a case-study of Karl, a boy of kindergarten age, who had long-standing problems of aggression, which involved frequent kicking and biting others. His teacher suffered particularly from his violent outbursts. He was enuretic and also indulged in much crying. The therapists set out to modify the behaviours of the mother and child as they interacted with each other. The mother was taught by instruction, modelling, and direct prompting. Positive reinforcement and extinction procedures were selected to improve Karl's interactions with people and to reduce his tantrums and separation anxieties. Their application produced a reduction in antisocial problems within fourteen days to a rate at which his mother and teacher agreed that there was no reason to continue the programme. There was in addition a significant increase in positive interactions between the boy and his peers.

Patterson et al. (1967) also describe how Earl, a 5-year-old, who was generally aggressive, negativistic, and uncooperative was treated. During his periodic violent emotional outbursts he would bang his head, explode violently, destroy toys, kick plaster off walls, crawl under the bed, sound like an animal and eat faeces. His mother understandably described him as a 'repulsive' child. Using a similar programme of parent training the authors applied social reinforcement and time-out procedures to the target behaviours. Considerable behaviour change was brought about in 6 weeks for Earl.

The operant programmes in both cases were essentially designed to reprogramme 'family systems' so that the parent–child interactions would become reciprocally reinforcing. In this way the children's prosocial actions would increase and negative behaviours would reduce in frequency. Patterson notes that the swiftness of the behavioural change that was achieved seems to indicate that the therapeutic programme was shaping up behaviour already available in the child's repertoire, but functioning at a low operant level. This, he modestly avers, means that the two boys had been previously socialized and the therapists could not take all the credit.

Russo (1964) has also reported the successful use of differential

208

reinforcement in reducing surplus and, in particular, aggressive behaviours in children. One, a 6-year-old girl, Sarah, behaved perfectly at school, but at home showed disturbing conduct problems such as fighting with siblings, invading their privacy, destroying their things, grinding her teeth, bed-wetting, and having sever temper-tantrums and general oppositional behaviour. Russo writes that the parents brought her to the clinic because their relationship was so poor and Sarah's actions so annoying and frustrating that the mother abstained from punishing her for fear of losing her temper and harming the youngster. The child was uncooperative and would not talk about herself or her activities. At school Sarah behaved very well. She got along well with the other children, did her work conscientiously, obeyed the teacher, and showed considerable respect and affection for her. It was concluded that the specificity of her misbehaviour to the home and the immediate neighbourhood made it probable that the problem was related to the family and its transactions with the child. Indeed, her 'antics' had been considered 'cute' and were a cause of merriment until she became so big and strong that she was harming her sisters.

Russo utilized differential reinforcement to increase the child's adaptive behaviour and extinguish her maladaptive responses. After some preliminary discussion of aims and methods the therapist took both child and parent to a playroom. During the early sessions the parent was a spectator and observed what the child and therapist did. Soon the parent began to take part in the activity and it became a three-way interaction. When this process was well underway, the therapist began to withdraw from the action until he became the spectator and the parent and child were left to interact with each other. Only in unusual incidents did the therapist take a hand in the activities. The parents learned to apply verbal and social reinforcement and generally to deal with the negative consequences of the maladaptive interactions between them, and were instructed in carrying out these procedures at home. It was possible to terminate treatment after 20 sessions.

SKILLS TRAINING

Bornstein et al. (1980) examined the effectiveness of social skills training with four highly aggressive children who were inpatients in a psychiatric setting. The children ranged in age from 8 to 12, were observed to manifest extreme levels of aggression with their peers, and were unable to express frustration and disappointment in an appropriate manner. More specifically, the children were found to exhibit a low rate of eye contact, an inability to make appropriate requests of others, and a high degree of hostile tone in their responses. These specific responses were measured on a series of role-play scenes.

Following pretreatment assessment, children received three half-hour sessions of social skills training for each of the three targeted deficits observed in the role-play assessment. Training was first applied to eye contact, then to hostile tone, and finally to appropriate requests. Training consisted of instructions, feedback, modelling, behaviour rehearsal, and reinforcement. The therapist presented one of the interpersonal scenes and instructed the child in appropriate behaviour; the child performed the response; the therapist provided feedback and reinforcement; a confederate modelled the appropriate response; the therapist provided feedback, reinforcement, and new instructions to the child; the child rehearsed the response for several trials until the criteria for the targeted response had been reached. Upon satisfactory performance, training proceeded in a similar fashion to new interpersonal situations. Throughout training, children were assessed on the role-play scenes approximately three times per week.

Elder *et al.* (1979) conducted a study with four highly aggressive, adolescent psychiatric patients but extended the test of generalization to untrained role-play scenes, natural settings, and ward behaviour. Training was conducted in a group and in an on-ward classroom. Further, training was conducted four days per week for approximately 45 minutes per day for a total of fourteen sessions. Hence, training was extended; it was conducted in groups in a natural setting; and an attempt was made to assess generalization from a number of perspectives.

Training proceeded in a standard fashion and included instructions, feedback, modelling, behaviour rehearsal, and reinforcement. Results of the Bornstein investigation indicated that positive effects of training were achieved for each target behaviour for each child. However, the changes noted in training did not generalize consistently to other settings. Thus, although the findings indicate that social skills training altered specific responses in specific role-play situations, the training did not generalize consistently to untrained prompts or to more natural situations. Still, the results of this study indicate that social skills training may be useful with aggressive children.

Results in the Elder study indicated that social skills training was highly effective and that all three targeted social skills were acquired by each of the adolescents. Generalization of the trained skills was evident in the untrained scenes and in the ward setting. The adolescents were observed to make fewer interruptions, to employ more appropriate responses to negative situations, and to make more appropriate requests of others. Furthermore, these changes in social skills were associated with ward changes.

COMBINED EXTINCTION AND TIME-OUT

Wolf, Risley, and Mees (1964) point out that under ward conditions, with personnel untrained in extinction procedures, it is far from certain that extinction will be reliably carried out. So they planned a procedure which was a combination of mild punishment and extinction for a particularly difficult child, Dicky.

Dicky was 3½ years old and had been diagnosed as retarded, brain damaged, and psychotic. The parents consulted the researchers after their son underwent cataract surgery which necessitated the wearing of glasses. Dicky had severe temper-tantrums, during which he showed self-destructive behaviour including

210

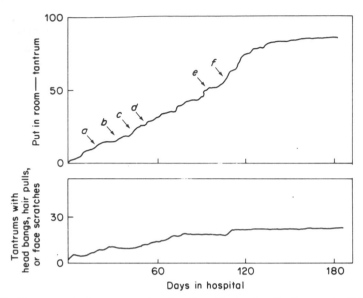

Figure 10 Two cumulative curves showing the effects of extinction and mild punishment (time-out) upon the tantrums and severe self-destructive episodes of a hospitalized pre-school autistic boy (Wolf, Risley, and Mees, 1964)

face slapping, head banging, and face scratching. Furthermore, he refused to go to sleep at bedtime, seriously interfering with household routine and keeping his parents up late at night, and did not eat in an age-appropriate fashion. His case became critical because he was in danger of losing his eyesight. Because of cataracts in both eyes, he had to have surgical removal of the lenses, and since he refused to wear glasses and habitually threw them on the floor, permanent retinal damage was very likely.

The research team recommended that the child re-enter the hospital before treatment was undertaken so that they could obtain better control of his total environment and thereby intercept the inadvertent reinforcement of the deviant behaviour which was occurring at home. They initiated careful record-keeping procedures to obtain base rates before modification began. Temper-tantrums, responsible for so much of Dicky's self-destructive behaviour, received highest priority for immediate treatment. Ward attendants, and later the parents, carried out the prescribed procedures under the guidance of the consultants.

Most of the serious recurrent behaviours, which obstructed any remedial efforts, were eliminated by combined use of extinction and time-out. In modifying the tantrum behaviour, e.g., whenever the boy slapped himself and whined, he was placed in his room for 10 minutes or until the disturbing action ceased. Under this contingency tantrums gradually declined and eventually disappeared. A cumulative record showing the frequency with which Dicky was placed in his room for tantrums and self-destructive behaviour is presented in the upper graph of Figure 10.

There are some artefacts in the record, which show a constant rate of being placed in his room for tantrums during the first 4 months. This would appear to indicate no improvement in Dicky's behaviour during this period — a phenomenon contradicted by casual observation. According to the authors several variables, each involving a sacrifice of experimental rigour, contributed to this discrepancy. These are worth detailing as they illustrate the exigencies of 'natural environment' work: (1) As Dicky's behaviour improved, the attendants lowered the original criterion (of two or more behaviours such as slapping himself or crying) finally to include any atavistic behaviour. The criterion change was encouraged by the authors because they believed this was to the distinct advantage of the child. (2) During the early weeks the attendants offered Dicky elaborate explanations as he was escorted to his room. There were also tender, practically tearful apologies and fondlings after the door was reopened. This pattern gradually became a perfunctory trip to the room with the door simply being reopened at the end of the tantrum, presenting a ward going on much as before. (3) By the beginning of the third month, temper-tantrums that lasted less than 5 minutes began to occur frequently, creating the likelihood that the trip to the room would become a socially reinforcing event. A minimum time-out of 10 minutes in the room was therefore brought to bear. (4) Dicky's contact with his family and home progressively increased during this time and this might be expected to precipitate some lengthy tantrums. The major changes are indicated in the tantrum curve. At (a) Dicky's parents were permitted their first 1-hour visit. Subsequently they made several scheduled visits a week, during which an attendant observed and instructed them in their handling of Dicky. At (b) the father put Dicky to bed on the ward for the first time. At (c) Dicky began wearing his glasses and at (d) the mother put Dicky to bed on the ward for the first time. Midway between (d) and (e) Dicky began short home visits accompanied by the attendant. At (e) Dicky spent his first night at home and at (f) he spent a second night at home. After (f) he spent an average of 3 nights a week at home, increasing to 5 nights a week during the final month.

Some estimate of the decreasing severity of the tantrums is indicated in the lower cumulative curve in Figure 10. Each step represents a tantrum, either during the day or at bedtime, involving head banging, hair pulling, or face scratching. After the first 2½ months this severe self-destructive behaviour remained near zero. The remainder of the tantrum record consists of face slapping, whining, and crying. Conditions for dealing with tantrums at the home were made comparable to those on the ward. The attendants coached the parents to deal with Dicky's tantrums by putting him in his room both on the ward and at home.

After about 10 weeks the severe self-destructive behaviours were substantially reduced, setting the stage for the modification of other deviant behaviours. The authors approached bedtime problems in a similar manner to that already described. The child was bathed, cuddled, and put to bed. If he got out of bed, he was returned to his room and the door was closed. If he returned to bed, the door was left open. This simple procedure resulted in a rapid decrease in bedtime problems as Dicky began to go to sleep when told after only about 6 days. Over the next 3 months, until Dicky left the hospital completely, he spent more and more nights at home with only minor disruptions.

The major challenge to the researchers was to try to get Dicky to wear his glasses. This required a systematic shaping procedure using sweets and food reinforcement. Initially, a conditioned reinforcer was established by pairing the clicks of a toy clicker with a small sweet or fruit. Before long the child learned to approach the bowl where the reinforcers were placed immediately after he heard the click. Initially, because the prescription of the lenses required was quite powerful and changed the visual field radically — a condition that might itself have been aversive — the child was rewarded for wearing the glasses *frames* only. Even this proved difficult; they could not be placed appropriately upon the child's head. Shaping involved the clicker being sounded (and reinforcement ensuing) when Dicky picked the glasses up, held them, carried them, or brought them close to his head. This was necessary because he became active and upset whenever anyone touched his head. The staff of the hospital ward were reluctant to deprive the child of food, so the sweets and fruit were rather weak reinforcers. To counter these problems. Wolf, Risley, and Mees (1964, pp. 309–310) report as follows:

> We attempted to increase deprivational control by using breakfast as a shaping session, bits of breakfast now being dependent upon approximations to the wearing of glasses . . . Later we added to the glasses . . . a 'roll bar' which would go over the top of his head and guide the pieces up over the ears.
>
> After wearing the glasses was established in these sessions, it could be maintained with often less manipulable reinforcers. For example, the attendants would tell Dicky, 'Put your glasses on and let's go for a walk'. Dicky was usually required to wear the glasses during meals, snacks, automobile rides, outdoor play, etc. If he removed the glasses, the activity was termined.
>
> At the time of Dicky's release from the hospital he had worn the glasses for more than 600 hours and was wearing them about 12 hours a day.

The success of these techniques encouraged the experimenters to use additional behaviour modification approaches to increase speech and language ability and to eliminate disruptive eating behaviour. As a result, much of Dicky's food throwing and food snatching was eliminated and imitative skills and verbal labelling were improved. The researchers note, with a well-deserved feeling of accomplishment, 'According to a report from the mother six months after the child's return home, Dicky continues to wear his glasses, does not have tantrums, has no sleeping problems, is becoming increasingly verbal, and is a new source of joy to the members of his family.'

Aversive control can be an effective method for managing aggressive behaviour in residential settings such as hospitals and Observation and Assessment Centres. However, it is unlikely to have much rehabilitative value in institutions for delinquent children and youths as they are constituted at present. If negative sanctions applied by staff members are strong enough to outweigh undermining peer influences, adaptive behaviour may be achieved and sustained as long as the institutional sanctions remain in effect. When aversive controls are removed, however, peer reinforcement serves usually to reinstate deviant patterns of behaviour.

PUNISHMENT OF AGGRESSION (OVERCORRECTION)

Foxx and Azrin (1972) developed a procedure that provided disruptive patients with re-education, removal of the reinforcement for the offence, time-out from general positive reinforcement, and an effort requirement. The offender was required by instructions or physical guidance to overcorrect the general psychological and physical disturbance created by the offence. The procedure was applied to one brain-damaged and two retarded patients, who displayed one or more of the following types of behaviour: physical assault, property destruction, tantrums, continuous screaming, and biting; all had resisted other treatments such as time-out, punishment, and social disapproval. The procedure reduced the disturbed behaviours of all patients to a near-zero level within 1 or 2 weeks and maintained this therapeutic effect with minimal staff attention. This method appears to be a rapid and effective treatment procedure for disruptive behaviour and emphasizes the individual's responsibility for his actions.

COGNITIVE CHANGE (WITH REGARD TO CONSEQUENCES)

Thoresen and Mahoney (1974) show that the probability of aggressive behaviour occurring at some future time may be influenced by its cognitive consequences — by symbolic self-reinforcement or self-punishment in the child's thought processes. He may praise himself when he behaves in ways which accord with his own values, while disapproved behaviour is followed by criticism of himself. In the latter case, aggressive behaviour may be suppressed even if there are no environmental consequences. Covert sensitization (Cautela, 1973b) is one such procedure. Aggressive behaviour in imagination is associated with fantasized aversive consequences. After a number of such trials the patient is told to imagine the aversive consequences immediately whenever there is a possibility of the aggressive sequence occurring in the natural situation. In this way he may be helped to pre-empt his aggression at an early stage. Conversely, alternative behaviour to aggression may be strengthened by cognitive self-reinforcement, such as feelings of pride or self-praise, even when there is no environmental reinforcement contingency (Thoresen and Mahoney, 1974). One of the methods of training in cognitive self-reinforcement is called 'covert reinforcement' (Cautela, 1973a). The child might be asked to imagine himself performing a series of behaviours which are prosocial alternatives to aggression in a provocative situation. At various points in the sequence he is instructed to imagine something that has previously been identified as reinforcing for him, so that his imagined performance of the alternative behaviour is reinforced in his own thought processes. Subsequently, he uses these rewarding images to reinforce his performance of the actual alternative behaviour in natural situations. There is sparse evidence about cognitive self-reinforcement, but Bandura (1973) suggests that it may be developed by programmes containing the following elements: (1) first, desired values and behaviour should be exemplified by models; (2) the imitation of these by the child should be systematically evaluated and reinforced by other people; (3) the child should gradually take over responsibility for evaluating his own behaviour, while others continue to reinforce it; (4) when accurate self-evaluation is established, then the child starts to reinforce himself as well; and (5) finally, external self-reinforcement is gradually replaced by cognitive self-reinforcement.

FAMILY BASED BEHAVIOURAL WORK

Patterson and his colleagues at the Oregon Research Institute have been a prolific source of ideas and data on the subject (inter alia) of predelinquent and delinquent disorders, notably aggression and stealing. They have developed a treatment package that involves training parents in child management skills (Patterson, Reid, Jones, and Conger, 1975; Patterson, 1982). It is difficult to summarize such an extensive contribution, but it is worth reporting the team's results with 27 conduct disordered boys referred to them and accepted for treatment from January 1968 to June 1972. Training the families took an average of 31.5 hours of professional time. The treatment programme (parents read a semiprogrammed text followed by a multiple choice test; staff teach parents to pinpoint problem areas and collect appropriate data on them; parents join a parent training group to learn appropriate change techniques; home visits occur where necessary) lasted on average from 3 to 4 months. Most parents opted to work on reducing their children's non-compliance to requests, but overall a further 13 behaviours in the conduct disorder syndrome were also pinpointed for treatment.

With regard to criterion measures such as the targeted deviant behaviours of the boys, an average 60 per cent. reduction from baseline level to termination was achieved. In 75 per cent. of cases, reductions exceeded 30 per cent. from baseline levels. In six cases the rate of problematic behaviour deteriorated. On another criterion — total deviant scores — the 27 boys showed a reduction from higher than normal overall rates (scores computed for normal boys over 14 'problem areas') to within normal limits. According to parental daily reports there was a significant drop in the level of reported problems during follow-up (data were obtained here on 14 families only). About two-thirds of the families reported marked reductions in the problems for which they were originally referred.

Follow-up data were obtained monthly for the first 6 months after termination of treatment, and every 2 months after that until a year after termination. Booster treatment programmes during follow-up took an average of 1.9 hours of professional time. It was soon discovered that improvements at home did not ganeralize to school, so a separate but paralleled package was prepared for use in classroom settings (Patterson, Cobb, and Ray, 1972). Patterson (1975) found that a substantial proportion of families (approximately one-third in his sample) requires much more in the way of intervention than child management skills; the parents need help with social problems, negotiation skills, depression, and resolving marital conflict (see Patterson and Reid, 1973).

A successful replication of this work was conducted by Eyberg and Johnson (1974) using the treatment package; a small-scale study by Ferber et al. (1974) showed only limited short-term results for three of the families, a figure reduced to one at the end of a year.

In a sample of 117 children with conduct problems accepted for family-based treatment at the Child Treatment Research Unit* (see Herbert and Iwaniec, 1981) a majority (83 per cent.) manifested problem behaviour beyond the realm of 'merely bothersome' and were causing serious disruption within the family. In many cases they were perceived by their parents to be 'out of control'. Using the framework for assessment in Figure 3 and a variety of behavioural methods (see below), 61 per cent. were evaluated as successful (improved on several criteria); 21 per cent. were moderately improved; and 18 per cent. showed no improvement. A median figure of 3 months (i.e. some 33 hours) of intervention to termination — but not including follow-up — was required.

Similar results were obtained with a further sample of conduct disorders drawn from 36 consecutive mixed cases referred to the unit.

Three children had reducing baselines and, after parents received advice, were discharged. A further 14 were deemed not to have relevant problems or difficulties severe enough to merit treatment as serious aggressive/conduct disorders; advice was given before discharging these cases. A group numbering 19 (15 boys, 4 girls) with an average IQ of 94.4 and an average age of 5 years 1 month received a full treatment programme. These children obtained high scores on a hyperactivity questionnaire compiled by the unit, and on the Behar Personal Behaviour Questionnaire.

There were no cases at termination in which deterioration was reported on any of the three criteria used – graphical record, structured parental report, therapist's judgement of child and family functioning — although temporary

*An account of the particular style of the unit — now the Centre for Behavioural Work with Families — is provided in Appendix B

exacerbation occurred as predicted in many cases with the initiation of extinction programmes. The overall rate of improvement, 84 per cent., is similar to that for the larger group mentioned earlier (82 per cent.); but rather less (53 per cent.) reached a fully satisfactory level, that is, the resolution of all target problems. There was no change for the better in 16 per cent. of cases. Twelve of the 16 children who improved with treatment maintained this improvement over a 6-month follow-up period; three of the four who deteriorated responded to booster programmes (which are nowdays made routinely and easily available as part of follow-up procedures).

Given that many of the families required some minimal support, or retraining during the follow-up, it suggests that the meaning of the concept of 'training' might best be extended to include retraining procedures necessary for long-term maintenance. In some cases, it seemed that regular retraining would be necessary throughout the entire history of a family. However, in the long run this may be less expensive than other alternatives, i.e. institutionalization.

CASE STUDIES

The successful use of cognitive and self-control training (along the lines described above) is illustrated in a child who was disrupting his home by violent behaviour Freddie B., aged 9 years 4 months, was assessed and treated by the present author. This was a crisis intervention because there was a distinct possibility of his beint taken into care. His parents could not cope with him because (they claimed) he was out of control at certain times. The behavioural assessment was made on the basis of visits to Freddie's home, a school visit to his School for the Blind, some 60 miles from his home village, and outings with him to a swimming pool. Freddie presented an intensely aggressive 'picture' on the first two visits, which belied his more general style. If we had made an assessment in generalized and global terms based on this session, it would have been highly misleading. A colleague saw Freddie initially, and he attacked her physically and then made himself bleed by putting his fist through a glass door. The author paid the second visit and was met by obscenities. These died away when Freddie was taken for a drive in the car and was allowed to manipulate the various controls at the end of the journey. Indeed, after this truculent and physically and verbally violent beginning. Freddie came over as a friendly and articulate boy. Despite his near complete blindness, he could get around places (e.g., the swimming pool) with remarkable ease and agility. He was robust, vigorous, and powerful. He gradually developed a warm and affectionate relationship with the author. Freddie tended (probably out of loyalty to his parents) to be reserved about some of his worries at home and at school, but, in almost imperceptible stages, he opened up about these. He lived in a terraced house with his mother (a woman of 45 with a serious heart condition) and his father (a man of 64, near retirement). Although he had no siblings, a girl of his age, Alice, lived a few doors away, was very much like a sister to him, and seemed as much at home in his house as he was.

Some of the refinements of a leisurely assessment had to be curtailed as the case was an emergency one. The parents were at their wits end and were arguing about whether or not to have Freddie at the weekends because of his difficult behaviour and its adverse effect on Mrs. B's deteriorating health. The parents were threatening to 'walk out' in relation to each other and in relation to Freddie. Social Services were involved in this and other issues (e.g., the family's financial problems).

An assessment of Freddie's difficult behaviour suggested that there was a 'halo effect' in the parents' reporting of his aggressive behaviour. In fact it was highly specific to a refusal to return in the school bus to his School for the Blind, on a Sunday afternoon. His behaviour leading up to, and particularly at, the point of being asked to go to the bus waiting outside his home consisted of what the parents called 'spasms'. These involved an escalation from grumbling, threatening his parents with words, fists, or a stick, to kicking the cat or a door, or throwing his cars or the radio at the parents themselves. An analysis of his behaviour showed that this tantrums were not so much frequent as frighteningly intense. Freddie would roar like a bull, adding to a very formidable scene. The parents were certainly daunted. The impending arrival of the bus to take Freddie back to school was the invariable (and main) trigger. There were minor (i.e. milder tantrums on a Saturday morning if Freddie was thwarted while playing with his friend, and again on Saturday evening at about bedtime when his parents were reading at a time of night when Freddie's radio programme had finished. In the case of these situations, the antecedents were either that Freddie was bored, frustrated, or thwarted (e.g., did not wish to go to bed). The analysis of the consequences of these sequences of difficult behaviour suggested that the parents were inconsistent and ineffectual. Freddie would generally get his own way if he had a tantrum. The exception, interestingly, involved his major problem. No matter how violent he was, he was made to return to school and (with the help of the driver) forced on to the bus.

It soon became clear from attempts to work out the broad outlines of a management programme with Mr. and Mrs. B. that practical difficulties would make for a doubtful outcome. It was decided to concentrate mainly on Freddie, helping him to learn self-control techniques. He took to the programme with remarkable enthusiasm. The therapeutic sessions were conducted in the context of swimming outings; the boy was only available at weekends and his home was unsuitable for quiet discussion or for rehearsing the exercises. Mrs. B. tended to interrupt and to interfere with the training.

Several observations were made of the family at home and of Freddie's behaviour at school. A consideration of his physical constitution and his home situation, together with the weekly separations that his way of life involved, led to the conclusion that despite the violent episodes—which were fairly specific— Freddie had really made an extraordinary adjustment to life. In a sense, his outbursts (although regrettable and requiring moderation) were wholly proportionate to the reality life-problems he had to solve. He certainly did not appear to be an emotionally disturbed child. The following themes were the ones which had a bearing on this conclusion:

(1) He was a premature baby (7 months, 3 lb 2 oz); the birth was an anoxic one. There was no heart-beat, he was severely jaundiced, and an exchange transfusion was required. He had gastroenteritis at 5 weeks and altogether was in hospital for 7 weeks. He was in and out of hospital after that as a hydrocephalic baby. He had a valve fitted at 4 months. In 1971 his vision deteriorated as a result of increased intracranial pressure from craniostenosis. He had an operation and a new valve was fitted. Freddie had epilepsy during his third year of life. He also suffered other vicissitudes in his formative years, including many separations from his mother while in hospital himself and when she was in hospital for psychiatric treatment.

(2) His birth was unwelcome as the parents were unmarried and, indeed, according to Mrs. B., she saw Freddie's disabilities as a punishment by God for her wrongdoing. She said she still bore a heavy sense of guilt that she was living with Mr. B. in an unmarried state, and this was made worse at weekends when Freddie pestered her about his sight, asking for it back and appealing to her to take him to other doctors. He sometimes said that he hated God for making him blind.

(3) Freddie's early separation experiences may well have sensitized him to overreact to the Sunday separation; he hated going back to school. He said to me that he wished that he could be at home all the time with his mother and father like other children.

(4) Freddie was refusing to accept his blindness; his teacher told the author that he had always overestimated the amount of residual sight that he actually possessed. It became apparent that he was frightened of losing what vision he retained and, from the way his mother talked about his reluctance to return to school, it seemed that the school represented the world of the blind (something he rejected) while his home village represented the world of the sighted (with whom he identified himself).

(5) In addition to these considerations, going back to school made Freddie insecure because he had been made to feel responsible for his mother's illness; it had been strongly suggested that his behaviour would be the 'death of her'. He understood that she had a serious heart condition and he confided that he *was* worried about whether she would be there when he got back. This insecurity was exacerbated by the frequent threats (in the past) by both parents that they would leave him or each other if he did not behave.

(6) The mother had not been a very good model of the sort of pacific behaviour she required of Freddie. He asked me (at one stage) if I would teach his mother self-control as she had thrown a chair at his father.

The object of therapy was conceptualized in terms of assisting Freddie to identify and focus his problem behaviour and to recognize the antecedent and outcome conditions which controlled it. A broader aim was to discuss with Freddie his perception of himself as 'sighted' and his rejection of everything to do with the blind — the special school, learning braille, etc. An effort was made to identify his strengths and possibilities, e.g., his swimming skill and musical appreciation. The first phase of treatment was a baseline assessment to indicate how Freddie behaved when no self-control measures were applied. Freddie was taken through a diary of events kept by his mother during 3 weekends and asked to comment on his behaviour, his feelings, and the situations in which they arose. Next, an attempt was made to increase his awareness of his feelings and maladaptive behaviours. This involved discussions in which we labelled the external and internal stimuli — situations and feelings — which led up to his violent outbursts. It also involved training him to monitor and 'talk-out' his feelings in role-played evocations of the 'return-to-school' situation. Later this was conducted in the 'real-life' situation (with the therapist present). 'Techniques' to help self-control such as 'playing turtle', 'counting to ten' and formulae such as 'think first, act later' were role-played for various situations at home and school in which he became angry. His reactions were rehearsed with him (see page 76). During this phase, Freddie's performance on weekends was discussed with him on the following weekend (based on his mother's recording and later on a self-rating). Parents were advised how to make life easier for Freddie by not threatening to put him into care, to separate, or to become ill as a result of 'bad' behaviour. Little was achieved in this aspect of the work with Mr. and Mrs. B. A good deal was accomplished in making his weekends less 'claustrophobic'. Where previously he had been cooped up indoors, outings were arranged. Freddie and the therapist discussed several issues such as Mrs. B.'s illness. Freddie's sight, school, and so on. The positive aspects of school were emphasized (aided by the teacher). Despite the absence of any real cooperation from the parents, Freddie's violent behaviour diminished in intensity within 2 weeks of beginning the self-control programme. There were only two setbacks over the period of over a year (once when Mrs. B. had a serious heart attack and another when Freddie's valve was blocked for a short period). Freddie's violent tantrums at home disappeared *completely* within 8 weekends of beginning treatment.

Skills training formed an important part of the treatment of a boy 'in care' who displayed several problems, including aggressive outbursts. Mark G. was treated by a member of the Centre team in his residential establishment. The case illustrates the need for a flexible use of behavioural methods in response to the exigencies that arise in the by-no-means smooth course of most treatments. Mark was 12 when assessment began — an illegitimate child referred for a multiplicity of problems. Mark was reported as having outbursts of aggression at Treetops Home together with 'vacant moods'. Assistant staff found him 'difficult'; he would often lie on his bed ignoring everyone. Social withdrawal and total non-communication when crossed were constantly referred to throughout his case notes. He did not appear to have developed social skills, being a consistently solitary child. His speech was poor and his play, which was considered immature, was exclusively with children younger than himself. When crossed, he would 'sulk' for long periods extending into hours. This behaviour was reported to be similar in three situations: at the Home, at school, and with his official 'aunt'.

Mark's family background was one of many vicissitudes. His mother had abandoned her husband and children. Mark was the fourth of a sibship of five. An older brother was also at Treetops Home. The remaining three children were at home with their mother. The three sisters had been discharged to the care of their mother and her cohabitee several years before. Mark and Jason now had no contact with either parent, nor apparently with their other siblings. The father had convictions for importuning and theft. His conviction for importuning appeared to have led to the fears concerning possible homosexuality in the children expressed in the files.

Treetops Home accommodated fourteen children (eight boys and six girls). Mark shared a bedroom with his brother and Alan (both aged 13). The running of the Home was somewhat disrupted during the assessment period because of a change of houseparent. However, there was a stable figure in Mark's life who knew him well, Mrs. J., a care assistant. Assessment of Mark's behaviour at the home and his school indicated that his problems were severe and merited treatment because of the distress they caused himself and others. The major difficulties appeared to be:

(1) outbursts of aggressive behaviour;
(2) gross deficiency in appropriate social skills in the area of age-peer relationships (these were presently complicated by peer rejection); and
(3) specific escape/avoidance behaviour ('sulks') in consequence of minor but specifiable difficulties, not limited to problems of peer interaction.

During the assessment stage and the early stages of treatment, the frequent changes in staff presented problems in that the succession of temporary staff members disrupted Mark anyway; it also disrupted the rest of the establishment. Then the new 'regime' was very different from the former, rather cold and authoritarian; procedures could not be followed consistently by different people. The varying levels of tolerance of the different staff members for Mark's behaviour varied, and this made it difficult to obtain any form of consistent recording of what was and was not an outburst. Mark was not himself consistent enough to self-monitor, although this was attempted.

Phase 1 of the treatment

Phase 1 of the treatment was started in June and comprised the following elements.

(1) Therapist reinforcement

The therapist reinforced Mark socially for: (a) periods free of outbursts (Mark being encouraged to 'beat his record' for the length of time he could remain free of them) and (b) reports of successful avoidance of outbursts or sulks in situations in which they typically occurred. As an aid to this procedure, a chart was kept on which outbursts were recorded (by the therapist) together with avoidances — instances where staff had expected an outburst. Incidents were also recorded if Mark spontaneously played with peers. These were recorded by Mark and were accompanied by praise. To secure a valid account of the week's events the therapist saw the housemother prior to discussion with Mark.

(2) Staff reinforcement

The staff caring for Mark were given four rules for giving him attention, the rationale being fully explained: (a) he was not to be 'coaxed' out of an outburst (to avoid the reinforcement of outbursts by staff attention); (b) he was to be given individual attention and specific praise as soon as he 'emerged' from a sulk or outburst, to reinforce its termination; (c) he was to be praised specifically on any occasion when he had been expected to lose his temper but had not done so (a DRO procedure intended to reinforce all ways he employed of coping with precipitating situations, other than by having an outburst or sulk); and (d) he was to be praised in private for all spontaneous activities engaged in with his age-peers. Although Mark's permanent housemother cooperated with this procedure, it met with serious obstacles which limited its effectiveness. Mark's outbursts were so disruptive and severe that staff found it hard to give him any praise later in the same day; a negative 'halo' effect coloured their judgement, to the effect that a day in which Mark had had an outburst became a wholly 'bad day' and any prosocial interactions or instances of self-control were overlooked or not reinforced with praise. One member of the case staff who spent much time with Mark rejected the programme altogether, and refused to implement it all.

(3) Social skill training

Swimming was selected as an activity particularly attractive to Mark, and one of the few in which he had some skill. Mark was taken by the therapist to the local swimming club on three occasions. Subsequently the boy went on his own. This was done in order to integrate Mark with a peer group having the following characteristics: (a) they were of a similar age to Mark, rather than the younger children he associated with exclusively, and (b) they did not know Mark. At the Home, his isolation from age-peers (and association with younger children) was considered to be due largely to their teasing and rejection of him. It was intended that Mark should be assisted in coping with his age-peers at the swimming club by means of role-play and direct instruction as it became necessary. Observation on the three occasions on which the therapist accompanied him to the club did not indicate that these more specific social-skill training techniques were essential. He proved to be a good swimming pupil and was readily accepted by the others. He entered fully into their activities. Although Mark achieved this (subsequently having some successful youth club experience) he continued to be isolated and rejected by the others in the Home. His behaviour continued to be too disruptive and odd for full acceptance there.

Phase 2 of the treatment

It had become apparent by November that progress towards reduction of outbursts was unsatisfactory and that, for the reasons already mentioned, it was not possible to increase the strength of the social reinforcement programme in the Home. Since it was the extreme intensity of outbursts rather than their frequency that constituted a cause for concern, and outbursts were always accompanied by muscular tension, particularly in Mark's fists and stomach, together with trembling, a new procedure was added to the treatment.

(1) Desensitization of anger

A relaxation procedure was used to counter-condition Mark's aggressive responses to provocative stimuli. While loss of self-control rather than anxiety was the response to be counter-conditioned, the use of the procedure was broadly analogous to classical densitization. The technique was considered by the therapist to constitute a self-control procedure. He found that cooperation was forthcoming for implementation despite the fact that the patient was an institutionalized aggressive adolescent — far from what is usually thought to be the ideal recipient of such an approach. Mark was taught muscular relaxation in the standard manner, and his degree of relaxation, ability to imagine scenes while relaxed, and overall cooperation with the procedure were considered adequate. During the therapist's weekly visits Mark was put into a relaxed state if an outburst had occurred since the previous visit. He was asked to imagine the internal and external events which had preceded the outburst, signalling to the therapist if he felt 'het up' (when the imagining of the scene would be terminated and further relaxation instructions given). Each chain of events antecedent to an outburst was imagined twice. It was not possible to identify typical precipitating stimuli for outbursts to incorporate into a hierarchy (as is usually done in desensitizing a phobia) and thus there was a need to desensitize to the particular antecedents of each outburst.

Desensitization was added to Mark's treatment in November. Throughout his treatment desensitization sessions were held, two of which related to known outbursts occurring at school.

On one occasion during this phase of treatment, the therapist arrived for his scheduled visit at the Home to find Mark in the midst of an outburst and being held under a cold shower to 'cool off'. The therapist terminated this somewhat unorthodox procedure and switched the shower off. Mark refused to leave the shower cubicle and continued to sob violently, refusing to speak and showing extreme muscular tension and trembling. The therapist withdrew, promising to pay attention to Mark when he left the cubicle. Ten minutes later he did so, running to his room and barricading himself in, shouting abuse to staff on the landing outside, and throwing clothing at the door. However, he admitted the therapist to the room and, with physical guidance only, agreed to lie on his bed. The therapist then began Mark's usual relaxation instructions, succeeding in securing some degree of relaxation within a few minutes, and then escorted Mark to the Home's office to continue the relaxation session in the normal setting. Within 1 hour of the therapist's arrival. Mark had terminated the outburst, apologized to the staff, and changed into dry clothing. In effect, the relaxation procedure had been successfully used '*in vivo*', almost as a 'first-aid' procedure, and had successfully inhibited severe tension and loss of self-control in Mark. The incident was considered important from the point of view of securing credibility in the eyes of staff for the therapeutic procedures being employed and also in providing a model of the use of social reinforcement for the termination of an outburst.

In order to further strengthen the therapeutic programme in use, a stronger operant programme was implemented from mid-January.

(2) Individual token system

A token reinforcement system was initiated in which Mark would be given a cardboard token each evening by the staff, provided the day had been free from outbursts, regardless of any other occurrences that might have occurred. This procedure constituted a DRO programme in which tokens were given to reinforce all activities other than outbursts. The value of the tokens to Mark derived from the fact that he could exchange them at intervals for a 'back-up' reinforcer that he desired and had negotiated with the therapist. These included cookery lessons with the housemother (he had an ambition to be a chef in the armed forces), being allowed to organize, prepare, and serve Sunday tea, and outings with a student social worker. In addition to tokens earned for complete outburst-free days, Mark was given quarter-tokens for succeeding in modifying any outburst that did occur in specific and negotiated ways. He could redeem a quarter of the token he had lost for having an outburst if (a) he did not hit anyone, (b) he did not throw or destroy any property, (c) he modified the outburst sufficiently for staff to accept his continued presence in the room or he voluntarily withdrew, breaking the chain of events until he had calmed down enough to return, and (d) he apologized to injured parties afterwards. On a number of occasions, Mark was able to redeem 2 or 3 quarter-tokens once an outbursts had commenced. The objection was made by various observers that Mark might discover that by having more than one outburst in any one day which were partially modified, he might earn more in quarter-tokens than was possible by controlling his outbursts for a whole day. Such loopholes can be seen in many token systems. The fact remains, however, that Mark never realized this or did not take advantage of it, and he never earned more than 3 quarter-tokens in one day. If he had done so, the system would have been amended. It had, in the first place, been established as a fair contract and any loopholes exploited could with equal fairness have been closed. It is often necessary when using token systems in the natural environment (as Morgan observes) to act as advocate for the child and instruct parents or staff not to withhold tokens the child has earned according to the agreed contract simply because he has not performed satisfactorily in some other, irrelevant, area.

The tokens were phased out in June, after 5 months of use, on the departure of the student who had been providing outings to back them up. This was agreed as acceptable from the start by Mark, and it was also agreed that the other back-up reinforcers could remain in force; the boy could, if he wished, continue his involvement in cookery in the Home, as his special activity, just as another child might regularly assist the staff in the garden or with the car.

The frequency of Mark's outbursts reduced markedly over the second phase of treatment. Their intensity also reduced overall. Procedures were phased gradually out from June. In August of that year Mark's mother renewed contact with him and some degree of disruption occurred in his situation generally. There was an increase in outbursts which led to reinstatement of the desensitization procedure in November. At the same time, assistance was requested for two other difficulties that had been present sporadically throughout treatment, but which had not been selected previously for specific intervention. One was Mark's occasional encopresis, together with hiding faeces and soiled underclothing around his bedroom; the other was his sexual interference with younger children of both sexes, which had on occasion included children outside the Home. Further analysis of his encopresis indicated that it was very infrequent and in fact it underwent spontaneous remission before the assessment had been completed. Mark's hiding of faeces, however, was treated, as was his interference with two younger boys in the Home.

(3) Response-cost procedure

A response-cost procedure was introduced to reduce Mark's hiding of faeces and inappropriate sexual activities, whereby he would lose a privilege in consequence of either of these behaviours. Initially, Mark would lose his right to a later bedtime each time he failed to follow the appropriate procedures for dealing with soiled clothing (procedures he accepted as reasonable) or his faeces in his room. Although this procedure was never followed, and his bedtime was permanently adjusted for other reasons outside treatment, only one incident of hidden faeces was reported subsequently. Once this had been achieved, a programme was agreed whereby, if he was found at any time in the bedroom of the two younger boys he had been accustomed to force into sexual activities, he would lose his right to sleep in his own single room without supervision the following night. Instead he had to sleep in a room under the supervision of his brother (who successfully prevented any such misbehaviour). This particular sexual difficulty did not occur again after this programme was initiated; the response-cost procedure was never implemented after its negotiation. The problem was basically one that was being overemphasized by some members of staff on occasion. It was essentially sex play that might have been innocuous in a younger child; it was of concern to the staff as Mark was pubescent and seeking unwilling partners considerably younger than himself. Much concern was also expressed at the homosexual component of his sexual interest, in the light of his father's conviction for homosexual importuning. It was apparent that those concerned in the case had become hypersensitive to sexual deviation, mislabelling sex play which was basically immature (and included both sexes) as early sexual deviation.

By November, therapy was discontinued and Mark's progress monitored at lengthening intervals. During April of the following year, however, after remaining free of aggressive outbursts for 2-months, Mark had one serious outburst in which he physically attacked another child and then the housemother, who sustained an injury to her hand on being hit with a chair. It was clear that Mark might not be allowed to continue in his present placement should any further outbursts occur. An intensive course of treatment was undertaken over the next week. Therapy took the form of one session of desensitization to the recent incident on five successive days, during which time no other outbursts or problems occurred. There were no more outbursts during a follow-up that had lasted 4 months when the report was written.

11

Persistent Non-attendance at School

For a large part of each weekday, the child lives in his classroom. His relationships with his teacher and with his classmates are major aspects in his adjustment to school. Indeed, as Robins (1972) shows, a child's attendance record at school is a very good predictor of his adult adjustment. Unfortunately, facts and figures are hard to come by in this area. It is difficult, for example, to check on the often-heard claim that school refusal is on the increase.

Parents take for granted the notion of their children leaving for and staying at school. So when a child opts out of this routine — either overtly or covertly — it is a shock to realize just how dependent they are on his voluntary cooperation in allowing them to fulfil their legal obligations. One sort of non-attender remains implacable in the face of threats, entreaties, and blandishments from all and sundry; and short of carrying the offender forcibly to school and chaining him to his desk, there seems little that harassed parents and teachers can do. Another child may *appear* willing to go to school, but he does not arrive or stay there. As with real 'rebellions', school refusal (of whatever kind) tends to catch those in authority by surprise. There is the age-old problem of what to do about the rebel once all the usual methods of persuasion have been exhausted. And there is the same feeling of impotence, for when the problem becomes really serious it can be fairly intractible.

Attendance problems can begin early in the child's school-going career. Indeed, the business of starting the child at school, and keeping him there — in a reasonably happy and receptive frame of mind — may be the first behaviour problem parents and teachers have to cope with. It is quite a widespread problem. In one study (Moore, 1966) of the difficulties ordinary children find in adjusting to school, researchers at the University of London Institute of Education kept track of 164 children (attending a large number of very

226

different London schools) from the ages of 6 to 11 years. The children's mothers were asked at various stages whether, during the past year, their children had told them about any problems or difficulties connected with school, or shown any reluctance to go. When they reached 12, the children themselves were asked what they had liked and disliked about their present and past schools. A reluctance to go to school affected, at one time or another, a majority of the 6-year-olds. This unwillingness decreased at 7, rose to a secondary peak at 8 (when there was a transfer from infant to junior school), and then dwindled steadily until the children's eleventh year. Even then, one boy in three was still showing some reluctance. In all, a vast majority of the children studied were found to experience difficulties in the infant school. Nearly one-half suffered problems of moderate or marked severity. At every age level, boys showed more negative attitudes than girls. Boys who were 'only' children tended to have most problems in adjusting to school. The specific problems of which children complained most were those connected with teachers and school work, though difficulties over school dinners and objections to the school toilets were also relatively frequent. Worries connected with other children and with problems in physical education were also expressed, but these were less often of importance.

Fortunately, most children's early fears and uncertainties vanish as a new routine is established and school life becomes more predictable. Observations (Slater, 1939) of 2- and 3-year olds during their first month of attendance at nursery school have shown that during the first days the majority of children displayed signs of uneasiness and apprehension. Tics, tears, postural tensions, facial anxiety, dreamy watching, and rejection of the other children were the sort of reactions frequently found. Subsequently these wore off and, in fact, by the end of the fourth week all but a few of the children had adjusted to the new situation. Some children begin their schooling with severe disadvantages, which may remain with them throughout their classroom years. This is a crucial consideration given to the association between truancy, delinquency, and academic failure (see page 248).

The inarticulate or non-talking child is not a rare phenomenon in the first term at infant schools. Such children are not physically mute. But they have never been given the opportunity of developing the habit of language, the practice of asking and answering questions, of communicating with the people around them. Overcrowding, high-rise flats, bad child-minders, isolated suburban homes, new-town loneliness — any one or all of these may contribute to the distressing problem of the non-talking child.

Most parents have had to cope — and successfully, by and large — with the occasional *reluctance* of their children to go to school. As many as 80 per cent. of ordinary, run-of-the-mill children experience difficulties at one time or another in adjusting to school (Moore, 1966), although the majority eventually come to say that they like, or at least 'don't mind' it. In any event there is little difference in the attendance records of children who like or dislike school (Mitchell and Shepherd, 1966).

SCHOOL PHOBIA

There is greater appreciation nowadays that some forms of school refusal constitute a very real emotional or conduct disorder, not simply a moral or disciplinary problem concerned with malingering. Some refusers may wish to go to school, but find that they simply cannot go through all the necessary motions of leaving home or entering the school. This type of school refusal has been called 'school phobia'. A phobia is an intense, unreasonable fear, usually directed at some specific environmental object. So the diagnosis of school phobia seems to imply a strong unreasonable fear of some aspect of the school situation. Although, strictly speaking, the phobias do not come within our subject matter, the issue of accurate assessment demands a working knowledge of these problems. There are also many mixed cases.

Obviously there are several fear-provoking possibilities inherent in the circumstances of school life, and any of these is capable of making a child fearful for quite objective and *reasonable* reasons. Some of the sources of children's anxiety at school are the size and routine of the school, examination stresses, experiences of classroom failure, disturbed relationships with teachers and schoolmates, parental pressures and expectations, and intellectual disability. American school children, aged 11, tend to worry about the following school situations, in order of frequency: failing a test, being late for school, being poor in spelling, being asked to answer questions, being poor in reading, getting a poor report card, being reprimanded, not doing as well as other pupils and being poor at maths and drawing. The point about a phobic reaction is that it is disproportionate to the objective 'distressing' situation. Most children manage to cope with the difficulties listed above without refusing to go to school. But the phobic child may not really be worried about any of these things, and this is what makes the term 'school phobia' rather clumsy. In many instances, it is a fear of leaving mother rather than something at school that is bothering him.

In attempting to identify the child who has serious emotional problems over school attendance, the parents will have been trying unsuccessfully, and for some time, to get the child to school. He is likely to be suffering from anxiety in connection with a number of other topics which most children cope with fairly well. His anxiety is apt to change shape — now attached to one object (say his mother's health), now jumping to another (perhaps a sarcastic teacher), and then another (possibly the playground bully). His apprehensions are not soothed by reassurances. He has recurrent physical symptoms, which tend to clear up at weekends, or even shortly after parents have reluctantly agreed to keep him at home. Is he, then, a malingerer or a rebel? The answer is 'neither'. Studies of children with attendance problems (see Hersov, 1960) show many of them to be neurotic, a large proportion of them being timid, fearful, and inhibited when away from home. A majority of these apparently timid children show a *reverse* 'acting-out' type of behaviour at home, being wilful and demanding and even dominating their parents by their stubbornness. Generally, school refusers are anxious because for some reason they cannot cope outside the home. When they *do* go to school, such children are well behaved, conforming (again, not rebels), and hard-working (some being successful, others backward), but usually they are socially maladjusted.

The school refuser's parents know he is absent; he *is*, indeed, at home. There is another group of problem children who are non-attenders; their parents do not usually know where they are — let alone about their absence. Truants, who go off elsewhere and amuse themselves, are much more like rebels. Their activities are frequently delinquent. And there are differences found in perso-nality, social and family background, and school performance (Hersov, 1960).

TRUANCY

The problem of truancy is distinguished from school phobia although the distinction is not always a clear-cut one. The truant is a child who absents himself from school without a legitimate cause and without the permission of his parents or the school authorities. Tyerman (1968) cautions against the attempt to classify persistent non-attenders as either truants *or* school phobics. He believes that this dichotomy is an oversimplification and that except for a minority of cases children who refuse to go to school do not fall clearly into either category. The conditions represent extremes which shade into each other.

A national survey conducted in the United Kingdom in 1974 found 2 per cent. of the secondary-school population to be absent without legitimate reason, compared with 8 per cent. absent through ill health. Absences over a 7-week period in Sheffield's 20 comprehensives and their feeder primaries have been analysed to see what light they shed on the dimensions and possible causes of the truancy problem. Up to the age of 12, no matter whether the child was in a junior or middle school or the first year of a comprehensive, persistent absenteeism (defined as missing half or more of all possible attendances without reason) never exceeded 1 per cent. Comprehensive 12-year olds had a rate of 0.5 per cent. But the rate steadily rose after that: to 1.3 per cent. at the age of 13, 1.4 per cent. at the age of 14, 2.3 per cent. at the age of 15, and 4.4 per cent. at the age of 16. In four comprehensives, over 10 per cent. of the 16-year-olds were persistent absentees (Galloway, 1976).

Fogelman and Richardson (1974) in an investigation of 16,000 children born in one week in March 1958 also found that 1.2 per cent. of their sample had truanted at some time, or were suspected of truancy. Percentages varied according to area, type of school, age of children studied, and many other factors. There are, in fact, many practical difficulties in ascertaining accurately the number of children truanting on a particular day. Although registers are kept in most schools, it is often the case that children (especially in large secondary schools where there is frequent movement and sometimes unsuper-vized private-study periods) will leave school after registration or half-way through the day. Some teachers may also turn a blind eye when a particularly disruptive member of the class is truanting, and parents may write notes to cover unlawful absence, again preventing detection.

Many more boys than girls become truants. Fogelman and Richardson (1974) had three times as many boys as girls in their sample, but different ratios are reported by different researchers. Education welfare officers (the old school attendance officers) and social workers are more reluctant to take official action against girls, and this might account for an even higher ratio of boys to girls when court cases only are included.

One of the startling facts about serious cases of male truancy in primary school is the finding (Robins, 1970) that 82 per cent. were frequently absent during their first 2 years at school. Robins observes that truancy begins very, very young, and thus the past clinical concentration on improving adult chances by trying to do something for high-school dropouts has been directed at the wrong age group. Excessive absence begins as a phenomenon of the very young; it continues into high school, but it certainly does not start there.

We have seen that in general, school phobics seem unable to go to school despite persuasion, recrimination, and sometimes punishment from the parents. In this type of absence the child refuses to go to school and instead wants to, or has to, stay at home because of acute anxiety about leaving home or going to school (see Herbert, 1974). The truant's absence from school is not usually known to the parents, until it is brought to their attention by the authorities. He does not go home until his usual time. Hersov's (1960) research indicated that truants tend to be children running away from difficulties, rather than the traditional representation of them as Tom Sawyer-ish adventure seekers. Many of the children in his group with truancy as the major complaint were wanderers from home as well as from school. This 'wandering from home' was one of the six items considered to be characteristic of a conduct disorder; the others being juvenile court appearance, persistent lying, stealing, destructiveness, and disapproved sexual activity. Hersov found that his truant group showed a significantly higher incidence of these items than either the control group or the school phobics, and he concluded that their truancy is an indication of a conduct disorder which often involves other delinquent behaviour.

Many other researchers have suggested there is a link of some significance between truancy and delinquency. As Kahn and Nursten (1964) point out, truancy almost inevitably leads to antisocial behaviour, e.g., lying becomes necessary to avoid detection, and also there are dangers associated with the amount of unoccupied time when the child should have been at school. Tyerman studied the records of 137 pupils whose parents were prosecuted for the child's truancy, and 64 of these children had police records by the end of the year. Also, when truants and general clinic cases were compared, a correlation of 0.56 between truancy and stealing was obtained. Again, in a study by Glueck and Glueck (1950) the proportion of delinquent children with records of truancy was found to be 95 per cent. The problem of truancy, not surprisingly, is often referred to as the 'kindergarten of crime'. Truants are characteristically beset by problems such as enuresis (bedwetting), lying, wandering from home, stealing, and aggression. Many of their delinquencies (such as shoplifting, stealing from cars, and so on) are committed by boys when they are roaming the streets during school hours.

Behind the truant's dislike for school lies a history of failure, often both academic and social. The child who is poor at schoolwork and who is constantly criticized by his teacher and called stupid, finds school a demoralizing experience. If he is kept down a year, he finds it exceedingly lonely and embarrassing to be with younger children and doing repetitive and familiar work. He is also likely to be bored (see Fogelman, 1976). Because over-age children generally fail to get social acceptance in the class, the repeater makes few friends and this increases his distaste for school. On average, truants are below the majority of their schoolmates in mental ability and attainment at reading, arithmetic and other school subjects (Fogelman and Richardson, 1974; Hersov, 1960). This is not always the case, and a few truanters may be of exceptional intelligence. Robins (op cit) found that truancy is as powerful a deterrent to high school success as a low IQ.

Studies of truants (Hersov, op cit; Tyerman, 1968) have uncovered certain features in the personality and behaviour of the children, and in their home life, which stand out because of their frequency. Often, home conditions are intolerable for the truant. Homes tend to be overcrowded and dirty, and parents may have little interest in their children's welfare. Hersov (1960) reports that maternal rejection occurred more frequently in the truant than in a school phobic and non-school-problem control group. Also, discipline was found to be inconsistent for these children, an observation which was confirmed by Tyerman, who also noted that supervision was ineffective and that control was mainly by corporal punishment. In a study of persistent truants and truants taken to court, unsatisfactory discipline by the parents was found in 87 per cent. of the cases of persistent truancy and in 92 per cent. of the court cases.

Many investigators report a lack of affection in the home and a general lack of interest in the child's welfare. Adriola, for example, whose studies are reported by Tyerman (1968), analysed records of 25 truants referred to a child guidance clinic and found that at least 18 of the children were obviously rejected by one or both parents. Also, truants often come from broken homes; studies such as that of Tyerman found the incidence of broken homes to be between a third and a half of the cases investigated. Often, when both parents are living in the home, it was found that there was marital disharmony, usually leading to rows and tension in the home. Hersov (1960) found that maternal absence before the age of 5 and paternal absence after the age of 5 had occurred more frequently for children in group T than the other groups. Their families tended to belong to the lower social classes and to be concentrated in uncongenial slum neighbourhoods. They tended to be larger than the families in the comparative groups.

The children in these families have histories in which many have slept out at night or run away from home. Children who truant tend to feel lonely and miserable, becoming unsociable and unable to persevere at anything. What the truant has learned, over a period, is that the best escape from tensions at home (so often the source of harsh punishment and the scene of rows and rejection) is to escape; in other words, the best way to cope with frustrations is to avoid their source. So he wanders away from school (where he feels he is disliked by teachers and children alike) in the way he wanders from home (where he also often feels unwanted). He may amuse himself as a solitary or he may look for congenial companions who also crave excitement and a distraction from their feelings of boredom, depression, and discouragement. The child who truants does not appear usually to experience great anxiety, but he does not receive sufficient reinforcement to continue school attendance.

Truancy appears to have a number of causes. Some children truant simply to demonstrate their independence of, or resistance to, adult authority. Other children are truants because they have adopted their parents' don't-care attitude to education and authority, and the parents may tacitly consent to their children's truancy. This is particularly found in some lower socioeconomic families where parents keep the children home to look after younger ones, to help with household chores, and so on. This is an important consideration in assessing the meaning of truanting behaviour of individual children. Although truancy is often regarded as maladjusted behaviour, there is a form of truancy which is a social norm for the group from which the truant comes. School attendance may actually represent a departure from the normal behaviour pattern of such a group, as it is regarded as neither necessary nor desirable. Such an attitude may not indicate any personal maladjustment to inadequacy, but is a reflection of the mores of a particular subculture.

The nature of a particular school is an important factor in juvenile delinquency considered as a general problem (Power, Benn, and Morris, 1972). We know that some schools seem to have a suppressive effect on the manifestation of delinquent acts in their pupils and to have a low incidence of such problems compared with other schools in the same area. It is widely believed that large 'impersonal' schools are a factor in the rate of delinquent activities such as truancy. Galloway (1976) found that when the overall absenteeism rate was correlated with school size — and this ranged from 560 to 1,779 pupils — the overall trend was negative. Small schools did not necessarily have more absentees, but they were more likely to have more, relative to the roll, than big schools. A high exclusion rate was also negatively related with high absenteeism. Schools with a reputation for 'toughness' were not particularly shunned.

What did tally with absenteeism, very strikingly, was the proportion of children in the school receiving free school meals. As this rose, so did the absence rate, with hardly any variation. When Galloway checked back he found that the primary schools from which these children had come also had high proportions receiving school meals and a high absenteeism rate (by primary standards).

But further investigation, with the aid of the education welfare officers, revealed that very little of this absenteeism could really be called truancy.

About 11 per cent. of the absentees were skipping school because they were bored and a further 4 per cent. were genuine 'school phobics'. Yet just under a quarter were at home with their parents' approval, and in just over a quarter of the cases the parent did not mind what the children did. It was convenient, it seemed, to have an able-bodied son or daughter around.

RUNAWAYS

An intensive study of a small group of runaways by Beyer et al. (1973 revealed that most of these youths came from broken homes and many were experiencing difficulty with their step-parents. About half the parents reported that they had had strong disagreements with the child for 2 years or longer. Conflict areas included number of nights allowed out and hours for returning home. Many of the runaways had a recent history of poor grades and absenteeism in school. In general, there was a strong suggestion that running away is a symptom of unstable and conflict-ridden family environments. Solutions lie in greater communication and understanding between parents and children, a willingness by both sides to accept some responsibility for the problem, and the development of a closer, more caring relationship between parents and child.

On the average, the runaways thought that the experience had been helpful, while their parents did not. The personality of the runaways was found to be impulsive (tended to do things on the spur of the moment) and depressed (frequent feelings of unhappiness). Many adolescents run away primarily to escape from the home, while others leave to experiment with independence or to manipulate their parents into changes that would make the relationship more satisfactory.

Riemer (1940) reports that his experiences with runaway youths indicate that their most pressing need is to be loved by their parents. When thwarted in this need, many seek to 'get even' by running away and thereby causing parental anguish and guilt.

TREATMENT: CONTINGENCY MANAGEMENT

A 16-year-old American girl named Claire was referred to a probation agency because of serious truancy (Thorne, Tharp, and Wetzel, 1967). In an attempt to correct this, her mother had stopped Claire's pocket-money, use of the telephone, and going out on dates, but had not made it clear how these privileges could be regained. When treatment started, the school attendance officer was involved; if Claire was present at all her classes during the day, he would give her a note. This note was exchangeable, with the mother, for certain specified privileges. It was stressed also that when Claire brought a note home her mother should praise her. Over a period of 7 weeks the improvement in behaviour was so marked that notes were gradually reduced and then stopped entirely. Before treatment, Claire was absent on 30 out of 46 days, whereas for 3 months after it commenced she truanted on only two occasions, and not at all during a follow-up over several months. Some improvement in her perform-ance, attitude, and interest in school was also reported. Another youngster treated by this team was Loren, aged 16 years. He was referred by the Juvenile Court following complaints of assault, uncontrollability, and habitual truancy. His stepfather and mother tried to manage these problems by withdrawing privileges, abusing him verbally, and threatening to call the police, but with no effect. Exactly what was expected of Loren and how he could regain his privileges were not clear to him. The treatment plan was based on a contract between Loren and his parents which would enable him to earn money for conforming to certain requirements such as being in at a prescribed time at night, while entailing losses of money and deprivation of the family car for failures to observe these requirements. During the first 35 days after the programme was instituted, Loren was rewarded an average of 81 per cent. in respect of the specified tasks, compared to an estimated 0 to 10 per cent. before intervention. Despite this progress, the stepfather was refusing to pay for the renewal of Loren's driving insurance, and a new contract was negotiated whereby he could earn a maximum of 50 points each week towards the 250 needed for his insurance to be renewed. In the first week he earned 22 points, followed by the full 50 points in each week thereafter. Loren re-entered high school, where he performed satisfactorily and did not truant for a period of 24 days. The parents concluded he was doing so well that the treatment plan should be abandoned. The treatment team thought this premature and strongly discouraged the parents, but they insisted on ending the contract. Loren truanted for the next 7 days and was arrested for burglary 11 days later. The authors conclude that the case indicates that problem behaviour can be changed by altering environmental consequences, while demonstrating the difficulty of achieving this with uncooperative parents.

Brooks (1974) has presented two case studies illustrating instances in which contingency management principles were used, successfully, to increase school attendance. One case, that of Mary, aged 15, is described here. She was a high-school sophomore, habitually absent from school during the first quarter of the school year. Her non-attendance included both periodic truancies and full-day truancies. Mary attended school only one or two full days a week during the entire quarter. During this period Mary was counselled at school and phone calls were made to her mother at home. She was warned that continued truancy would result in suspension from school and the filing of a petititon with the probation department, which would subsequently result in her being placed in a juvenile detention establishment. In addition, Mary experienced restrictions at home from her mother. She was required to report home immediately after school and was not allowed to go out of the house until she left for school the following day. Her mother also reported that she 'blistered her with a belt' and threatened to remove her from school and keep her home. All of these measures failed to have any effect on her truancy. Her counsellor eventually realized that he was spending at least 2 hours a week working with this one pupil and to no real effect. So he arranged a conference with Mary and her mother, during which he briefly explained the principles of behaviour modification and contingency contracting. A major part of the conference was spent in determining what reinforcements could be used to help Mary increase her going-to-school behaviour. The conference concluded with the drawing up of a contingency contract, which was signed by Mary, her mother, and the counsellor.

Mary followed the provisions of this contract and received the rewards specified in it. After 6 weeks written contracts were no longer used, and Mary continued to attend classes regularly. The author notes that at the time the contracts were discontinued, it appeared that several attitude changes seemed to be taking place in both Mary and her mother. First of all, Mary reported that she felt school was not so bad after all and that she even liked a few of the teachers. Second, she stated that she thought she would like to start planning for her future and that she was now considering going on to a junior college. Finally, Mary's mother appeared to have a more positive attitude towards Mary and was very pleased that Mary was attending school.

The present author also made use of contingency contracts together with several other procedures, to get three adolescents back to school, in each case after prolonged absences. In making an assessment of a complex problem like school refusal it is helpful to have a guide to the factors that require investigation. The first conceptual aid is to assess the push-pull factors in school attendance. Many children feel reluctant at times to go to school. Their parents 'push' them into going, sometimes simply by their being there, i.e., they do not have to exert undue pressure. But there are 'pull' factors: the authority of the school, the presence of friends at school, the interest provided by a good school (and conversely the boredom of being at home or elsewhere on one's own). In any assessment of persistent non-attendance at school the presence or absence, strength or weakness of these push-pull factors need to be evaluated (see case study of Barry later in this chapter).

Alexander, Corbett, and Smigel (1976) have studied the effects of individual and group consequences on school attendance and curfew violations with seven predelinquent adolescent youths. The consequences involved the use of token reinforcement backed up by lunch-money contingent on individual or group class attendance of the boys. They were in the custody of a county department of family and children services. The treatment was conducted in a residential treatment centre. Youngsters referred to the centre were considered by the court to be in danger of becoming habitually delinquent because of repeated charges of truancy, absconding, assault, theft, unmanageability, and violation of probation.. The students attended three different high-school settings for five periods during the school day. Each student was told that he could receive 1 dollar for lunch-money for every day that he attended all five periods. One dollar was given to all of those students who attended 100 per cent. of all their classes for that day. Packed lunches were provided for those youths who failed to meet the 100 per cent. criterion. Baseline conditions were again implemented for a week. The individually contingent reward was put aside during this phase. On Sunday, each student was told that no lunch-money would be available for that week; however, each student was given an attendance card for the week and asked to have each teacher in their classes sign the cards.

Group consequences 1

On Sunday evening, each student was told that lunch-money would be available for that week; however, for anyone to receive the money, every student had to attend 100 per cent. of his classes for any given day. Everyone would either receive 1 dollar or no one would receive money. Attendance cards, praise, and feedback were managed as the other phases. When everyone had 100 per cent. school attendance for a particular day, each person received 1 dollar.

Baseline 3

The baseline conditions were re-established for 1 week and group contingent lunch-money was removed.

Group consequences 2

All conditions in the group-contingency phase were replicated.

The use of individually-based contingent reinforcement increased class attendance over baseline measurements; however, group contingent reinforcers increased class attendance to the highest levels. (In another phase of the study, the authors were able to demonstrate the effectiveness of a group contingent response-cost system compared to an individual response-cost contingency in reducing curfew violations.)

COMMUNITY PROGRAMME

Fo and O'Donnell (1974) developed the 'buddy system', a community-based programme for youth, using local non-professional people as agents of change. Adult residents in two American communities served as 'buddies' of youths referred for behaviour and academic problems. They met regularly with youngsters in their natural environment and attempted to guide and influence them to engage in socially appropriate behaviour. The authors state that such intervention with youth is in keeping with the current trend in the helping professions towards establishing community treatment programmes and calling for assistance from the resources of the community. It is becoming widely acknowledged that the greatest potential for fostering behavioural change resides in the community (Smith and Hobbs, 1966).

The triadic model served as the operational basis of the buddy system. The professionals, graduate students (behaviour analysts) and their supervisors (consultants), provided training and consultation to the local non-professionals

(mediators). These buddies intervened directly in altering the deviant behaviours of youths (referred for a wide range of problems, including truancy,
poor academic achievement, classroom disruption, curfew violation, and
fighting) through the establishment of friendships. The researchers saw as their
primary aim with the buddy system the changing of behaviour and, in particular, increasing school attendance. A second major objective of the project was
to demonstrate the use of non-professional residents as effective change
agents. The aim was to equip non-professionals with the requisite skills and
techniques for successful behavioural intervention with youth, thereby increasing the number of skilled and experienced helpers in the community.

Youngsters of both sexes were invited to participate in the buddy system if
they were residents of the Model Cities neighbourhoods and between 11 and 17
years of age. Buddies ranged in age from 17 to 65, included both sexes, and
represented a diversity of ethnic and occupational groups. They ranged in
education from the fourth grade to completion of master's degrees, with a
median educational attainment of the twelfth grade. Each youngster participating in the project received the friendship and companionship of an adult
resident in the community. Each adult buddy worked with three youths and
extended to them a relationship of mutual affection, respect, and trust. The
buddy met with his youngsters individually and at the appropriate times, as a
group; they engaged in such activities as arts and crafts, going to rock concerts,
camping, surfing, and so on.

Buddies were paid up to 144 dollars per month by earning points for
engaging in certain specific behaviours such as making a weekly contact with
each of their assigned youngsters, attending bi-weekly training sessions, and so
on.

Training of buddies consisted of six initial 3-hour weekly sessions followed
by bi-weekly sessions for the duration of the project year. The emphasis of the
training programme was on equipping buddies with the knowledge, skills, and
techniques of contingency management — for developing a warm and
meaningful relationship. Modelling and role-playing procedures were also
used extensively in teaching buddies the requisite human relations skills and
intervention techniques for helping their youngsters. These adults were trained
to engage in the following role behaviours: (a) meet weekly with each of their
target youths and participate in social and recreational activities with them: (b)
establish a warm, positive, and trusting relationship with their youngsters; (c)
identify problem areas and specify them in behavioural terms; (d) count the
frequency of occurrence of the targeted behaviours and submit weekly behavioural data to the behaviour analyst; (e) draw up and carry out intervention
programmes aimed at ameliorating the youngsters' target behaviours; and (f)
serve as an advocate for the youngsters in their dealings with persons in their
environment.

With a 4 × 3 research design, the effects of four conditions — three
experimental and one control — were compared across three time periods:
baseline, first intervention, and second intervention. Youngsters eligible for

participation in the buddy system were randomly assigned to one of four conditions:

(1) *Relationship* Buddies were instructed that a warm and positive buddy–youngster relationship that is always present (i.e. non-contingent) is most effective in producing behaviour change. In addition, the youth's monthly allotment of 10 dollars was to be spent in a non-contingent manner.

(2) *Social approval* Buddies were instructed that a warm, positive relationship contingent on the performance of desired behaviour is effective in obtaining the greatest amount of behaviour change. As in the relationship condition, the 10-dollar monthly allotment was to be spent on the youngster in a non-contingent fashion.

(3) *Social and material reinforcement* This condition was similar to social approval except that the 10-dollar monthly allotment was to be spent contingent on performance of the desired behaviour.

(4) *Control* This condition consisted of youngsters who were referred to the buddy system, met all criteria of acceptability, but were not invited to participate in the project.

Each buddy was assigned three youngsters and instructed to respond differently to each youngster in accordance with the three treatment conditions. Behavioural frequency data were collected on a total of 42 youngsters: 26 with school attendance as the target behaviour, 6 with assorted target behaviours, and 10 with academic achievement as the target behaviour.

Implementation of the social approval and social and material reinforcement conditions during intervention I resulted in substantial reductions in truancy rate from baseline. There was correspondingly little change from baseline for the relationship and control conditions. In addition, both the social approval and social and material reinforcement groups had lower truancy rates during intervention I than the relationship and control groups. While both contingency conditions (social approval and social and material reinforcement) were effective in increasing school attendance from baseline, there were no reliable differences between them in their truancy rates during intervention 1.

During intervention 2, the truancy rate of the social and material reinforcement group was again significantly reduced. More importantly, the truancy rate for the relationship group, which received social and material reinforcement treatment during intervention 2, decreased significantly. The truancy rate for the control group showed no reliable change throughout the three time periods. As a result, the truancy rates at the conclusion of intervention 2 were significantly lower for youngsters in each treatment condition than for those in the control group.

In addition the authors classified each youngster with respect to absolute improvement exhibited during each intervention period. Improvement was defined as a decline in truancy of 10 percentage points or more. With one exception, all of the youngsters in the contingency conditions improved from baseline to intervention 2, with improvement ranging from 13 to 92 percentage points, while only two youngsters in the control group and one in the relationship group improved.

In the case of Barry, an only child aged 15, the author had to intervene over a wide spectrum as many of the push-pull factors in his life were absent or minimal. This meant, *inter alia*, enlisting the help of a kindly neighbour to wake him up. When his mother was alive she'd had to 'drag' him out of a deep slumber. The father was on early shifts with a bus company and could not supervise the early morning routine. A series of school visits was also required to mobilize the personal interest of a teacher and educational psychologist in the fate of this lonely boy. The school was an extremely large and impersonal place. The programme also involved discussions with the boy about his future plans, his social life (he was introduced to a youth club) and his grief over the loss of his mother. Joint meetings were arranged between the author, Barry and his father to iron out misunderstandings, to work out a rota for household chores, and to arrange a contract (see below) involving a loan for a moped if Barry returned to school and gave proof of his intention to attend regularly.

In the case of the two girls, aged 14 and 15 respectively, a central theme in their problems was a sense of helplessness (see Seligman, 1975), purposelessness, and apathy. A carefully structured 'timetable' of events and activities was constructed in order to help them to face life again. Incorporated within this was a controlled and gradual re-entry into school. Social skill training helped the girls to overcome their lack of social confidence.

Contract

Between Barry K, and Mr. K.

Son agrees to:
1. Get up and make ready for school when aroused by the next door neighbour (every weekday).
2. Catch the 8 a.m. village bus to school.
3. Stay at school during school hours.

Father agrees to:
1. Lend Barry £20 toward the purchase of a moped.

Both parties agree to the following conditions:
1. The loan will be paid after Barry has been back at school for 1 month.
2. The penalty for missing school after that date will be the loss of the use of the bike for each day missed (unless there is a legitimate reason for absence from school).
3. The money will be returned at the rate of £1.50 per month out of Barry's paper round money.

Signed: ——————————
Father

Signed: ——————————
Son

12

Delinquent Behaviour

The 'face' of delinquency is changing dramatically. The number of juvenile crimes, detected and adjudicated in the United Kingdom and the United States, has increased markedly. There is a change in the sex ratio with regard to criminal acts, too; an almost complete male reserve has given way to substantial numbers of female offenders. The average age for the first court appearance of youngsters has declined, and there is a movement in the kinds of offences committed towards more violent activities. Delinquent behaviours of young people range from theft and vandalism to brutal sexual assaults and murders. Small wonder we get the 'Armageddon outcries' of doom and disaster. In Chapter 2 we considered some of the factors associated with the development of delinquent patterns of behaviour.

Criminology suffers from an embarrassment of riches when it comes to theories as to why individuals become delinquent (see Feldman, 1977). They can generally be subsumed under the following headings: sociological, biological, and psychological. We have already discussed one of the latter theories — a learning approach. Sociological explanations of delinquency are likely to be couched in terms of the attributes of the *society* in which the delinquent lives, as is the case with subcultural theories of delinquent acts. They may take the form of a social control approach which focuses on the nature of social roles and rules, the activities of rule enforcers and the consequences of social relationships for the labelling of deviants (Becker, 1963).

This sociological approach can be contrasted with those biological and psychological theories which seek to explain how *individual* differences in genetic make-up, central or autonomic nervous system functioning, upbringing, and personality cause some youths to be prone to delinquency and others to be apparently immune. The interactionist approach in sociology argues, for example, that deviance does not exist objectively in either people or situations but is a status conferred on particular people in particular situations (see Hardiker, 1972).

Among the biological theories are those which propose genetic influences which some theorists believe to be crucial. Others (e.g., Rutter, 1972) conclude that the evidence shows that delinquent behaviour is not inherited as such, but rather that personality disorders in the parents probably lead to antisocial problems in the children through their association with deviant models and with family discord and disruption (see Herbert, 1980).

DEVIANT MODELS

Belson (1975), for example, found in his survey of London boys that the onset of stealing was highly correlated with exposure to social models of offending — that is, associating with boys already stealing (see also Knight and West, 1975). Feldman (1977), after reviewing the evidence, concludes that failures in learning not to offend during childhood are not as *exclusively* significant as suggested by earlier research. As he puts it, 'certain social settings favour the positive acquisition of criminal behaviours by exposure to relevant persuasive communications and social models, as well as by direct experience'.

L. Berkowitz et al. (1978) report three experiments that demonstrated that a diet of aggressive films increased aggression in adolescent male juvenile delinquents during the movie week and in the following period as well. Some of this influence was clearly imitative in nature. The controversy over the effects of television viewing on conduct problems such as aggression continues — although the evidence (e.g., Bandura, 1973) would seem to be tilting in the positive direction, that is, that exposure to certain categories of television violence occurring in particular settings increases the likelihood of violent actions from some observers.

The causes (short term and long term) and maintenance of problematic behaviour are dependent on many contributary influences (see Figure 2).

Wolkind and Rutter's (1973) investigation of a sample of 10-year-old boys drawn from the general population indicates that short-term admissions to a foster home or institution are followed by a markedly increased risk of antisocial disorder. The authors show that these admissions tend to be brief periods in a long history of adverse influences acting on the child. They point out that children from unhappy backgrounds are vulnerable to stressful separations, and the short exposure to residential care increases their risk of developing antisocial problems. Most important, probably, is the long duration of family discord and other aversive influences. There are high rates of mental disorder, particularly personality disorder of aggressive type, among the parents, especially the fathers; parents show an unusual amount of rejecting, hostile, and critical behaviour towards their offspring.

Rutter (1978, 1979) points out that single chronic stresses are surprisingly unimportant in the genesis of conduct disorder in childhood; the factors —

family processes and community influences and school conditions — are multiple and interactive. Genetic vulnerability and environmental stresses seem to interact in such a manner that each potentiates the other's deleterious influence. The intriguing question, as always, concerns those children who emerge unscathed despite the apparent hazards in their lives (Rutter, 1977b).

FAMILY VARIABLES

The family is likely, in a high proportion of cases, to be broken up through divorce or separation and the children to have had periods of being placed 'in care' at times of family crisis (Power et al., 1974; Rutter, 1972). There are several investigations which have shown that delinquency tends to be commoner in unhappy unbroken homes (i.e. where there are quarrelsome neglectful parents) than in harmonious but broken ones (McCord and McCord, 1959). Rutter (1972) in an excellent review on parent–child separations concludes that the evidence on 'broken homes' is surprisingly straightforward. Although parental death may play a part in the pathogenesis of some disorders (Rutter and Brown, 1966) delinquency is mainly associated with breaks which follow serious parental conflict rather than with the loss of a parent as such. Even within the group of homes broken by divorce or separation, it appears that it is the discord prior to separation rather than the rift itself which was the main adverse influence. Rutter's own findings suggest that separation as such is of negligible importance in the causation of delinquency. He does not deny that genetic factors have an influence on the antisocial behaviour of children, although he questions the major role some theorists give to heredity. Rutter claims that they are of importance with respect to temperamental characteristics which render certain children more susceptible to psychological stress.

To summarize the available evidence on family variables, children with persistent conduct disorders come most often from families notable for their disharmony and quarrelling, for an absence of affection, and for inconsistent discipline which is ineffective and either extremely severe or lax (see Figure 11). The links between these global influences and actual delinquent behaviour are delineated in the following model by Stuart, Jayaratne, and Tripodi (1976) as follows: (1) within the family, parents (and, at school, teachers) inadequately cue and/or reinforce positive behaviours by youths, (2) while they inadvertently strengthen deviant behaviours by overattending to these responses, (3) at the same time that peers differentially strengthen problematic behaviours at the expense of prosocial responses. This model is based upon empirical research (see Patterson and Reid, 1970; Stuart, 1971b). As a result of this kind of formulation, several theorists recommend projects to reduce delinquent behaviour by changing the behaviour of parents (Patterson, 1971; Patterson, Cobb, and Ray, 1973) and teachers (Hall and Copeland, 1972; Patterson, Cobb, and Ray, 1972; Stuart, 1974) through educational programmes.

The same formulation leads logically to criticisms of residential institutions (detention centres, industrial and training schools, community schools) for

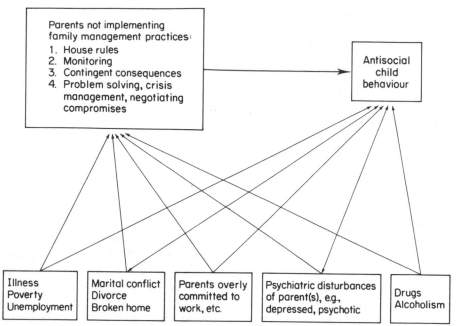

Figure 11   The relation among family management practices, crises, and antisocial child behaviour (Patterson, 1982)

juvenile offenders. As Stumphauzer (1970) observes, they can so easily become settings in which to learn delinquent behaviours rather than environments for learning socially acceptable modes of living. In a sense these places are colleges of further education in which the 'learning programmes' are provided by other inmates, some of whom may be powerful models to emulate, thus encouraging antisocial behaviour. Rewards (social approval and tangible goods) and punishments (physical intimidation and withdrawal of approval) also shape deviant patterns. There is evidence to support this depressing formulation. Patterson (1963) made fifteen 2-hour observations of a group of delinquent girls in a detention home. Descriptive accounts were obtained of each episode of social conforming behaviour (e.g., talking of going to college) and each episode of antisocial behaviour (e.g., rule breaking). The immediate consequences of these behaviours were noted and classified into positive reinforcement and punishment. Data clearly indicated reward and approval from peers for rule infractions, criticism of adults, and aggressive behaviour. The peer group was most likely to punish behaviour which deviated from delinquent norms and conformed with society's values. Admittedly, the observation is limited to one observer, one group, and one institution. However, an extension and replication of this work has been conducted by Furniss (1964) using a method called 'interpersonal communication analysis'. Observers recorded interactions of the residents of four cottages in a state institution for girls. Data were coded independently by two judges into (1) level of communication (verbal, non-verbal), (2) delinquently appropriate or socially appropriate, and (3) peer responses (reward or punishment). In all cottages, delinquent behaviour was reinforced by peers and socially conforming behaviour was punished. Non-verbal levels of communication transmitted rewards and punishments significantly more than verbal communication. Another study (Buehler, Patterson, and Furniss, 1966) focused on peer groups but also examined the reinforcement contingencies dispensed by institutional staff members. An observer recorded the interpersonal transactions of six cottage inmates, including transactions with staff members. It was apparent that peers dispensed reinforcements at a higher rate than did the staff and were more consistent in providing rewards and punishments. Peers tended to reward delinquent behaviour and punish moves towards socially acceptable behaviour while staff alternately rewarded and punished the girls for the same acts. The authors comment that the peer group appeared to be running their own behaviour modification programme — indeed, more efficiently than the staff. Sadly, the results indicate that institutions may encourage and maintain, through inconsistent staff but consistent peer reinforcement, the very behaviours which lead to incarceration.

These findings about inappropriate contingencies and poor socialization in the youth's various social settings link up with a taxonomy of delinquent disorders first developed by Hewitt and Jenkins (1946). It is a formulation in which the presence or absence of self-control in the child is related to affectional and disciplinary patterns within the home and other social environments within which he interacts. Essentially, the authors put forward a control theory in which the concept of inhibition is made to account for three categories of delinquency found among children.

PATTERNS OF DELINQUENT DISORDER

The main subdivision usually made within the overall group of delinquent disorders is that between socialized delinquency and unsocialized, aggressive behaviour. The authors distinguish between the following types of disorder: (1) overinhibited neurotic behaviour, (2) socialized (pseudosocial) delinquency, where the child may truant and steal but is on good terms with his peers, and (3) unsocialized aggressive behaviour, where the child is openly at odds with others.

These categories, as we shall see, are related in large part to parental attitudes and practices. The *neurotic* delinquent (to put it in terms of a profile based upon empirical studies) is sensitive, overinhibited, lonely, and anxious, and he has strong feelings of inadequacy and inferiority. His delinquencies tend to fit a pattern of compulsive and solitary stealing, furtive sadism, and sexual problems such as exhibitionism and voyeurism. He tends to be submissive, apathetic, and dreamy. Unlike the third category of delinquent, he does feel guilt for the wrongs he commits. He is usually well behaved at school and reasonably obedient and truthful at home. Wright (1971) provides a portrait of his home background: the neurotic delinquent tends to come from a small and intact family, where attachments to parents are strong, where the mother is overprotective and overanxious, where there is some emotional instability in either or both of the parents, and where the parents set austere and uncompromising standards for their children. Sanctions against the child are predominantly psychological, in the sense that they threaten rejection or withdrawal of approval or love. These are the conditions which in psychoanalytic theory are said to lead to strong identification with the parents and the development of a harsh, rigid, and irrational super-ego or conscience. When they do not result in neurosis or compulsive delinquency, they produce the highly conscientious and tense character, who leads an impeccably respectable life, but whose own instinctual satisfactions are severely curtailed, and who cannot tolerate 'immorality' in others. They are also conditions and effects which can be explained in other (e.g., social learning) terms. (See Chapter 2 for a discussion of the internalization of rules and values.)

For another type of child, brought up usually in run-down overcrowded slum areas, delinquency may almost be a way of life. Take the so-called *pseudosocial* or *socialized* delinquent; he is a loyal gang member and is described as having a normal shell of inhibition. But he demonstrates it only towards members of his own group. There is minimal restraint of antisocial tendencies in relation to the out-group. Though he is suspicious, defiant, and hostile to those in authority (e.g., parents, teachers, and the police), he is not a victim of violent uncontrollable impulses, but adjusts well to other members of his peer group and is thought to have no psychiatric disorder as such. It would appear that he has acquired standards which are at odds with society at large although in keeping with those of his often-neglectful or broken home and immediate peer group. The socialized delinquent shows towards his deviant peer group or gang a loyalty and obligation commensurate with it being for him a substitute family. It provides him with an emotional anchorage.

Scott (1966) suggests a modification of the socialized delinquent category. He points out that it really includes two two subcategories: those who have failed to acquire any consistent set of standards and those who have a well-developed set of standards which happen to run counter to those of most other people. The youths without consistent values tend to come from disorganized families in which gross inconsistencies of discipline prevail and in which the parents demonstrate minimal self-control and lax standards of behaviour. The patterns of delinquent behaviour manifested in this context begin early and are varied in kind. They are seldom destructive or aggressive and consist largely of evasions of things unpleasant and sporadic stealing. These youngers require help in connection with their lack of direction and lack of internal controls. They need an opportunity to gain their own coherent set of values and to learn responsibility.

The *unsocialized aggressive* youth seems to suffer from a more far-reaching conduct disorder, as evidenced by his emotional disturbance and poor interpersonal relationships. He (and eventually society) becomes the victim of his poorly developed self-control and lack of compassion (or, in the terminology of Hewitt and Jenkins, 1946, his 'inadequate shell of inhibition'). The underdevelopment of inhibitory processes contribute to a fairly characteristic profile of a youth who is malicious, defiant of authority, sullen, and frequently hostile and coercive to the people around him. He tends to be extrapunitive — always blaming others and, in the process, feeling hard-done-by and persecuted. He is relatively unmoved by praise or punishment (a practical problem in planning behavioural treatment) and he shows little guilt or remorse. He tends to give free rein to his impulses and he is often unpopular because of his cruelty and vengefulness. Nevertheless, while he is feared for his violence and malice, he is likely to be respected as a leader. He needs his gang around him, not because of the friendship it provides but for the self-esteem its subservience gives him. These typologies are all very well; they are based on empirical studies and are useful for theoretical discussion. However, the nomothetic methods upon which they are based mask many crucial individual differences and situational variables which would be helpful in planning a treatment programme for a particular youngster. The danger of these typologies is their implication of therapeutic nihilism. Terms like 'psychopath' or 'unsocialized aggressive delinquent' connote a gloomy prognosis, pessimism about any cooperation from the client and the prospect of a thankless and abrasive intervention.

Studies of unsocialized aggressive delinquents (see Wright, 1971) suggest that they most often come from families in which the parent–child interactions are marked by mutual suspicion, hostility, and rejection. The parents are severely punitive, inconsistent, and unjust. It is difficult for the child to identify with such parents, and thus the aggression they provoke is not directed against the self (intropunitive) as it is in the case of a child with a well-developed conscience. It is turned outwards and vented on members of the community and on objects — as in the vandalism of property.

The unsocialized delinquent can be conceptualized as an individual whose behaviour has developed under conditions of learning that failed to establish the internal controls which keep most people in his culture from committing antisocial acts. Bandura and Walters (1963) were among the first proponents of an explicit socialization explanation of delinquency based on principles of modelling and reinforcement. They, like Andry (1960), report the pattern of parental rejection combined with a harsh punitive father (or a father whose criminality provides a criminal role model) commonly found in aggressive or delinquent boys. Physical assaults, carried out persistently, against a background of no affection tend to provoke retaliatory aggression in the child. This, in turn, can be the first stage of a slippery slope toward the juvenile courts. The absence of a father, or the presence of a father with whom there is a disturbed relationship, is a further factor related to the incidence of delinquent behaviour. The often-repeated finding of a background of inconsistent discipline (over a long term) in the families of conduct-disordered youths is another crucial theme.

But why should inconsistent discipline play such a part in delinquent patterns of behaviour? Wright (1971, p. 99) explains this as follows:

Not only will the delinquent be confused over what is right and wrong, but he will be angered by injustice and he will learn that whether or not he is rewarded or punished is not predictably related to his own behaviour. This last point is of great importance. In a home where parents are consistent, the child learns that his own behaviour to a large extent determines how others respond to him and this is a crucial element in his general feelings that he can exercise some control over how others behave towards him. If, on the other hand, the child learns to dissociate his own behaviour from the rewards and punishments that come from others, he will feel that bit more powerless to influence his social environment. This in turn will contribute to that general alienation from society which sociologists have noted to be a feature of delinquents. Many students of delinquency have observed the prevalence of fatalistic attitudes among delinquents. To them it seems that the only way they can elicit a predictable response in others is through provoking their angry indignation by acts of theft and vandalism.

It has been found that the chances of a youth on probation re-offending depend to a great extent on his family and, in particular, are reduced when (1) the father's discipline is firm, (2) the father demonstrates affection for his son, and (3) the father is supported in his discipline by the mother (Davies and Sinclair, 1971).

Of course, there is no one-to-one relationship between these various background variables and delinquency. It is naive to maintain that all delinquents have a common background or that background factors found with relatively high frequency among delinquents will clearly demarcate delinquents from non-delinquents. Investigations always reveal that a large percentage of delinquents have the background commonly found among non-delinquents and, conversely, that there are non-delinquents with backgrounds commonly found among delinquents. What other factors, then, must be taken into account?

EMOTIONAL DISTURBANCE

A popular viewpoint is that emotional disturbance of 'maladjustment' predisposes the offender towards delinquent behaviour. Delinquent behaviour is regarded as the outward and visible sign, or an 'acting-out', of a variety of psychological problems (e.g., intrapsychic conflicts) and can be reduced only as a result of their resolution. Although some role is given to the individual's current environment in maintaining delinquent behaviour, it is stressed that this is primarily internally motivated. It is for this reason that it is believed that delinquent behaviour will continue to occur so long as the sources of the maladjustment are not sought out and removed. Stealing from the mother (for example) is said to symbolize the restitution of the affection that is rightfully the child's, but which has been denied him. Such ideas are notoriously difficult to validate (Lee and Herbert, 1970). What practical implications flow from such theories for (say) the probation officer who has to work with juvenile offenders? Must he learn to psychoanalyse his clients? Apart from the implications for their training the suggestion would be totally impractical given his or her caseload.

EDUCATIONAL FACTORS

We have already discussed some of the main psychological and biological determinants of delinquent behaviour in Chapters 2 and 3. Educational correlates are also of great significance. Serious educational backwardness is an almost invariable concomitant of conduct disorder. About a third of antisocial boys have specific reading difficulties, a rate many times that of the general population. There is no clear explanation for this association. There may be several mechanisms at work. First, the temperamental characteristics which lead to conduct disorder bear a remarkable similarity to those which predispose to reading problems. Second, the adverse family situations which make the child vulnerable to conduct disorders are often associated with those linked with reading difficulties. The large size of families is linked with both. Children with conduct disorders are more likely than other children to come from families with at least four or five children. Then, again, several surveys have shown that large families are much more likely than others to live in poor-quality, overcrowded housing and to have financial difficulties.

An important determinant of underachievement is the existence of emotional problems in the child. The National Survey of Health and Development demonstrated (Douglas, Ross, and Simpson, 1968) a close relationship at 8, 11, and 15 years of age between adjustment, on the one hand, and ability and attainment, on the other. Children who are divided at 15 years of age into the categories 'well adjusted' (27 per cent.) and 'least-well adjusted' (28 per cent.) showed marked differences in school performance; the least-well adjusted (i.e., maladjusted) children had the poorest results in terms of non-verbal ability, verbal ability, reading, and mathematics. Chazan (1959) found that even highly intelligent maladjusted pupils tend to have real difficulties in school performance. Underachievers at school have poorer self-concepts than normal achievers and reflect feelings of defensiveness, loneliness, and undue restriction on their freedom (Ausubel et al., 1954).

SELF-ESTEEM

Self-esteem plays an important part in the conduct and delinquent disorders. Bandura (1969) points out that most instances of human behaviour result not only in environmental consequences but also in self-evaluative reactions. The extent to which we see ourselves in control, guiding our own lives, is an important determinant of self-esteem. Research has shown that lower-class children and delinquents tend to be externals (i.e., they believe that things happen to them rather than their having any control over their own destinies) (Rotter, 1971). Cohen (1955) has argued that the delinquent gang permits working-class boys to recoup self-esteem lost through defeat in middle-class institutions. A reasonable agreement between the self-concept ('myself as I am') and the concept of the ideal self ('myself as I would like to be') is one of the most important conditions for a favourable psychological adjustment — at school and in other aspects of the child's life (Ausubel et al., 1954; Crandall and Bellugi, 1954). There is clear evidence that all human beings old enough to have acquired even a rudimentary self-image need to see themselves in at least a moderately favourable light. There are wide variations in the ways this need manifests itself, particularly in the case of the neurotic person. But, in general, the desire for an acceptable self-image appears to be one of the most critical and significant motivating factors in childhood behaviour. From a very tender age, children discover and make use of complex *defensive strategies* designed to protect and enhance their gradually evolving self-image. Marked discrepancies (i.e., negative self-concepts) arouse anxiety, unhappiness, and general dissatisfaction with life (Crandall and Bellugi, 1954).

Delinquent boys tend to be poorly motivated for achievement. This may result from their lack of success in school, their low social standing, the self-fulfilling prophecy resulting from the labels ascribed to them by significant others, or the lack of successful role models (especially parents). Research has shown that boys in homes where the father is absent tend to be: (1) low in self-esteem and (2) poorly motivated for achievement (Bronfenbrenner, 1967). A favourable self-image (or its opposite) is shaped by the significant people in his early life. It is their attitudes towards him, their opinions of him, which become part of his view of himself. After early childhood, persons outside the family, teachers, classmates and friends, assume an increasingly important role in forming this self-concept. At the same time, the child's self-image is modified as he repeatedly lives up to parental expectations — or continually fails to do so in the case of overcritical or ambitious parents.

Coopersmith (1967) provides evidence that the optimum conditions required for the achievement of high self-esteem in children are a combination of firm enforcement of limits on the child's behaviour, together with a marked degree of freedom (autonomy) within these limits. As long as the parentally imposed constraints are backed up by social norms outside the home, this provides the youngster with a clear idea of an orderly and trustworthy social reality which, in turn, gives him a solid basis for his own actions.

A child as he grows up has to assume responsibility for changing and maintaining his own behaviour. Although environmental controls are essential in the beginning stages, eventually the new behaviour has to be carried out in the individual's daily life in the absence of parents and teachers or other adults. During the formative years there is a balance in the influence of adult figures and peer group in the shaping of the child's value system and behavioural

250

repertoire which, if tilted in the direction of a preponderant control by peers, usually leads to serious problems (see Wright, 1971). Here lies one of the dangers of academic underachievement. It seems that in some children the very fact of educational failure leads to disillusionment, boredom, and resentment, which throws the child into the arms of a deviant peer group. Their search for excitement, adventure, and resolution of different tensions and needs leads them into a variety of rebellious, aggressive, and delinquent acts, such as truancy, theft, and vandalism.

SOCIAL SKILLS

Furnham (1986) in a review of skill deficits in adolescents is of the opinion that difficulties in establishing and maintaining relationships with peers and authority figures reduces the quantity and quality of potential and significant learning experiences available to them. And it *is* a matter of concern to them. The most commonly cited problems concerned employment, self-confidence/social adequacy, and school/academic concerns. Peer acceptance seemed to concern most adolescents, more so than problems regarding authority and control. Many of the problems clearly concerned skill deficits; 66 per cent. of girls and 48 per cent. of boys reported being afraid to speak out in class; 40 per cent. of girls and 37 per cent. of boys wondered why people are not nicer to them; 35 per cent. of girls and 46 per cent. of boys were too shy to go to dances.

There is a fairly considerable and consistent literature on social skills training (SST) with delinquents and young offenders (Spence and Marzillier, 1981). The literature has in fact been extended to delinquent girls court-adjudicated probationary youths, and pre-delinquent youths (Henderson and Hollin, 1983; Kifer et al., 1974).

Social skills training has had a number of aims — to reduce delinquent behaviour, to improve specific skills such as interview skills, and to increase the effectiveness of penal staff–delinquent interaction. Henderson and Hollin (1983) critically reviewed 15 studies on social skills training with young offenders and concluded:

both practitioners and administration must recognise the limitations of the technique; it cannot cure the 'causes of crime' and it is naive to assume it can; to press for its adoption as such is both misleading and damaging. Misleading because it will raise false expectations of its results, and damaging because of the adverse consequences when these expectations are dashed. SST techniques may have a role to play for some young offenders' development, but considerable experimental investigation is required before any firm commitments for the intervention can be made.

There appears to be a consensus about which areas of skill deficit are important in adolescence and early adulthood: viz. assertiveness, heterosexual interaction, dating and friendship formation, parent and other authority figure (teacher, professional) relationships, job interview skills, and coping with loneliness.

THEFT

Stealing is a widespread social problem and one which young people engage in to a growing extent according to police statistics. Of course, children 'take things' that do not belong to them in the course of learning the complex rules about possession and property. Even after the child has learned that it is wrong to steal, the seriousness of stealing is interpreted differently at different ages. Those acts of theft which become less serious in the view of the child as he grows older involve hoodwinking persons in authority, keeping found property, and using the belongings of brothers and sisters. Obviously, there are different types of juvenile theft.

Rich (1956) concluded, after a study of 200 youths admitted to a London remand home, that the offences involving theft could be divided into four categories. There is, first, the 'marauding' type — an unplanned affair involving several boys. It depends very much on circumstances (an unlocked car, attractive goods on display and within snatching distance, or an open window) and is committed by those who are not essentially deviant in personality. Nothing particularly harmful or abnormal can be found in their home backgrounds. As they come chiefly from the lower socioeconomic level of society, it is possible that their attitudes to property may be less reverent than those of the middle and upper classes. Conforming to the group seems to be an important element. Rather immature boys, who are not essentially antisocial in their outlook, tend to get involved in these escapades. The groups are loosely formed — hardly even gangs — and are normal for the early adolescent age range; their delinquency is, in a sense, whimsical or accidental. Another category of stealing is the 'proving' type of offence. This is usually carried out by a boy alone, or with one other, and consists of stealing, breaking, and entering, or taking a car and driving it away. Sometimes the objects stolen have a value which is symbolic rather than practical. The boys involved in such offences tend to be older than the marauders and from homes higher up the socioeconomic scale.

Rich states that this stealing is often neurotic in its origin, in that the boy is trying to prove something to himself; the act may be one of rebellion against his father or one of emancipation from an overpossessive mother. The 'comforting' type of stealing (mentioned earlier) is associated with a history of separation from, and rejection by, the mother. It is a type of theft which spreads outside the home and persists into adult life. There is a fourth category of stealing — for gain — in which the robberies are planned and measures are taken to avoid detection. Some of these thefts are committed by those from deprived backgrounds who are getting older and who will go on to form part of the population of persistent offenders.

We have already seen that antisocial acts begin early. Almost 60 per cent. of adolescent delinquents commit their first offence (although it may not be detected then) *before* the age of 10 years (Robins, 1966). And this early oneset applies to theft in particular. There seem to be two distinct cycles in juvenile law-breaking. The first involves theft, mainly petty in kind. It starts at about the age of 9 or 10 years and persists to 14 or 15. The second stage in juvenile law-breaking begins at about 15 or 16 and persists until about 18 or 19. This stage involves rowdyism, some violence, taking away and driving cars, and so on. A child can only be described as delinquent if stealing becomes a *habitual* activity, particularly as a gang pastime. This has to be 'measured' against normative studies like those of Belson (1975). His survey of 1,425 London boys showed that 88 per cent. had at some time stolen something from school and 70 per cent. from a shop; 69 per cent. had at some time received stolen goods and 33 per cent. had stolen from a stall or barrow; 32 per cent. had stolen from somewhere they had worked, 18 per cent. from a telephone box, and 17 per cent. had taken a letter or parcel; 11 per cent. had stolen from a meter and 5 per cent. had taken away a car, lorry or van. When trivial thefts were excluded from the tally, the above percentages become respectively: 63, 53, 60, 20, 25, 11, 7, 9, and 5 per cent. In addition, the report presented percentages based only upon those thefts where the items concerned were valued at 1 pound or over. With regard to the factors that contribute to stealing, the great bulk of findings related to the causal factors that operate in the initiation and development of juvenile stealing.

Five of the causal hypotheses came through the testing procedure as highly tenable, namely those concerned with permissiveness in relation to stealing, association with boys who are already stealing, a desire by the boy for much fun and excitement and a tendency to go out 'just looking for it', truancy from school, and a belief on the part of the boy that the police would not catch him for stealing. Other hypotheses were also confirmed, but to a lesser degree. The principal causal factors in these hypotheses were the existence of home conditions that make the home an unpleasant place for boys to be in, frequent boredom on the part of the boy, and a state of affairs in which the boy's wants exceed his legal means. On the available evidence several factors appeared to work appreciably *against* the development of continuance of stealing: getting caught for stealing by the police or knowing about mates getting caught, frequent church attendance, Jewish denomination, and having a grandparent living in the home.

VANDALISM

A major problem, these days, especially in urban environments, is the wanton destruction of property. A lot of minor vandalism is extremely prevalent among school children (Marshall, 1976). However, it sometimes reaches a level of seriousness and persistence, where it forms one manifestation of a more general conduct disorder. Among the different categories of vandalism are, first, a type of damage emerging from playfulness. It is a feature of all children's play to undo things, bang them, climb trees, throw stones, or draw on doors and walls. Not surprisingly, damage occurs willy nilly during such play activity. Play 'vandalism' of this kind is common among children and predominates among children up to the age of 12 years. These children, in general, do not go on to commit any other crime.

Peer-group pressures play a part in the next category of vandalism. From the age of 13 to 16, boys become increasingly involved with their contemporaries; play becomes secondary and activities take on an element of daring. This is a means of winning prestige. Among the 'daring' activities may be deliberate damaging of property. This kind involves, according to a British estimate, some 30 to 40 per cent. of older schoolboys — the ones who are most committed to their group of friends (Marshall, 1976). Many of them get involved in other types of delinquency as well, such as shoplifting and gang fights. Their vandalism, consisting of competitive activities to see who can disfigure or break up park benches or road signs most effectively or who can break most windows in an empty factory, tends to be a group phenomenon.

Another category of vandalism involves lashing out at society out of resentment and frustration. The destructive behaviour is still motivated by a search for status among their peer group, despite the fact that for most youngsters over 16 years this need is becoming less pressing. Most other boys of this age are now spending more time with girl-friends, or are already married, with steady jobs. The 'outsiders' may feel inadequate by comparison, and it is this which may contribute to their increasingly wanton and arbitrary vandalism. Marshall states that this is the most persistent form of vandalism. The youth who gets caught more than once or commits more serious damage is more likely than other vandals to commit offences of others sorts (especially burglary or theft). He is also more likely to come from a broken home and, if he has left school, to be out of work.

A further type of vandalism has been called 'instrumental'; the damage caused is less for enjoyment and more a means to some other end. Included here are acts of damage where the object is to steal, as in breaking into cars to steal radios, damaging telephone kiosk coinboxes, stripping lead from buildings, and so on. Marshall states that what is most worrying is the serious damage done by a small number of children and adolescents. As they usually commit a wide range of other offences as well, they are really part of a general crime problem. The frequency and seriousness of their offences leads eventually to their apprehension by the police.

TREATMENT OF DELINQUENT PROBLEMS

There is a dearth, in quantity and quality, of *hard* evidence concerning the effectiveness of behaviour modification in the area of juvenile delinquency. Today, there is a growing literature (see Braukmann and Fixsen, 1975; Davidson and Seidman, 1974; Henderson and Hollin, 1983; Stumphauzer, 1970) but we are still a long way from definite conclusions based on objective and painstaking empirical studies. Comprehensive programmes have not yet been evaluated in adequately controlled trials. What, then, has been achieved by behaviour modification?

Assuming that some treatment intervention is judged to be necessary, this is aimed at the prevention or reduction of delinquent behaviour and the promotion of more acceptable alternatives. The direct approach is used to bring about a cessation of the antisocial activities which have been deemed illegal. Strangely enough (although understandably given the difficulty of tracking illegal and therefore furtive actions) there is a dearth of such studies. Another approach is to examine the effect of interventions on the problem of delinquent behaviour indirectly, by using educational or programme performances as success criteria. To achieve both ends, new learning experiences are provided in treatment by systematically altering those contemporary events which instigate or maintain delinquent acts or their alternatives. These changes constitute certain specific treatment procedures, including:

(1) Stimulus change
(2) Covert sensitization
(3) Modelling
(4) Punishment
(5) Positive reinforcement of prosocial alternative behaviour
(6) Non-reinforcement of delinquent behaviour
(7) Competence training

The first of these procedures (e.g., removing the child from temptation) of itself achieves only a temporary decrease in delinquent behaviour for so long as it continues in operation. The remaining procedures are designed to produce a more enduring decline in antisocial behaviour, together with the acquisition, performance, and reinforcement of alternative behaviour. In day-to-day practice (outside the residential token economies designed for groups) several specific procedures are likely to be combined into a comprehensive and individualized treatment programme for implementation in the context of good care and concern for the child.

COVERT SENSITIZATION

An attempt is made to increase emotional reactions in specified situations. Maladaptive approach responses (e.g., stealing) are repeatedly paired with noxious experiences. The procedure is much like aversive conditioning except that it takes place in the patient's imagination. Cautela (1967) has used this approach in the treatment of certain delinquent problems such as breaking and entering, glue-sniffing, and motor-car theft. Juvenile offenders are trained to imagine, for example, a shoplifting scene. As they approach the counter of the supermarket they are to imagine becoming increasingly nauseous and find relief only when they cease their act of theft. Through repeated pairings it is hoped that an aversion to shoplifting will develop. Although Cautela reports good results, his data are based on only a few subjects with no measured changes in rates of these maladaptive behaviours reported. A major problem in the modification of behaviours such as theft is the difficulty in monitoring the behaviour; another obvious one concerns the uphill task of obtaining contingency control with adolescents. They roam far and wide, away from supervision. They are often under the sway of the peer group and resent adult authority, not to mention being poorly motivated for change, so that they do not use aversive imagery as a means of self-control in natural situations.

MODELLING

Modelling (and role-playing procedures) have been designed to teach new, constructive behaviours as alternatives to antisocial repertoires. Such a programme can be administered while the youth is still in custody in order (hopefully) to build up his behavioural repetoire before he is confronted and seduced again by aggravating or beguiling situations in the outside world.

One programme of this type has been developed by Sarason (Sarason, 1968; Sarason and Ganzer, 1973) for use with juvenile delinquents. Sarason used modelling experiences to counter the inadequate learning experiences that he sees as the basis of some forms of juvenile delinquency. In this particular study, he and his affiliates investigated the effectiveness of modelling procedures, compared to traditional group discussion approaches, with institutionalized male delinquents. They analysed the effect of modelling experiences and traditional role-playing on subsequent behaviours as reflected in (1) their self-reports, (2) staff ratings, (3) the semantic differential, and (4) Wahler's self-description inventory. The sessions took the form of demonstration, role-playing, and group discussion. Each session had a particular theme, such as applying for a job, resisting social pressure from peers to engage in antisocial behaviours, and delaying immediate sources of gratification in order to obtain more valued goals in the future. The groups met four times a week for a 1-month period. In the modelling groups, consisting of four or five youths, two models (graduate students in psychology) acted out a script which demonstrated appropriate behaviour in these problem situations. Following the modelling sequence, the observers were called upon to summarize and explain the main points of what they had just observed. Each youth then enacted the same scene with either another boy or a model as a partner. The method was found to be highly effective as assessed by the attitudinal and behavioural adjustment measures. What effect it has (and this applies to other indirect interventions) on subsequent resistance to delinquent actions, remains an unknown quantity.

PUNISHMENT

The words 'crime' and 'punishment' go together like salt and pepper. Probably for a majority of people the gut reaction to vicious delinquent acts is the wish to punish the perpetrator — to see him atone for his wrongdoing by suffering. Walker (1972) provides an excellent account of the penal philosophies that underlie the penal system. Ideas of deterrence and rehabilitation put a gloss on the retributive functions of some of the penal institutions for juvenile delinquents. By teaching the juvenile offender a trade and the habit and routine of steady work, it is hoped to reform him. Walker notes that some institutions deny that they are intended to act as deterrents, claiming that their effectiveness is reformative and that they do not penalize but rather educate delinquent youths. As Walker puts it: 'the fact that their inmates regard them as deterrents, and persist in talking about their "sentences", is dismissed as irrelevant' (p. 99). Whether we are discussing the deterrent effect of punishment at the institutional or person-to-person level, there is scant evidence to go on. As Stumphauzer (1973) notes in a comprehensive review of the literature, punishment (although in common use) has met with relatively little controlled research with delinquents. Several of the papers reviewed use it in combination with positive reinforcement, as part of a general contingency management programme. What can be said is that many criminal acts go undetected and unpunished; and if punishment is remote and uncertain it is unlikely to compete with the immediate rewards of, say, stealing. We shall deal with individual programmes first and then examine the efficacy of institutional corrective measures.

Earlier (page 204) we saw how Tyler and his colleagues used a punishment procedure — time-out from positive reinforcement — with successful results. In a similar fashion, Buchard (1967) used a 30-minute time-out procedure combined with loss of tokens to reduce the incidence of fighting, property damage, physical and verbal assault, stealing, and lying. This work involved retarded delinquents who were institutionalized. Using a reversal design Buchard found only a small change in the behaviour of the youths that was attributable to the use of the time-out procedure.

In a study with a similar population and using a counterbalanced design, Burchard and Barrera (1972) examined the use of varying time-out and response-cost procedures in reducing the occurrence of swearing, fighting, destroying property, and disobedience. Eleven institutionalized male delinquents were alternately exposed to the loss of 5 tokens, 5 minutes of isolation, 30 tokens, and 30 minutes of isolation, contingent on the undesired behaviour. Each of the four conditions was in effect for 12 days. Only two conditions reduced the undesirable behaviours below baseline levels. They found a substantial improvement when either a 30-minute time-out or a loss of 30 tokens was contingent on the behaviour. The 30-minute time-out condition and the 30-token response-cost condition were essentially equally effective in reducing the youths' inappropriate behaviour. However, the authors and White, Nielson, and Johnson (1972) point out that time-out procedures are not effective for all youths and in some cases even increase levels of inappropriate behaviours.

Brooks and Snow (1972) describe the case of a boy, Jim, who stole and was frequently absent from class; he received a great deal of attention from his peers for these behaviours. In the modification programme he received points for attendance and academic assignments. These points earned free time for the whole class. The boy also received a small cash reward. Inappropriate behaviour resulted in a response-cost penalty. The group contingency had an immediate effect on Jim's behaviour, and the target behaviours were reduced to zero. Academic work rose to a level consistent with the boy's ability.

Several studies have reported procedures that contain components of the restitution procedure. Kraft (1970) successfully dealt with a case of compulsive shoplifting by requiring the client to send the correct amount of money for a stolen item to the pilfered shop. Other studies involve the provision of predictable consequences for acts of theft.

Reid and Patterson (1976) found with ten cases of childhood stealing (defined as at least one theft per two weeks) that the parents typically denied or overlooked the stealing and lacked the motivation to continue treatment. The children were often left unsupervised for long periods each day because both parents were working. The first step in treatment involved teaching the parents correctly to identify, label, and record the incidence of stealing. Stealing was defined as the possession of an object not clearly (in the parents' perception) belonging to the child. The parents were to confront the child with each stealing incident and not to allow any explanations of how he came into possession of the object. The parents then implemented a behavioural management procedure involving close monitoring, and setting consequences (loss of privileges and time-out). Daily phone calls were made to the parents to encourage their cooperation. The results with the first seven families treated were remarkably successful.

Holland (1969) helped parents to eliminate fire-setting behaviour in their 7-year-old son Robert. The first step was to suppress fire-setting behaviour through a response-cost method so that new and adaptive behaviour could be learned. The treatment programme involved:

(1) Suppressing fire-setting by making it a discriminative stimulus for effective punishment. It was made plain to Robert that the next fire would result in destruction of his new and highly prized baseball glove. At the same time, procedures were implemented so that adaptive behaviour might occur.
(2) A system of monetary and social rewards was designed to strengthen the behaviour of bringing matches to his parents, to prevent fire-setting. The idea was to condition a response incompatible with fire-setting. The father told Robert that if any matches or match covers were found, they were to be brought to him immediately. He deliberately placed an empty match packet on a table. The packet chosen was an empty one, so it was assumed that the boy would comply with his father's request. When he brought the packet to his father, he immediately received 5 cents and was told that he would be taken shopping. He was allowed to spend the money as he wished. During that same evening and on subsequent evenings the father

placed packets containing matches around the house; they were promptly returned to him. The boy was reinforced each time — a total of eight times. The value of the reinforcers varied from 1 to 10 cents. Next, the father was advised to tell his son that he should not expect money all of the time. In other words, a variable-ratio schedule was introduced. Match-finding occurred with remarkable frequency! It was clear that even matches and match covers found outside of the house were saved and given to the father during the evening.

(3) Non-striking behaviour in the presence of matches had to be strengthened. There was a strong possibility still that if the child found matches away from home (when neither parent was there) he might take the opportunity to start a fire. A procedure to strengthen non-striking behaviour in relation to matches was initiated approximately 1 week after the programme began. In a game with his father, Robert was allowed to strike a whole packet of matches if he wanted but was given a cent for each match he did not strike. His father told him that if he wished, he could strike a packet of matches while being supervised. During this time, the father placed 20 cents by the packet of matches. Robert was told that for every match he did not strike he would receive 1 cent. Every time the child struck a match, a cent was removed. On the first trial, the boy struck ten matches. During the second evening he earned 17 cents; during the third trial he received 20 cents. After that the child would not strike matches. The father told Robert that he would not know how much money he would receive or even if he would obtain any money if he did not strike a match. The reward varied from no money to 10 cents. Social rewards were always paired with the tangible reinforcers, and the father, on his own, faded out the monetary reinforcers, replacing them with praise and approval. The reduction in scheduled reinforcements led to no repetition of the problem behaviour.

Holland indicates that some generalization of training may have occurred since the parents reported success in dealing with other deviant behaviours of their child as well. There was little formal or sophisticated education in learning theory principles. Nevertheless, the parents helped design the programme and were primarily responsible for its application. Holland did not see the child. At the end of the fifth week, the child's fire-setting behaviour was eliminated. Upon follow-up at a point in time 8 months later, the child's fire-setting behaviour had not recurred. During this 8-month period, the father continued to use a ratio schedule of reinforcement.

Welsh (1968) treated a 7-year-old boy's fire-setting by *satiation* techniques — transforming a stimulus that initially has reinforcing properties into one that is aversive. This was achieved by the repeated presentation of the stimulus — controlled, lengthy and exhausting sessions of lighting matches, holding them at arm's length (hand unsupported) and blowing them out. Eight session were required to extinguish the lad's fascination for setting light to objects in the house.

BEHAVIOUR CHANGE IN INSTITUTIONS

How effective at producing beneficial change is the practice of removing a delinquent from his home environment to a large institutional setting? The evidence indicates unambiguously that 'reformatories' (and institutions by other names) have not been widely successful (Cornish and Clarke, 1975; Harlow, 1970; Martinson, 1974). The success rates of individual approved schools in the United Kingdom differ considerably, the variations being attributed to differences in intake (Dunlop, 1975). Notwithstanding this, overall success rates calculated over a 3-year period range between only 30 and 35 per cent. (HMSO, 1972). These rates are based upon the percentage of youths who have remained free from reconviction, and cover the after-care supervision period. Reconviction data collected over longer periods show even lower success rates. Granted that these are crude criteria for the assessment of outcomes, they reflect nevertheless, failure. Of course, punishment is not the *stated* rationale of most penal institutions. Current institutional programmes, whether 'treatment' or 'training', rely on a 'disease' model of delinquency and a 'medical' model of intervention.

One explanation for the failure of institutional programmes is a model of human deviance that places the main source of behavioural variance within the individual. The primary thrust of therapy is in changing the individual; the hope is that a change in behaviour in the institutional setting represents a fundamental change (e.g., in personality, maturity, character, or self-discipline) and will therefore accompany the individual upon return to the community — no matter what its temptations, deprivations, or other disadvantages.

BEHAVIOUR CHANGE IN FAMILY SETTINGS

Alexander and Parsons (1973) describe behavioural family therapy with delinquent adolescents. During the project families were referred to the Family Clinic at the University of Utah. The adolescents' offences included absconding, being ungovernable, chronic truanting, shoplifting, drug possession, and so on. Families were randomly assigned (as near as possible) to either the treatment programme, comparison groups, or a no-treatment control condition. The treatment group (46 families) involved a short-term family intervention programme. The goal was to modify the interactions of deviant families so that they would approximate those patterns characteristic of 'normal' or 'adjusted' families. Therapists emphasized the removal of the circumstances (interactions) that elicited the behavioural offence, substituting for them a process of contingency contracting. Therapists modelled and prompted, and reinforced all the members of the family where they manifested (1) clear communications, and (2) clear presentation of 'demands' and alternative solutions, leading to (3) negotiation to the point of compromise. The behavioural group showed a recidivism rate (6 to 18 months following termination of treatment) of 26 per cent. compared to 50, 47, and 73 per cent., respectively, for the no-treatment, family groups (comparison) programme, and the eclectic psychodynamic family programme.

Behaviour modification — in cases where temporal and situational generalization are not planned for — provides no panacea. In a carefully designed study, Jesness (1975) investigated the short-term and long-term outcomes for 904 adjudicated delinquents randomly allocated either to an institution based on behaviour modification or to one based on group therapy methods derived from transactional analysis principles. The behavioural programme tended to do better on various behavioural outcome measures, whereas the programme of transactional analyses produced better results on various psychological outcome measures. Nevertheless, these differences disappeared when it came to an overall evaluation in terms of recidivism rates in a 2-year follow-up after release, as assessed at periods ranging from 3 to 24 months. The parole violation rate — regrettably not the most desirable measure of effectiveness of rehabilitation — proved to be the same for both institutions. However, the recidivism rate at 12 months for both programmes was 32 per cent., which differed significantly from the rates during a baseline period (45 per cent. mean) and from the rates of two other institutions (43 per cent. mean). At 24 months the recidivism rate for both institutions was 48 per cent.

A variety of residential projects have emerged in recent years that adopt a less sanguine view of the permanence and internalization of change. Many make use of behaviour management principles, and a growing number emphasize the need for integrated programming with the subject's family and local community in order to enhance the likelihood of success. One of the best-known schemes, Achievement Place — a community-based, family-style group home for six to eight predelinquent or delinquent boys under the direction of teaching-parents — has enjoyed positive results (Wolf, Phillips, and Fixsen, 1972). Behavioural methods are used. The boys can remain largely in their usual community, and through carefully phasing their return home, the improvements in social and academic skills and in self-control appear not only more frequent but also more enduring than in traditional regimes. Wolf and his colleagues have described the results for the first 41 boys to be admitted (average age 13.8) — mainly from very deprived social backgrounds, all with serious conduct disorders. There are many ways to evaluate such a programme. To take one criterion, reconviction rates and later institutionalization of the first 18 boys in the experiment: 3 were placed in other institutional care in the 2 years following treatment — compared with 9 of the 19 local reformatory boys in the contrast group. Court contacts decreased among Achievement Place boys during the treatment, but increased among the boys at the reformatory.

According to Cornish and Clarke (1975) the more traditional models of residential care inevitably put the primary focus of therapy on changing the individual because the main source of behavioural variance is seen to lie within the individual. As Cornish and Clarke (1975, p. 36) put it:

The residential programme is seen to serve a similar function with regard to delinquency to that of the hospital in the treatment of physical or mental diseases; thus the individual is temporarily removed from an environment in which therapeutic measures cannot be satisfactorily organised. In the 'hospital' are provided both a temporary isolation from disease-provoking stimuli and, perhaps, more positive treatment facilities through which the 'disease' itself can be cured, and subsequent attacks prevented by the building up of an individual's resistance.

One explanation for the failure of institutional programmes which is some-times put forward is that the penal system is often naive about the extent to which changes in behaviour in one setting represent fundamental changes (e.g., in personality) and which, therefore, will accompany the youth when he returns to society — no matter what its temptations and deprivations. Ideas about punishment, discipline, training, rehabilitation, and treatment for the offender (as a rationale for his incarceration) seem to get hopelessly confused, in the theory *and* practice of these establishments. Whatever the stated theories or harsh expediences behind the rationale for herding offenders together in an institution, the power and influence of the deviant subculture thereby created are depressing obstacles to overcome.

CONTINGENCY MANAGEMENT

It has been conceded that the poor results quoted earlier mask some differences between types of residential treatment, some of which (as we have seen above) are more effective in dealing with offenders than others (Dunlop, 1975). Tutt (1976) believes that the variations are marginal. Sadly, the reality has to be faced that as matters stand at present there are not always alternatives to institutionalization available. In the wake of the failure of institutional environ-ments to provide effective amelioration, treatment of predelinquent and delinquent youths (in the United States in particular) has shifted increasingly to community-based settings. As we saw on page 236, recent years have also witnessed a growing awareness of the potential of local non-professional people in producing beneficial change (Cowen, Gardner, and Zax, 1967; Fo and O'Donnell, 1974).

A number of non-residential programmes have been implemented through parents and youth counsellors. This approach uses a triadic model of interven-tion. The successful application of a model of community intervention with youngsters in which non-traditional community workers functioned as agents of change (Tharp and Wetzel, 1969) involves direct modification of a youth's behaviour by changing the likelihood of its being performed. Behaviour modification techniques are used to manipulate the reinforcements which follow the forbidden activity in order to reduce its status in the individual's response hierarchy. The problem with most therapeutic interventions is that the antisocial activity may remain available as a potential response every time the individual is placed is an environment similar to that in which the original response was made; a return to old haunts may ensure that it comes to be strongly entertained again as a source of satisfaction. The novelty of the work of these authors is that they go into the youth's natural environment to counter this difficulty. They have implemented non-residential programmes using parents (as we saw in Chapter 6) but also youth counsellors, teachers, and friends.

A large-scale study was made with the single individual working as a consultant in an Appalachian community (Wahler and Erickson, 1969). Thirteen volunteers were trained to collect data prior to the following intervention for the 66 treated families. The volunteers treated a wide range of problems. On referral, the child, his immediate family and anyone else closely involved were interviewed by the clinic staff. The focus was on specifying the problem behaviours, and where possible their consequences. The psychologist then discussed the interview data with a volunteer consultant. Again the behaviours considered deviant were the focus, and the theory that these were being maintained by the responses of others in the child's environment was emphasized. A general discussion of reinforcement theory, extinction and punishment followed, and the psychologist would indicate his own hypotheses as to the maintaining reinforcers in the case under review, and ways of changing these.

At least two one-hour observations of the child in his natural environment were made by the volunteer consultant, using a check-sheet to record occurrence or non-occurrence of specified problem behaviour and its consequences in successive 20-second intervals. It was possible to carry out reliability tests with a second observer for half the volunteers: average agreement of 20-second observations exceeded 85 per cent. in all cases.

The volunteers and a staff member conducted a second interview with those members of the natural environment who 'seemed to provide clear and potentially modifiable contingencies for the child's deviant behaviour.' The specification of problem behaviours and the potentially reinforcing nature of social attention were explained to them, and they were instructed to ignore the problem behaviours but respond as usual to other behaviours, especially those which seemed incompatible with the problem ones. A time-out contingency was suggested for highly aggressive behaviour or behaviour otherwise impossible to ignore. It was explained to the parents that the volunteer worker would pay weekly visits to observe their interaction with their child, and suggest modifications.

While the volunteer was inexperienced these joint interviews with mediators took place every fortnight; when the staff member felt confident in the volunteer's understanding of the case, joint interviews were discontinued. The staff member and volunteer now met for supervision once a fortnight, with the focus on the child's progress and the mediators' maintenance of appropriate contingencies. Finally, the volunteer carried out two one-hour observations in the natural environment (as above) just after termination.

The presenting problems were classified in five categories: classroom disruptive behaviour (including shouting, fighting and disobedience); classroom study behaviour (attending to teaching materials or teacher); school absences; home disruptive behaviour (including fighting with siblings, parents or others, destructiveness and disobedience); and home study behaviour.

The 66 individual children often showed problem behaviours in several of these categories, thus a total of 197 behaviours were tackled. On average, occurrences of problem behaviours in the classroom-disruptive and home-disruptive categories fell (by termination) to one-third of their baseline levels. Classroom study behaviour was almost twice as frequent per time-period as at baseline, and home study behaviour was four times as frequent. School absences fell to just over a fifth of their baseline level.

All of these differences were statistically significant, so that some confidence can be placed in the reliability of measured improvement in all categories of behaviour. As the authors note, the lack of a control group means that the precise role of the therapeutic techniques and volunteer strategy cannot be asserted with the same confidence, though the results can be treated as tentative evidence for their effectiveness.

The cost in professional time, and the number and duration of cases, were amenable to a direct comparison with more traditional practice, since the two authors had seen children at the same clinic during an earlier year and employed traditional dyadic assessment and therapy. Twice as many cases were seen annually using the triadic model, and the number of weeks between screening and termination averaged 9 as compared with 19 during dyadic practice. The input of professional time per case was halved using the triadic model. Comparison of the effectiveness of the two approaches was not possible since there had been no evaluation of the dyadic practice.

Although Wahler and Erickson caution against interpreting their results as evidence for the effectiveness of behavioural intervention in the absence of a control group, some weight must be given to their study in the context of a coherent theory linking techniques and predicted effects, and in the context of a cumulative body of similar empirical findings. The distinctiveness of their project as a whole is the use of volunteers from the local community as consultants, who received if anything less training than Tharp and Wetzel's behaviour analysts; and who received all of their training in a form of apprenticeship. Unfortunately no follow-up data were collected.

One strategy in working with delinquent youths is to concentrate on increasing the youngster's repertoire of socially desirable behaviours. This may be carried out on an individual basis or in a group context. The number of behaviour modification group homes for predelinquent and delinquent youths is growing. In these projects the organizers have attempted to construct therapeutic micro-environments, which provide acceptance and the opportunity for new learning.

After all, the behavioural model which is thought to apply to most delinquents (see Stuart, 1971a) has three main elements: (1) inadequate reinforcement of positive behaviour within the family; (2) reinforcement of antisocial behaviour among peers, and (3) inadequate programming in school. What guarantees are there that these factors will have changed in any essential way when the boy leaves his special (and artificial) environment? Even the best treatment programmes may be doomed to failure given the lack of follow-up control over the youngster in his own environment after he completes treatment, and the relative absence of programmes to 'internalize' change (in institutions) by utilizing self-reinforcement programmes (see page 96).

GROUP PROGRAMMES

Two types of incentive system are used in structuring predictable consequences to behaviour in most behavioural treatment programmes for delinquent and predelinquent youths: the token economy and the behavioural contract. Points are earned in accordance with specified criteria or on the basis of staff ratings. These token economy programmes are fixed rather than flexible. There is a maximum number of points that can be earned in each of several categories, such as social behaviour, academic behaviour, and 'convenience' behaviour (behaviours deemed necessary for the smooth functioning of the programme). Points can also be earned by delinquents for improvements in their individual behaviour problems, behaviours which are often specified in a contract between the youth and his therapist (Cannon et al., 1972; Jesness and De Risi, 1973).

Achievement Place

There are programmes which have been designed to take into account several of the methods described above and to apply them systematically in planned environments. There has been a trend in the United States and elsewhere, away from the use of large penal institutions toward the establishment of small residential units. An outstanding example of such a unit as we saw earlier, employing token economy principles with delinquent and predelinquent boys is Achievement Place.

The rationale for this work is that the delinquent behaviour of these boys is the product of inadequate social learning experiences. As Phillips et al., (1971) put it:

> The cause of this disturbing behaviour is that the past environment of youths has failed to provide the instructions, examples, and feedback necessary to develop appropriate behaviour . . . and this general behavioural failure often forces the youth to become increasingly dependent upon a deviant peer group which provides inappropriate instructions, models and reinforcement that further expand the behaviour problems.

In trying to reverse such developments, the most important role of teaching-parents is educational. They teach youths a variety of social, academic, vocational, and self-help skills to equip them with alternative, more adaptive behaviours. The aim is to increase their chances of survival and success in the community. A very powerful and comprehensive token reinforcement system is established to develop specific social skills such as manner and introductions, academic skills, and personal hygiene habits. Unlike many treatment programmes with global objectives, the specific treatment aims are specified in great detail.

An advantage of operating a community-based programme is that it allows the teaching-parents to work directly with a young person in natural settings, such as his home (to which he typically returns on weekends) and the school (which he continues to attend). It is hoped that this increases the likelihood that prosocial behaviours acquired in these settings will persist even when he leaves the programme. Being community-based, this approach also allows the teaching-parents to monitor and, if necessary, to provide additional treatment for the youth after he moves away from the programme.

The evaluation of procedures has played a significant part in the development and refinement of the Achievement Place model. The majority of the original research publications evaluating Achievement Place were intraindividual reversal designs (ABAB) or variations on this theme (see Appendix A).

An evaluation of the Achievement Place model has been carried out at the programme level (Fixsen et al., 1972). Pre- and post-treatment comparisons were made *post hoc* between the first 16 youths treated at Achievement Place and 28 other youths who, in the opinion of the probation officer, could have been candidates for Achievement Place. Of these, 13 youths had been placed on formal probation and 15 had been placed in the state industrial school (Kansas Boys School, an institution for 250 boys). It should be noted that these data are only suggestive since these youths were not randomly assigned to the two groups. The preliminary follow-up results indicated that youths who participated in the Achievement Place programme were progressing better than comparable youths who were placed on probation or sent to the state training school. For example, only 20 per cent. of the Achievement Place youths required further treatment within 1 year after their release as compared to 44 per cent. of the training school youths and 55 per cent. of the probation youths.

Achievement Place youths and youths assigned to the Kansas School for Boys were most similar in terms of their prior offences, whereas the boys placed on probation had fewer offences than those assigned to Achievement Place or Kansas Boys School. While it is possible that other differences may have existed between boys assigned to the latter two facilities, the post-treatment differences in their recidivism and school attendances was dramatic — a tenfold difference in their school attendance.

Hoefler and Bornstein (1975) provide an evaluative review of the work carried out at Achievement Place. The model of 'teaching parents' and a family-style (but, nevertheless, controlled) environment has proved to be an ever-evolving system. Achievement Place has provided a refreshingly detailed account of procedural details so that other communities can establish similar facilities utilizing principles based on empirical data rather than arbitrary decisions. It should be possible to replicate the work and evaluate whether other 'teaching-parents' can produce beneficial changes similar to those of the first Achievement Place parents. This is a crucial matter because, although a good relationship between the youths and their teaching-parents is important, it can also be argued that this is not enough. Half-way house, family-style living arrangements, foster homes, and variations thereof have existed for years, but their efficacy with delinquents has not been demonstrated.

Case I and Case II projects

One of the pioneering efforts to deal with the enormous problems presented by delinquents was made by Cohen, Filipczak and Bis (1967) in projects called CASE I and II (contingencies applicable to special education) at the National Training School for Boys in Washington, D.C. Eighty-five per cent. of the subjects were school drop-outs with crime records including rape, car theft, and homicide. A special educational programme was made available to sixteen young men. Academic work, in the form of programmed learning, provided opportunities for the youths to earn points. These points could later be used to buy food-treats, material from a mail-order catalogue, admittance to the lounge, or to rent a private office with a telephone. Careful measurement of academic progress and time spent in the various activities afforded a demonstration of the success of the project. Although academic progress was the major preoccupation, changes in social behaviour were also noted.

The half-day programme — a pilot study — lasted from February 1964 to October 1965. Significant increases were found in academic progress and a significant mean gain of 12.5 IQ points on the 'revised beta' was found as well. In addition, social and attitudinal changes were found. There was a new pride of ownership in personal belongings and in living quarters. No discipline problems developed while subjects participated in the project, and the youths were found to be modelling the behaviour of the staff. They went so far as to acquire clothing similar to the staff's with some of their points.

The success of this programme convinced Cohen and his associates that a 24-hour programme (CASE II) would be a logical next stage. The basic premise of CASE II was that educational behaviour is functionally related to its consequences and that — by creating a situation in which appropriate consequences are made contingent upon changing behavioural requirements — these behaviours can be established, altered, maintained, and transferred.

The authors established a token economy programme in a four-storey hall on the grounds. The 41 young men in the new programme ranged in age from 14 to 18 (mean 16.9 years) and had been convicted of homicide, rape, thefts, and housebreaking. They spent an average of 18 months in this programme. The project emphasized training in social, vocational, self-help, and academic skills. (The 41 students were compared with a similar group of students from the standard training school programme.) They spent 6 hours a day working on programmed instructional material. A major way a student inmate could earn points for money was by studying. As Cohen and Filipczak (1971) put it, the model was 'that of a student research employee who checks in and out of various activities for which he is paid or for which he pays. As a Student Educational Researcher, the student was hired to do a job and paid to learn'. Points were received (token reinforcement) for completing the material at 90 per cent. accuracy. The points allowed them to purchase such back-up reinforcers as store items, the use of a lounge containing a television and jukebox, the use of a private room, and the use of a private office. Though the training school was a penal institution, choice in CASE II was maximized and arbitary orders from authority figures were kept to a minimum. In addition, in CASE II, a student-inmate coould receive points for exemplary social behaviour from officers. A learning environment which guaranteed privacy was available for students where they could work on self-contained, programmed instructional materials.

Effectiveness of CASE II as a learning environment was evaluated in terms of the youths' performance over time on standardized achievement and IQ tests. Cohen and Filipczak (1971) report that on two different achievement tests (Stanford achievement test) the youths averaged 1.5 and 2.0 grade level increases per year, respectively. Most of the youths located for this part had maintained or increased their achievement test scores. Thirty-one of the 41 youths who participated in the programme were located in a 3-year follow-up of the project. Twenty-seven of the located youths had been in the project at least 90 days. Eleven of these 27 youths were released directly from Case II and the remaining 16 were released from other penal programmes between 1 month and 2½ years later. Four (36 per cent.) of the 11 youths released directly from CASE II and 11 (69 per cent.) of the 16 youths released from other penal programmes required reinstitutionalization. Thus, 15 (56 per cent.) of the 27 youths had been reconvicted over the 3-year period. The first year following release the recidivism rate was two-thirds less than the norm for inmates at the National Training School. Unfortunately by the third year the total rate of recidivism appeared to be near the norm. As the investigators concluded, CASE delayed the delinquents' return to incarceration, but a special programme to maintain their lawful behaviour is necessary for the CASE programme to have effects after 1 year.

Hobbs and Holt (1976) have documented the effectiveness of a large-scale token-economy programme focusing on social behaviour (peer interaction), rule following, and task completion of 125 adolescent delinquent youths. The programme took place at the Alabama Boys Industrial School and was sequentially introduced in a multiple-baseline design in three independent cottages. A fourth group served as a comparison group. Appropriate

268

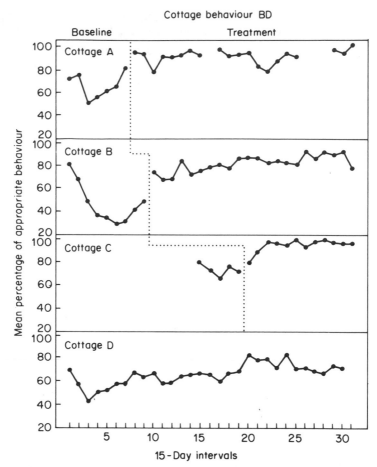

Figure 12   Cottage behaviour BD: mean percentage of appropriate behavour recorded during the 2-hour afternoon period. The time period extended from the group's return from school (or vocational assignment) to the evening meal. Each data point represents the mean percentage for a 15-day interval (From Hobbs and Holt, 1976)

behaviour increased from baseline means of 66, 46.7, and 73.2 per cent. to treatment means of 9.16, 80.8, and 94.2 per cent. for cottages A, B, and C respectively. An example of the improvement in behaviour during the activity period is given in Figure 12.

The behaviour change was maintained for periods ranging from 7 to 12 months depending upon the cottage involved, but the data do not apply to periods after release from the programme. So the generalization of treatment effects from a programme to a non-programme environment remains an unresolved issue. The authors discuss the financial costs of the programme as well as other 'costs' — ethical issues involving conflicts of interest between needs of staff and students.

The problem of 'phasing' members of a programmed environment back into the larger society was tackled by Martin et al., (1968). A group of nine adolescent delinquents displayed problems ranging from temper-tantrums to sexual promiscuity, and, in addition, they experienced difficulty over school-achievement. In the initial programme, they met in a special problems-class for 1 to 3 hours a week. The class utilized a token system in which points, earned by school progress, could be exchanged for canteen items. Five students were phased into full-time school by gradually increasing demands and decreasing concrete reinforcements. The amount of schoolwork increased while disruptive behaviour began to diminish. Moreover, both students and parents accepted the procedures and enjoyed the results. A 6-week follow-up found that school-appropriate behaviour was maintained and home adjustment (as indicated by parent reports) had improved. While Martin and his associates illustrate one approach to the problem of returning 'programmed subjects' to the natural environment, their conclusions are based on only five subjects.

A series of three studies (Bailey, Wolf, and Phillips, 1970) demonstrated the efficacy of home-based reinforcement contingent on school performance with five delinquent boys in the group home described on page 287. The authors developed a reinforcement procedure that did not require additional classroom personnel. The method consisted of giving a boy a 'daily report card' which was to be checked by the teacher. The card listed several categories of behaviour that were suggested by the teacher. Examples included: acceptable use of class time, following classroom rules, assignment completed on time, a grade of a certain level on an assignment or a quiz, and overall classroom behaviour. At the end of class the youth turned in the 'daily report card' to the teacher who simply marked each category ('yes' or 'no') to show how well he had behaved in class that day. The youngster then gave his completed card to the home staff. Privileges in the home were contingent on the teacher's judgement of his class performance. Using a reversal design, Bailey and his colleagues found that the youths' appropriate classroom behaviour improved from about 40 per cent. to approximately 90 per cent. when the daily report card was made use of in school. The report cards and reinforcement contingencies could be gradually faded out with no apparent decrement in performance. A rather sad study is provided by Kirigin et al. (1973). They evaluated several strategies to improve the independent reading behaviour of delinquent girls. These were point consequences for reading, point consequences plus tutoring, and finally a 'tutor-avoidance' condition where the girls could avoid the tutoring session through independent study. The only condition that produced an effect was the 'tutor-avoidance' condition, which suggested that for some individuals tutoring is an aversive event that can be used as an avoidance contingency.

SELF-GOVERNING BEHAVIOUR

Fixsen, Phillips, and Wolf (1973), as we saw on page 265, developed a system of self-government at Achievement Place in order to teach delinquent youths some of the social skills involved in group decision making and problem solving. The youngsters were taught to establish many of their own rules on a democratic basis. If one of them violated a rule they had to determine his guilt or innocence and decide on the consequences. These discussions occurred during daily 'family conferences'. In one of the experiments designed to evaluate how well youths participated in this system of self-government, it was clear that more boys took part in the discussion of consequences for a rule violation when they had complete responsibility for setting the consequences during family conferences than when staff determined the consequences for each rule violation before the family conference. An analysis of rule violations revealed that the boys reported more transgression than were reported by the teaching-parents, school personnel, or natural parents.

In a series of experiments reported by Phillips, Wolf, and Fixsen (1973), the researchers analysed several procedures for involving the youngsters in the routine administration of household chores in the home. Each method was evaluated in terms of its effectiveness in accomplishing the tasks and in terms of the preferences expressed by the youths. It was found that the procedure that met both criteria involved a democratically elected peer 'manager' who had the authority both to give and take away points for his peers' performances. The 'manager' could also earn or lose points depending upon how well the tasks had been accomplished.

VOCATIONAL SKILLS

The possession of vocational skills is important (as is academic performance) in the long-term adaptation to social living. An unusual study of vocational performance was conducted by Schwitzgebel (1964) and Schwitzgebel and Kolb (1964). They developed a Boston area street-corner research project. Twenty 15- to 21-year-old delinquents, each with multiple arrests and court appearances, were recruited from the streets and were paid an hourly wage to participate in taped interviews. The treatment was described to the delinquent youths as an experiment whose purpose it was to find out how teenagers feel about things, how they arrive at certain opinions, and how they change. The specific 'job' of the delinquent was to talk into a tape-recorder for which he was paid 1 dollar per hour. Each youth was also informed that other previous 'employees' had changed their minds about many things, but that such changes were not a job prerequisite. In the beginning of the treatment, these youths (with an average of 15.1 months of incarceration and an average of 8.2 arrests between them) were reluctant to come to the laboratory, and thus they were shaped to arrive there by having the experimenter meet the employee at various places which were successively closer to the laboratory. Thirty other delinquents served at matched controls. The treatment methods involved (1) avoidance of punishment and (2) modest reinforcers of cigarettes, small change, or food given intermittently for attendance. For 90 per cent. of the subjects, attendance became dependable within 15 appointments and prompt within 25 appointments. The tape-recorder interviews lasted for 1 hour, two or three times per week. Generally, the experimenter suggested topics to discuss and shared some personal experience with the youth. He reinforced the youth for particular types of verbalization with praise, small cash bonuses, or unexpected privileges. Advice giving was decidedly avoided. The youngster was encouraged to talk about his own experiences with emotion and in great detail. Through successive approximations and positive reinforcement these young men were taught social skills such as coming to work on time, being dressed appropriately, and limiting hostile statements in their conversation. All these could be helpful in holding down a job. In addition, they were taught to solder and other similar technical skills before they were helped to find jobs in the community. Termination of employment was gradual and individual; if a youth got an outside job which went well, the interviews were gradually dropped. If an outside job went poorly, interviews were increased. Generally, youths were associated with the project for 10 months. On follow-up 3 years later the arrest and conviction record of the first 20 subjects was about half of that of the control group. Unfortunately, the *number* of persons returned to prison or a reformatory did not differ. In other words, the project was associated with a reduction but not an elimination of delinquent behaviour. Of note, however, is the fact that the youths who participated in the experimental project seemed to have less serious offences and were arrested less frequently.

Schwitzgebel and Kolb (1964) do not choose delinquent behaviour as their target behaviour for direct modification. Instead of simply reinforcing delinquents for staying out of trouble the delinquents are taught behaviours which will be reinforced elsewhere or given legitimate jobs. As Schwitzgebel and Kolb (1964, p. 288) observe:

> The tone of the project was clearly not one of 'fighting' delinquency or delinquents but rather one of sympathy, firmness and sharing. The experimenters attempted to establish conditions in which subjects could become secure enough to share experiences, to express honest opinions, and to explore new ways of feeling and living — in short, to become good employees.

Ayala et al. (1973) worked out a set of procedures to improve performance by youths on a part-time job. Training consisted of instructing them in how to carry out tasks, demonstrating appropriate behaviour, and having them practise the appropriate behaviour. Feedback was provided during training and each day on the job. The results showed that training and feedback were effective in producing substantial improvements in the youngsters' behaviour at work. The research team found that with continued training the improved behaviour generalized to other work settings.

Braukmann et al. (1974) developed an 'instructional package' to teach job interview skills to delinquent boys in a group home. It contained a detailed description of appropriate interview behaviours and a detailed description of a training procedure consisting of instructions, demonstrations of appropriate behaviours, and differential feedback to the youth on his performance while rehearsing these behaviours during training. The authors conducted three experiments and found that the 'instruction package' was effective in training each youth appropriate interview behaviours.

Eitzen (1975) has made a study of the effects of behaviour modification on the attitudes of delinquents. We have seen how Achievement Place teaches delinquent youths some of the skills thought desirable by society. Eitzen notes that the dependent variable for behaviour modifiers has been limited to overt behaviour. Providing the behaviour of the youngster becomes more socially acceptable, it is of little importance to most therapists if there is a concomitant shift in attitudes. Eitzen challenges this indifference on two grounds: (1) an attitude change corresponding with a change in behaviour is likely to increase the probability of a lasting effect and (2) such an eventuality will make the case for behaviour modification more compelling to community agencies contemplating the direction to take in their efforts to attack a particular social problem. In order to assess whether the Achievement Place experience brings the attitudes for former delinquent boys in line with average boys, all eighth-grade boys from a Lawrence junior high school were given the same questionnaire. Eighth graders were selected because the average age of Achievement Place boys is 13 years. The junior high school chosen was sited in the school district in which most families of Achievement Place youngsters lived.

A questionnaire was designed which included scales of achievement orientation, internal–external attitudes, Machiavellianism, and self-esteem. It was administered to each boy at the beginning of his stay in Achievement Place, after 4 months, after 9 months, and at the completion of his stay. The findings are based upon responses from 21 boys, a few of whom did not participate in all of the testing phases. A children's version of Rotter's internal–external scale was used in this research. Upon entering the programme, the delinquent boys, as expected, tended to be externals, but by the time they left the average score had dropped below the mean of the control group in the internal direction. Some critics have speculated that children in a behaviour modification setting may become more manipulative and deceptive in their own social relationships because of their experiences of being the objects of modification by others more influential than themselves. The data on Machiavellianism, however, demonstrated that the Achievement Place experience did not lead to greater Machiavellian attitudes among the boys. As a group they entered Achievement Place with a mean slightly less Machiavellian that the control group and they remained remarkably consistent across time.

To determine the degree of self-esteem a semantic differential scale was included in the questionnaire. The youth was asked to rate himself on each of ten sets of bipolar adjectives (e.g., I am: good . . . bad, useful . . . useless). The data on self-concept showed that the Achievement Place experience was conducive to a good self-concept. As expected, the mean score of the entire group was significantly more negative in self-esteem than the control group mean. The greater the length of stay in Achievement Place, however, the less negative the self-concept. The post-test group mean was not only significantly different from the pre-test mean but those completing the programme also differed significantly from the control group, this time in the positive direction. When the data were analysed across time for each boy it was discovered that 88 per cent. of the boys improved in self-concept. Analysed in another way, 80 per cent. of the boys entering Achievement Place were *above* the control group mean (i.e. had a more negative self-concept), while 75 per cent. of the boys at the post-test administration of the questionnaire were now *below* the control group mean. The longer the stay at Achievement Place, the greater the improvement in self-concept. Accompanying the behavioural changes of these delinquent boys are positive shifts in attitudes. The greatest shifts in attitudes were from poor to good self-esteem and from externality to internality. The author poses the unsolved problem: are these positive attitudinal changes a function of the treatment model or the result of placing troubled boys in stable environment with caring 'parents'?

No matter how enlightened and apparently effective a therapeutic programme may be within an institution, a custodial sentence carries with it two inescapable problems. As Walker (1972, p. 99) explains:

One of these is the difficulty, under conditions so unlike those of real life, of telling whether, and if so when, reformation has been achieved. Conformity under the strict regime of a prison is no indication that the prisoner has become law-abiding. It is true that there are custodial institutions — especially for the young — where the regime is designed so as to test the offender's responsibility, self-control and other qualities that will help him to lead a law-abiding life outside; but the staff of such establishments are the first to admit that they are often wrong in predicting subsequent success or failure for individual inmates. The other inescapable problem is the unwanted by-products of custody. The inmate loses his job, is separated from his family and is compelled to associate with other delinquents. Even in the best-run systems, prison work is seldom more than a way of reducing the economic burden which prisoners represent, and of weaning them from idleness: it is only in the exceptional case that the prisoner learns a trade which he afterwards takes up.

Walker points out that these are ancient and hackneyed arguments and do not constitute conclusive arguments for the total abolition of custodial sentences. The evidence from the smaller community-based homes is at least promising, but the perennial problem of a reversion to old ways when the offender returns to his own environment has not been resolved. Cornish and Clarke (1975) argue, therefore, for more home-based or home-linked therapy of the behavioural kind.

Walker (1972) argues that the reduction of prohibited conduct must be the main aim of any penal system, but must be tempered by both economic

274

considerations and humanity if the system is to be practicable and tolerable. He concludes that the aims which raise serious difficulties are retribution and denunciation. If we accept this prescription and his recognition (commonly held among criminologists and clinicians) that efforts to bring about change are more likely to work when the offender is young, then a dispassionate, non-elitist (i.e., economic) therapeutic programme would seem to be called for — one which operates as close to his natural environment and as early in his path towards delinquency as is humanly possible.

EVALUATION

Despite some promising findings, a realistic assessment of the overall results of behavioural work with juvenile delinquents must concede their somewhat disappointing nature. It is true that behaviour modification programmes employed to enhance a variety of prosocial activities and to reduce several classes of antisocial actions in juvenile delinquents have been found generally effective (Brauckmann and Fixsen, 1975; Burchard and Harig, 1976; Davidson and Seidman, 1974; Farrington, 1979; Ollendick, Elliott, and Matson, 1980). However, the major gap in our knowledge has to do with prognosis. A majority of the experimental studies reviewed by Davidson and Seidman (1974) and Stumphauzer (1970) fail to report any subsequent follow-up of their subjects.

Person variables such as locus of control cannot be disregarded. Jesness and De Risi (1973) demonstrated that juvenile delinquents who have a capacity for insight and responsibility and who are internally oriented with regard to locus of control respond most favourably to behavioural programmes. Ollendick et al. (1980) used a fixed token economy and a flexible behavioural contracting system in a treatment programme for 90 delinquent adolescents. Although the overall programme resulted in a relatively low recidivism rate (38 per cent.), the findings relating to locus of control are particularly significant. Internally oriented youths committed fewer offences during the institutional programme and manifested lower recidivism rates 1 year after discharge; externally oriented youths derived less benefit from the programme and evidenced higher rates of reconviction.

The authors state that 'such findings tend to affirm the basic principles underlying the social learning approach to treatment; namely, that behaviour is learned and maintained through a reciprocal interaction between the person and his environment' (p. 261).

What seems clear is that adolescents, in a general sense, are more difficult to treat than younger children, because they are more self-directed and yet, at the same time, more under the influence of the peer group. Life is more open-ended for the young adult than the child, and therefore it may be difficult to manage the contingencies in his environment. These factors, however, can be capitalized upon. The budding self-direction may become the cornerstone of a self-control programme; the tendency to emulate admired peers may be harnessed by providing peer models of desirable behaviour. Feldman (1977), cites the failure of a home-based behavioural programme (Weathers and Liberman, 1975) with 28 adolescents on probation, and notes that any natural environment programme, to be successful, must involve peers as well as parents.

Where there *is* the possibility of structuring the youngster's environment through the systematic application of operant and classical conditioning procedures (i.e., in the institutional environment), that very capacity to exert far-reaching control over rewards and punishments does promote prosocial behaviour, but the gains prove ephemeral. This failure of 'treatment' programmes (of the token economy kind) during institutional interventions is due to the problem of generalizing behaviour gains to the post-institutional environment or of countering their extinction there. The possibilities of self-reinforcement have yet to be given a proper trial.

What we have, at present, are numerous reports of behavioural approaches to juvenile offenders that indicate, at the least, an encouraging level of success in improving several classes of behaviour, such as academic achievement and related school behaviour, socially cooperative behaviour within specially designed treatment centres, and some conduct and delinquent problems in natural settings (Davidson and Seidman, 1974; Herbert, 1987a; Henderson and Hollin, 1983).

CASE STUDY

Wetzel (1966) describes the use of a response-cost procedure in the treatment of a problem of compulsive stealing. A 10-year-old boy named Mike had a long history of uncontrollability and stealing. After he had been placed in a Home for mildly disturbed children, his behaviour improved somewhat, with the exception of his stealing and bed-wetting. Dinsmoor (1966), in a paper published in the same journal shortly afterwards, commented on the historical importance of Wetzel's treatment/research design. He modelled his study on the single-organism, within-subject design that had become traditional in recent years in 'free operant studies' of animals. The main comparison was between the performance of the same individual during two or more periods in time and not between the performance of two or more groups of subjects. This eliminated the contribution of individual differences in the confounding of the comparison. Unfortunately it also raised new problems such as sequence effects. One might also add that it is one thing to elaborate intra-subject designs with animals, but quite another matter to play the laboratory scientist with human beings.

However, to return to Mike's problems, the target behaviour was his compulsive stealing. It had been occurring with substantial frequency for at least five years. This knowledge provided an indirect base line. The history was supplemented by a period of direct quantified observation. The proposition put forward by Wetzel was that if a child behaves in more or less the same fashion, within narrow limits, for a considerable period of time, and then

276

changes when conditions are altered, neither *random variation nor environmental accident* seem likely to explain the change in behaviour. Such an argument is strengthened if repeated changes can be produced in the child's behaviour by repeatedly changing the 'experimental conditions', that is to say, the treatment.

The child care workers were told that whenever the property of another person, the school, or the home was found on Mike's person, in his locker, or in his room, and it was determined that the property had not been legitimately given to him, they were (a) to record a stealing incident on a daily chart and (b) when the time came, report the incident to Maria, the cook in the Home. Maria was instructed to keep a record of sessions she missed with Mike because of his stealing. (Dinsmoor (1966) comments that the range and sensitivity of the record could have been increased by plotting the number — rather than only the presence or absence — of stealing episodes per day).

Once a week the charts were collected and transferred to a cumulative record. Each step up represented one or more stealing incidents for a given day. The period of observation covered approximately 5 months and 1 week. The 4 days around Christmas which Mike spent out of the home were not recorded since observation was impossible.

A programme of response-cost was applied to his problem. A deliberately fostered relationship between Mike and Maria was made use of in the treatment. Conventional punishment of the stealing was not thought desirable. Mike had shown himself resistant to the usual consequences of stealing. Scoldings and disapproval by the child-care workers, the anger of peers, and the return of the objects all had no effect on the stealing rate. The history indicated that assorted punishments (including spanking and isolation) prior to his admission to the Home had been ineffective. The general policies of the Home, moreover, encouraged only the most minimal and judicious use of punishment. There was no doubt that a great deal of attention was paid to Mike's stealing. He had developed an extensive repertoire of excuses and explanations which could hold the attention of a child-care worker often for an hour. Mike's relationship with Maria, although friendly, was only a casual one, so it was necessary to intensify it to give it effective reinforcing value. It was explained to Maria that she seemed to play an important role in Mike's life at the Children's Home and that it would be helpful if she could become even more important to him. She was also asked whether she would eventually help Mike with his main difficulty, stealing. Maria agreed to cooperate in creating opportunities for this relationship to form the basis of social reinforcement for appropriate behaviour by the boy. A plan was devised whereby she saw Mike daily. He was invited into the kitchen, prepared Mexican foods, and was taken to Maria's home for visits. Maria mended his clothes, and took him shopping and to church. In a few days, Mike apparently was looking forward to his visits and Maria, in turn, became especially fond of him. Four weeks were allowed for the relationship with Maria to develop. The child-care workers were instructed to continue the recording they had begun in the training sessions during this time. They were told, also, to handle the stealing in their customary way. Although there was a reduction in stealing behaviour immediately following the beginning of the visits with Maria, the rate soon returned to its original level. During the treatment phase, it was arranged that Maria would be told whenever Mike was found to have stolen something; as soon as possible she would then say to him, 'I'm sorry you took so-and-so's . . . because now I can't let you come home with me tonight'. She would not enter into any further discussion of the matter with him. This constituted the 'cost' of stealing.

In the later stages of the programme, a positive reinforcement programme for non-stealing was added. This proved a difficult criterion to schedule, however, and the only solution seemed to be to reinforce at certain intervals as long as he did not steal. The problem was resolved on 'bank day' when the children banked part of the money they had earned for chores, or had otherwise accumulated. At a certain point in treatment, instead of banking, Mike divided his money between two boys, stating that it was to replace some articles he had previously taken and lost, and announced that he was 'not stealing any more'. It was the first instance of definable 'non-stealing' be-haviour and was strongly reinforced by the supervisor and child-care staff with praise. According to the records kept, after 3½ months on the regime, stealing had stopped completely, and this continued during another 2 months of systematic follow-up. As so often happens outside the laboratory (that is to say, in the hurly burly of practice in the natural environment), the staff made errors in the administration of the programme and this places a question mark on the cause–effect relationship. However, Dinsmoor (1966) observes that a long horizontal segment on the graphical record covering the last month-and-a-half of the study indicates that a substantial and persistent change had occurred in the child's behaviour. Wetzel (1966), in discussing this case, raises an impor-tant issue. He points out that the successful application of behavioural techni-ques to the modification of deviant behaviour probably depends on several conditions not specified by principles of reinforcement. For example, in the middle of this study Mike was shown the charts and informed of how his stealing eliminated a visit with Maria for the day. Although this event was not dictated by reinforcement principles, it might very well have influenced the effectiveness of the contingency. As we saw on page 89, it has been demons-trated that the reinforcing value of a stimulus may be a function of whether or not the subject perceives the reinforcement to depend on his own behaviour (skill) or the whims of the environment (chance) (James and Rotter, 1958). Likewise, contingency management in a natural setting tends to produce several changes in the relationship between an individual and his environment (and Maria and Mike are a case in point) well beyond the scope defined by the target behaviour. The nature of these changes and their contribution to the outcome are not always described or assessed in studies of environmental manipulation. Wetzel (1966) remarks that though the technique of interven-tion may be the establishment of a particular reinforcement contingency, several other factors must be considered if the success of the technique is to be evaluated. So far, these additional conditions have been 'ad libbed' or managed on the basis of 'clinical intuition'.

13

General Issues

All forms of therapy — and there are many — are in the business of producing change. They all probably contain a learning element. Indeed, Goldstein, Heller, and Sechrest (1966, p.213) propose the following definition of psychotherapy:

Whatever else it is, psychotherapy must be considered a learning enterprise. We need not specify too narrowly just what it is to be learned in psychotherapy; it may be specific behaviours or a whole new outlook on life, but it cannot be denied that the intended outcome of psychotherapy is a change in an individual that can only be termed a manifestation of learning.

In behavioural therapies the learning element is central and it gives rise to two fundamental questions: (1) how effective is a learning-based therapeutic method in generating change and (2) what are the ethics of the means and ends involved in such an approach?

THE EFFECTIVENESS OF BEHAVIOUR MODIFICATION

No treatment procedure can be said to be effective unless the stability of improvements has been demonstrated over time. This calls for systematic follow-up studies. These are sparse in number, not only for behaviour therapy but for all kinds of psychological treatment of problematic behaviour in children.

The task of validating behaviour modification — an approach encompassing so many specific techniques and, in practical application, many uncontrolled

280

non-specific variables — is highly complex. There is little doubt in the author's mind (and hopefully this book provides some evidence) that the field of behaviour modification has developed a powerful technology for changing a variety of child problems in the home (Kazdin, 1979; Patterson, 1975; Wahler, 1976) and classroom (O'Leary and O'Leary, 1976). The outcomes of such interventions are positive and can be replicated. They provide substantial support for the efficacy of a behavioural approach to child treatment.

O'Leary, Turkewitz, and Taffel (1973) found (for the behavioural treatment of 70 cases in an out-patient training clinic) that the average improvement rate as reported by therapists (87 per cent.) and parents (90 per cent.) was substantially higher than that reported by Levitt (1963) in his survey of child-clinic psychotherapeutic outcomes (65 per cent). Furthermore, the specific problem-improvement rate reported by parents (77 per cent.), on average 6 months later, was strikingly higher than the improvement rate (54 per cent.) reported by Gluck et al. (1964). The authors note that although it is not possible to specify the improvement rate of control subjects with problems similar to those in this sample, the improvements measured were high. The parents in this sample specifically attributed these improvements to their contact with the clinic, as opposed to ordinary process of maturation, in 71 per cent. of the problems.

But what constitutes an improvement? How much of an improvement will suffice? Should a problem behaviour be eradicated altogether in all situations and for ever? Or should the therapist be satisfied with a more modest reduction in the frequency of deviant behaviour, say a 25 per cent. or 50 per cent. decrement. There is no simple answer. It depends on the problem behaviour, its implications, the context within which it occurs and so on. As with the criteria of what constitutes a problem it is more a value/social question than a scientific one.

There is a great deal of unpredictability in the effects of behavioural interventions. The therapist soon learns that techniques which yield the most impressive results are not always effective with all types of problem or with all children. Furthermore, to his (and everyone else's) frustration, a given technique may, on one day, produce complete control in the case of a particular child, but on the next have no apparent effect at all. With regard to places, numerous studies have demonstrated that behaviour modification procedures can be applied successfully in such varied settings as clinics, mental hospitals, schools, homes, and residential facilities for delinquent or handicapped populations. However, only rarely is there an 'automatic' transfer of improvement from one situation to another (a matter we return to shortly).

The weight of evidence in favour of the efficacy of behavioural treatment is cumulative. Although success has been reported in a wide variety of individual cases, there is a relative lack of studies using 'no-treatment' or 'other-treatment' control groups to which subjects are randomly assigned. Relevant control groups are undoubtedly difficult to find. Therapies and therapists are difficult to equate and a sufficient number of cases with the same problem behaviour are rarely available. In most of the work reported so far, each child has acted as his own control, being assessed before and after the intervention. Such designs provide useful correlational support for an association between the therapeutic intervention and the outcome, especially (some would claim) if the reinforcement contingencies are reversed in an intrasubject replication design. However, they cannot establish definitive evidence (although they may collectively provide support) for the existence of cause–effect relationships. The issues involved in research designs for assessing treatment are discussed in Appendix A.

Unfortunately, the studies that illustrate the unpredicted counterproductive effects or non-effects of differential social attention procedures in the treatment of conduct problems have failed to offer satisfactory explanations for them. The point has been made by many theorists that demanding children (they are proactive as well as reactive) create situations in which their hapless mothers — and fathers — feel themselves forced to follow virtually every childish action with attention. That means, in effect, that the therapeutic use of differential attention consists almost entirely of removing social attention following unwanted behaviour, rather than increasing the rate of reinforcement (attention) for prosocial behaviours, or shifting attention from undesired to desired activities. Then again, categories of child behaviour targeted for modification in each of these investigations tend to be global categories (e.g., disruptive, negativistic, deviant, inappropriate behavioiurs) rather than clearcut, precisely defined actions. Thus behavioural techniques are applied in a hit-and-miss manner to multiple, diverse behaviours of an unacceptable kind — providing an ambiguous learning situation for both parents and child.

The elusive goal still remains the one of achieving a long-term maintenance of change after the termination of treatment. There is a paucity of research on the temporal generality of therapeutic effects. What evidence exists is somewhat equivocal, with reasonable maintenance reported by some workers (Patterson and Fleischman, 1979; Wells, Griest, and Forehand, 1980) but discouraging returns to baseline, or worse, reported by others (e.g., Wahler and Fox, 1980).

Coercive children and many of the members of their families (as we saw earlier) lack self-control skills. A strategy that has been successfully used to assist in maintaining positive change is to instruct the parents in self-control (Brown et al. 1976; Wells et al., 1980). The central issue in self-control is a temporal one: coercive children show an excessive orientation towards immediate reinforcement and an inability to foresee, or be motivated by, longer-term consequences. The use and development of self-control procedures has flourished (S. G. O'Leary and Dubey, 1979) and may contribute to long-term improvements.

Bandura (1969) reminds us that learning theory shifted the focus of causal analysis from hypothesized inner determinants to detailed analysis of external influences on responsiveness. Human behaviour was increasingly examined in terms of the stimulus events that evoke it and the reinforcing consequences that change it. Researchers repeatedly demonstrated that response patterns, generally attributed to underlying forces, could be induced, eliminated, and reinstated simply by varying external sources of influence. Mischel (1968) emphasized the large component of specificity in behaviour. Indeed, situation specificity is the key to assessing therapy. In a sense there are two therapeutic objectives in working with children:

(1) To enhance a child's responses to the controlling factors in his environment without deliberately altering the latter. Assuming a family environment to be essentially satisfactory, one might attempt to adjust a child to it.
(2) To change the controlling factors in an unsatisfactory learning environment as a means of modifying problem behaviour.

Where the latter strategy is predominant the therapeutic objective is to programme the environment so that it sustains the child's (and parents') 'improvement' after the formal programme is terminated. The long-term purpose of this phase of therapy is to help parents to become more systematic in their own behaviour so as to be more effective in managing their children. The data reviewed in this book certainly suggests that parents can learn to control their own behaviour, which in turn helps to maintain the levels of desirable behaviour in their children.

It must be admitted that there are special problems in assessing the success of therapy in young children. There could easily be a double standard at work in the behaviour modifier's stringent criterion of stability of 'improvement' in his child patients, which he would not apply to changes in behaviour in (say) his or her own offspring. Depending on the age of the child, parents have to go on and on repeating themselves in the attempt to socialize their children: rewarding them, instructing them, and rehearsing them in prosocial behaviours, while applying sanctions and chiding them for 'deviant' behaviour — month in and month out, and sometimes year in and year out. This goes on until the child has certain crucial social behaviours (or the control of antisocial behaviours) as habitual (internalized) parts of his repertoire. Others behaviours will always remain, to varying degrees, under the control of external contingencies. Time-scales vary, depending on the age and maturity of the child and the nature of the behavioural task, but parents should not (and usually do not) expect the child to acquire and maintain certain lessons without setbacks and frequent reminders. Although some therapists pay lip-service to returning the child to an environment which will 'naturally' maintain the target behaviours, precise attention is not always paid to whether this actually happens. And when it does not, the therapy of the child has somehow failed. What has failed is the modification and maintenance of an environment that will promote the new behavioural repertoire of the once-deviant child. The easy availability of brief booster sessions as a routine post-treatment procedure would seem to be essential. A promising and increasingly popular approach to the generalization problem is represented by attempts to provide the child with self-regulating strategies which can be applied across a number of situations. At the highest level of functioning, mature individuals regulate their own behaviour by self-evaluative and other self-administered consequences. Self-instruction training (Meichenbaum, 1973) has led to changes which are maintained once training is terminated. Tangible self-reinforcement and symbolic rewards can be used to maintain new patterns of behaviour until they become a source of personal satisfaction. While this may be a desideratum of treatment, especially with more mature individuals, the behaviour of children is very much under the control of external contingencies and the relative generality of responses (implicit in self-regulation) is the exception rather than the rule.

Society puts a high value on the inhibition of certain behaviours, such as aggressive or sexual impulses, because these are difficult to enforce by continuing external controls. A survey (Herbert, 1974) of research and theory on the mechanisms of socialization reflects the centrality of this issue for understanding the transition of the infant from an impulsive, uncontrolled organism into a social being who is able to exert a reasonable degree of self-restraint. Early manifestations of self-control are encouraged during childhood training by many parents, especially in middle-class families. In Chapter 2 we discussed the use of guilt to control socially undesirable behaviour. The common disciplinary and other child-rearing methods for developing resistance to temptation were reviewed. Just as the development of self-regulation has been viewed consistently as one of the most important objectives of the socialization process, therapeutic procedures which can be brought under the control of the individual himself are most beneficial (see Jehu et al., 1972). There are several advantages such as the possibility of (say) a delinquent maintaining or modifying certain aspects of his own actions by symbolic rewards or sanctions which are relatively independent of the contingencies operating in his present environment. This may be crucial if it is a deviant environment.

In day-to-day life, much of the reinforcement that maintains behaviour is self-reinforcement or internalized feedback that the person gives himself for his activities. We are not dealing with an 'empty organism', but human beings who think and enjoy an *inner life*. Various discriminative stimuli serve as a means of self-reinforcement in addition to being cues or signals. In the case of a young child they are frequently things that are observable, but for the adult or older child they are often internalized. The kind of approach which encourages self-regulation is particularly helpful when desirable environmental consequences are unavailable, likely to be postponed or simply outside the control of the therapist. If these problems obtain, self-management is likely to be an important means of achieving the generalization and persistence of therapeutic changes.

There is evidence to suggest that such changes are enhanced if the person perceives them as to be generated by himself rather than by the therapist or anyone else (Brehm and Cohen, 1962). Goodlet and Goodlet (1969) and Bolstad and Johnson (1972) have shown that aggressiveness can be eliminated (by having boys reward themselves for reductions in aggressive behaviour) as well as or better than by having adults evaluate and reward their improved conduct. Another pressing reason for fostering self-control as a goal of treatment is the fact of life that the therapist is not a clairvoyant, and therefore cannot foretell all the circumstances in which the youth will find himself. Therefore he needs to provide the youngster with a repertoire of self-regulation so that he will be able to cope with circumstances as they arise. A major limitation in using self-control procedures, as Jehu (Jehu et al., 1972) points out, is their restriction to motivated and cooperative clients who are capable of monitoring,, reporting, and manipulating their own behaviour and the situations in which it occurs. These constraints apply particularly to younger children. Children at different levels of development, with different types of problems, will, of course, require different programmes. Self-regulation (or self-management) interventions are not always appropriate.

If the goal of treatment is the maintenance of improvement after the termination of therapy, then a well-designed behaviour modification programme will involve a specification of the environment in which the individual normally lives and a provision for establishing and strengthening behaviour that is desired or useful in that environment. This is the 'functional' criterion mentioned on page 18). Of primary concern is a *planned* transition between the therapeutic programme and the natural environment. Generalization of behavioural changes needs to be programmed (Baer, Wolf, and Risley, 1968; Kazdin and Bootzin, 1972). There is evidence that treatment effects tend to be specific to the setting(s) in which they are produced; that is to say, that 'unprogrammed' generalization of treatment effects to non-treatment settings is the exception rather than the rule (Davison and Taffel, 1972; Wildman and Wildman, 1975). Herein lies the theoretical superiority of intervention in the natural environment; it circumvents (at least partially) the problem of generality and persistence of change that occurs in institution-based treatment.

Wahler (1969b) argues that the lack of generality can be explained in terms of the environmental antecedents and consequences that operate in different settings. If there is congruence between the settings events and contingencies in a child's home and school environments (to take one example), then his behaviour in these two settings are likely to show greater similarity. Alternatively, if there is a poor 'match' in these setting events and contingencies, his behaviour in the two settings would understandably be less similar. Thus, if stimulus variables and/or reinforcement contingencies are altered in order to change behaviour in one setting, one would not necessarily expect the changed behaviour to generalize to other settings in which these variables have not been altered.

Gelfand and Hartmann (1975) admit that preventing the child's behaviour from reverting to pre-treatment patterns soon after the cessation of treatment is one of the most intractible problems associated with behaviour modification programmes. They point out that if such a reversion occurs, the child will have benefited only briefly from the programme; he and his family might become unduly fatalistic and disillusioned about the possibility of his ever improving. In other words, in some instances an untimely relapse might exacerbate an already fraught situation. What then can be done? It may be possible to promote stimulus and response generalization by making the treatment setting as similar as possible to the child's natural environment. This involves stimulus generalization; similar situations tend to elicit the same behaviour, and the more parallel the situations can be made, the greater is this tendency. With regard to the response side, it has been shown that a situation which elicits one response is likely to evoke similar responses. There is a gradient of response generalization according to the degree of similarity between responses. One way to programme response maintenance and transfer of training is to develop the target behaviour in a variety of situations and in the presence of several individuals. If the response is associated with a range of places, individuals, situations, and other cases, it is less likely to extinguish when the settings vary.

Goocher and Ebner (1968) varied stimulus settings in developing appropriate classroom behaviour in a deviant child. At first, training was carried out in the presence of a single experimenter in a special room set aside for training. The child was praised and given sweets for paying attention to a task. Gradually, planned distractions such as television and other individuals passing by were introduced. Training was transferred to the classroom itself in the presence of other children. Throughout training, maladaptive behaviour increased whenever distracting stimuli were introduced, but it quickly extinguished. Appropriate behaviour was maintained in the classroom for 9 months after training had been terminated.

It is possible to reinforce behaviour in other ways which are likely to facilitate its persistence. An intermittent schedule of reinforcement might be used, as behaviour which has been reinforced in this way requires fewer reinforcements to maintain it and it takes longer to extinguish after the cessation of reinforcement. Similarly, we have seen how artificial reinforcers in treatment such as tokens or material rewards are gradually replaced by others like social attention and approval which are more likely to apply after treatment ends. An abrupt transition from a rich reinforcement schedule in a behaviour modification programme to a lean one following treatment (or indeed, one in which *no* provision is made for the administration of reinforcers) is often the equivalent of placing the desired target behaviour on an extinction schedule. A gradual modulation is possible using *fading procedures* or other scheduling techniques. A fading procedure changes the environmental stimuli so that they approximate more closely those natural conditions that are likely to prevail following the end of formal treatment. Reinforcement schedule transitions have to be introduced *gradually over a period of time*.

Gelfand and Hartmann (1975, p.251) offer advice on how to proceed in order to maintain the level of behaviour achieved during the therapeutic intervention at that critical termination juncture:

> The wise therapist incorporates increasing intermittency of reinforcement into the treatment whenever circumstances permit . . . If you have

been applying a fixed-interval or fixed-ratio schedule, introduce a less predictable variable schedule prior to termination. The variable schedule more nearly matches most naturally occurring schedules and so blends well into the child's everyday routine. If you have applied a variable schedule since the inception of treatment, increase its intermittency until the natural environment's schedule is closely approximated . . . It is advisable to thin the schedule gradually. Sometimes the process of thinning the reinforcement schedule produces a performance loss. This problem is relatively easily remedied, however. Should the target behaviour decrease appreciably in rate following an increase in performance requirements to earn each reinforcer, you must revert to the immediately preceding schedule, restabilize this behaviour, and then introduce a less dramatic schedule change. (Note that this procedure is similar to that employed whenever introduction of a new performance requirement disrupts the process of shaping). In so far as possible, avoid large magnitude and sudden reductions in the frequency of reinforcement of the desired behaviour.

In another approach the therapist fades out special and perhaps artificial discriminative stimuli used in the behavioural programme so that the targeted behaviour is evoked in situations where the control is exerted through appropriate cues. These should be present in the child's natural environment (see Hawkins et al., 1966). It is not always necessary to arrange special measures for the purpose of prolonging treatment effects; the intervention may strengthen skills or remove inhibitions so that the client gains access to existing sources of reinforcement, or it might reduce the aversiveness of his behaviour for himself or others and thus entail reinforcing consequences.

Overlearning is another protection against relapse; it involves plentiful (and redundant) practice well beyond the point at which the child has acquired new behaviours and skills.

An example of behaviour patterns that tend to persist once they have been produced are peer interactions among children (see Allen et al., 1965). Baer and Wolf (1970) have formulated the concept of a 'behaviour trap' — a behaviour pattern which, once begun, produces environmental consequences that maintain the behaviour. Guiding children into such traps appears to be highly desirable if behaviour change is to persist in the environment. Having claimed that it is unlikely that techniques designed to delay extinction or relapse can have permanent success unless the changes are supported by the environment, it underlines the necessity for developing procedures for training parents to deal with their problem children.

A novel and useful elaboration in the training of parents as 'behavioural modifiers' is reported by Brown and his colleagues, arising out of their work at a reeducation school in Kentucky (Brown et al., 1976). They note that while the effects of contingency management have been shown to be effective in training parents, little attention has been given to the maintenance of these effects. The results are often short-lived. The positive behaviour change tends to fade as contact with the therapist is lessened. They suggest that one method of helping maintain therapeutic effects is to transfer the control from the therapist to the client; the cardinal feature of self-control, after all, is that it is the individual himself who is the agent of his own behavioural change. Brown et al., describe the classic choice situation which invites a self-control approach; given any problem behaviour on the part of the child, the parents have the choice of either suppressing undesirable behaviour or encouraging appropriate behaviour. While the suppression of undesirable behaviour is an immediate way to handle a specific problem (sometimes with an immediate pay-off) parents who really make use of self-control techniques will be more likely to use praise or positive reinforcement to increase the probability of continued positive behaviour in the future. The parent can choose either the immediate punishing contingencies in attempting to suppress the problem behaviour or the distant contingencies, which will probably have greater long-range benefits for the parent and the child. Here then are the three important features of self-control phenomena: (1) they always involve two or more alternative behaviours; (2) the consequences of those behaviours are usually conflicting; and (3) the self-regulatory pattern is usually prompted and/or maintained by external factors such as its long-term effects. The authors take into account these features in systematically training parents to produce desirable behaviour in their children — a project which has produced encouraging results.

Self-reinforcement procedures are implemented for the mothers once contingency management procedures have demonstrated their effects in improving the rate of desirable behaviour, or reducing the level of maladaptive behaviour in their children. The primary purpose of this phase is to help parents become more systematic in their own behaviour; it is hypothesized that they will then be more effective in managing their children. Parents are instructed to present themselves with a reward after having exhibited a desirable behaviour. For example, a parent might say to herself 'I am a good mother' each time she praises a child's desirable behaviour or ignores deviant behaviour. In addition, parents choose to treat themselves with a cigarette or a cup of coffee, contingent upon a desired performance.

SYMPTOM SUBSTITUTION

Many theorists and practitioners regard as symptoms (the outward and visible signs of underlying disorder) what the behaviourally oriented therapists regard as the focus of treatment. It is often argued that a failure to deal with underlying problems (e.g., intrapsychic conflicts) leads to 'symptom substitution'. Just how one defines operationally such a construct is never made clear. Without measureable indices of 'substitution' — a clear-cut way of specifying the links, symbolic or otherwise, between symptoms — the criticism is impossible to prove *or* disprove. Studies (e.g., Baker, 1969) designed (*inter alia*) to investigate whether *other* problems appear when behavioural programmes have successfully removed symptoms (such as enuresis, a problem often found in association with conduct problems) do not indicate that such an eventuality occurs. Indeed, Baker reports that children who have been treated behaviourally often show improvements in areas that had not been specific targets of the behaviour therapy.

It may be that serious problem behaviour blocks the child from engaging in behaviour that might be a source of positive reinforcement for him from parents and peers, the absence of which hinders his socialization and development of a prosocial repertoire of behaviours. The answer to fears about symptom substitution is to avoid metaphors such as 'underlying' and 'deep-seated' causes, but to carry out rigorous and comprehensive assessment into *all* the contributary causal factors which have a bearing on planning successful treatments. The safety net is to engage in thorough and systematic follow-ups after therapy is terminated.

RELATIONSHIP

In evaluating the effectiveness of any therapeutic procedure, it is important to consider the non-specific factors that operate not only in the behavioural approach but also in most other forms of treatment. These non-specific factors include placebo influences and the therapeutic relationship. Shapiro's (1975) review of the literature on psychotherapy research suggests that the findings do not justify, and may indeed make untenable, the view that social relationships have no place in the modification of psychological disturbances. He states that the client-centred therapeutic conditions of empathy, warmth, and genuineness (Truax and Carkhuff, 1967) may serve as a useful adjunct to behaviour therapy. Two studies have found the level of the Truax conditions offered by interviewers to effect their efficacy as behaviour modifiers (Vitalo, 1970; Mickelson and Stevic, 1971). An interesting use of relationship to foster behavioural change is reported by Persons (1966). He conducted a group therapy aimed at providing a sequence of (1) establishment of supportive relationship, (2) interpretation and differential reinforcement, including role-playing, (3) induction of stress concerning antisocial behaviour, and (4) discussion of difficulties in returning to the community. This sequence appeared to involve establishing a relationship in which the therapist acquired influence over the patients and then systematically exercised the influence via modelling, shaping, and persuasion techniques. Records kept during institutionalization showed most beneficial effects in the treated group, who also showed a lower recidivism rate over a 1-year follow-up period than both the untreated group and the base rate.

Bandura (1969) regards non-specific factors as facilitative rather than sufficient conditions for the production of therapeutic change by behavioural treatment. He notes that it is an article of faith for many that 'relationship' factors are the primary agents of behavioural change, and consequently that the specific methods employed are of secondary importance. As he puts it (pp.76–77):

> This view — which is somewhat analogous to relying on 'bedside manner' rather than on specific therapeutic interventions in the alleviation of physical disorders — can be seriously questioned . . . Let us assume that two children have been referred for treatment, one passive and nonaggressive, the second exhibiting a hyperaggressive pattern of behaviour. Since the goal is to increase assertiveness in the passive child and to decrease the domineering tendencies of the hyperaggressive child, should the therapist employ the same methods? Clearly, the answer is in the negative. Based on established principles of behaviour change, procedures aimed at reducing inhibitions . . . the provision of assertive models . . . and the reinforcement of assertive response patterns . . . are most appropriate and effective for promoting increased assertiveness. These methods, however, would be clearly inappropriate in the treatment of the hyperaggressive child since they would simply strengthen the already persistent deviant behaviour. Withdrawal of rewards for aggression . . . combined with modelling and positive reinforcement of nonaggressive frustration responses . . . is highly effective for decreasing aggressiveness. Although in both these hypothetical cases warmth, interest, understanding and other relationship factors would apply equally, it is unrealistic to expect these general factors to increase aggressiveness in one child and to reduce it in the other. Nevertheless therapists often adhere to a single set of therapeutic conditions, disregarding the nature of the client's deviant behaviour . . .

In the author's opinion, a reliance on relationship rather than carefully planned specific measures leads to the 'Micawber syndrome': if one develops a good relationship with a child, some benign change is bound to turn up. It seldom does; not even 'spontaneous remission' is on the side of the serious conduct disorders. This philosophy is an extension of the 'love is enough' fallacy in child rearing. Conduct disorders *do* occur in 'loving' homes in which the detailed and sometimes burdensome socialization-training tasks are neglected — in the name of a romantic 'noble savage' concept of childhood. A highly-charged relationship is not a desideratum for therapy and in any event would exclude a majority of clients from treatment.

Relationship, when elevated to a mystique, seems to assume, with some degree of arrogance, that the therapist should be one of the most significant figures in his client's life. In behavioural work no such intense relationship is required. It is only necessary for the client to have enough trust and confidence in the therapist to accept treatment in the first place. A closer relationship may, of course, develop and will be of value but it is not central.

INSIGHT

Psychotherapists stress the part played by insight in producing behavioural change in patients. In a behavioural approach this factor is not overlooked, but the nature and contribution of a client's insight are different from those assumed in the more traditional approach. Practitioners of behaviour modification commonly put forward two main criticisms of insight as a basis for therapy. One has to do with the validity of the hypotheses underpinning psychodynamic approaches — in particular, a scepticism about the therapeutic value of delving into 'causes' of behaviour which lie in the past in the search for understanding (see Lee and Herbert, 1970). The other involves the traditional assumption that insight is a necessary condition of meaningful therapeutic change. Bandura (1971a) re-analyses the psychodynamic interpretive insight-giving process as an instance of social influence or brainwashing, rather than genuine self-understanding and revelation. He contends that patients in the emotive ethos of this kind of therapeutic relationship are highly amenable to persuasion and conditioning (often unwitting). As he sees it, suggestive probing and selective reinforcement of a client's verbal reports lead to a self-validating interview in which the patient imperceptibly but increasingly replaces his own opinions and ideas about himself with the therapist's views and interpretations. The more impressive the authority of the therapist, the more likely is the patient to alter his self-concepts to fit with the therapist's theories, despite the possibility that they may seem far-fetched or even false. Given the nature of the explanatory concepts used they are often inaccessible to proof or disproof but depend upon 'faith-validity'. And who is to say that *that* has no therapeutic value? However, there is evidence for a form of verbal conditioning. Truax (1966) has shown that Carl Rogers selectively but subtly reinforces certain classes of desirable behaviours and that the 'unconditional positive regard' which should be accorded to the client is *by no means unconditional*. Psychotherapists can unwittingly guide the patient to learn new methods of tackling problems; they reinforce conformity to their own ideas and opinions by giving cues (verbal and non-verbal) as to what they approve of in the patient's output. In Bandura's view, insight into the hypothesized psychic determinants of interpersonal responses is, on the one hand, of questionable validity and, on the other hand, has little practical effect on behaviour (Bandura, 1969, p.98). One might add that such a view would be argued (by the critics) even more powerfully when young children are the subjects of therapy. Jobbs (1962) is of the opinion that insight is often defined in psychotherapy in a 'heads I win, tails you lose' *ex post facto* manner. If change occurs, then the insight has been demonstrably genuine; if not, then it was erroneous. There are many instances of successful therapies without insight being invoked, and examples where insight having apparently been obtained has had little effect on behaviour. It can be argued that insight is a consequence rather than an agent of beneficial change. Cautela (1965) suggests that changes in verbalizations during psychotherapy, commonly called 'insight', frequently *follow* rather than precede behavioural changes. As relief of tension and difficulties proceed, insight as to their causation may develop.

Yelloly (1972, p.147) makes what seems a fair comment on this vexed question:

> . . . awareness may operate in a number of ways. The sheer provision of accurate information may correct a false and erroneous belief and bring about considerable change in behaviour; prejudice, for instance, may be diminished by new information which challenges the prejudiced belief. And in human beings (pre-eminently capable of rational and purposive action) comprehension of a situation, knowledge of cause and effect sequences, and of one's own behaviour and its consequences, may have a dramatic effect on manifest behaviour. Thus to ignore the role of insight is just as mistaken as to restrict attention wholly to it. It would seem that the relative neglect of insight by behaviour therapists until recently has occurred partly in reaction to the over-emphasis on it in traditional psychotherapy, and partly because of their preoccupation with directly observable behaviour. . . . the potential of symbolic factors for therapeutic change has not been fully exploited although classical behaviour therapy procedures rely heavily on cognitively-produced effects; for example, symbolic rehearsal of behaviour in imagination forms part of systematic desensitization and of some aversive techniques. Such imaginative rehearsal or fantasy is surely evidence of the powerful effects of symbolic arousal on manifest behaviour. Even so it would appear that the use made of higher-order processes in behaviour therapy is relatively unsophisticated by contrast with the wealth and richness of the human symbolic processes and inner mental experience portrayed in language and art.

ETHICAL ISSUES

It is perhaps a backhanded compliment to the effectiveness of behaviour modification that its many critics pay more attention to its ethical implications than is the case with other therapies. It may be that critics get most hot under the collar about this kind of intervention because they suspect that it *really works!*

Nawas (1970) notes that the behaviourist's approach is considered to be sterile by some and downright dangerous by others. Behaviourism is said to be futile because it fails to get at the 'real' person, assuming him to be a passive bundle of stimulus and response connections. Other perjorative descriptions include its being deterministic and dehumanizing.

Therapies are always what they seem, or how they are seen, by the commentators on the outside. Caricatures of theoretical and practical therapeutic models are set up as 'straw men' for the zealots (often poorly briefed) to knock over. Psychoanalysis has suffered the same fate, often at the hands of behaviour theorists, so it is rough justice that the latter should now be on the receiving end. There is, in any event, a case to answer (see Stolz, Wienckowski, and Brown, 1975).

Leung (1975) observes that, whereas the medical model provides a reasonably unambiguous ethical rationale for treatment by an *a priori* standard of 'health' and 'pathology', behaviour modifiers tend to construe abnormality as not in itself different from normal behaviour. This means that they face ethical decisions with which the medical model has not been confronted. As he explains, if abnormal behaviour is considered learned, the therapists are involved in making, or at least concurring with, a value judgement that some other behaviour would be preferable. They are responsible not only for the cessation of one set of behaviours but also for the behaviours that replace the previous ones. Furthermore, instead of believing in 'sickness' or 'health', behaviour modification is in sympathy with the idea that the evaluation of abnormal behaviour is usually a social judgement. This will immediately lead to the rhetorical question: to whom is the behaviour undesirable and is it really in need of change? Of course, all therapists are trying to produce change, no matter what their orientation.

Tharp and Wetzel (1969) note that, far from assuming an authoritative posture and considering the art of therapy as a secret cult, behaviour modification is more willing to rally the support of non-professionals like parents, housewives, university students, etc., to participate in the treatment programmes. Nawas (1970), too, has a rejoinder for those who single out behavioural methods for these criticisms. As he puts it (p.367):

> In actuality, behaviour therapists are prone to be less judgmental and to impose their own values less than those who accuse them of wanting to 'control' man. The clarity of the behaviour therapists' operations, and their well-defined role as modifiers of explicitly stated complaints by the client himself, allows them to guard against imposing their own values on the client and to give him the freedom to go in the direction *he* wants to go. A therapist is a humanist to an extent inversely proportional to his (a) professing to know what is good for man in general; and (b) attempting actively to help the client achieve this imposed aim. In these terms, no other orientation can be said to have a greater claim on humanism than behaviour therapy, and behaviouristically oriented therapists are closer to the spirit of humanism, as commonly conceived, than most outspoken defenders of humanism, from Rollo May to Carl Rogers and from Abraham Maslow to Victor Frankl.

Many of the processes of change that take place in the psychodynamic therapies are somewhat mysterious and invisible to the patient or client (and, one might add, *all* therapies are like this for young children). At the Centre for Behavioural Work with Families it is policy to explain to the children (and allow them to be privy to) all the proceedings in working out a treatment programme. Another crucial principle involves the therapist acting as advocate for the child, in the sense of representing his point of view. No safeguards are foolproof; in the end, all therapies are open to abuse because they depend on trust and good sense, and therapists (of whatever persuasion) are human. Stolz, Wienckowski, and Brown (1975) note that some mental-health professionals attack behaviour modification on the grounds that its underlying assumptions are at variance with their basic values and tend to dehumanize man (e.g., Carrera and Adams, 1970). Again, it is misleading to categorize behaviour modification as a monolithic system. Behaviour modification *does* have a 'human face', and it might be argued (to take but one example) that the approach illustrated in Appendix A returns dignity to demoralized parents and provides increased choices for restricted and unhappy children.

However, the author has reservations about the use of behavioural methods is closed institutions and with detained clients. The most sensitive and worrying moral dilemma is the use of behavioural methods to deal with the rebellious and non-conformist behaviour of youths in penal institutions. Stolz, Wienckowski, and Brown (1975) rightly observe that the behavioural professional is often placed in the position of assisting in the management of inmates whose rebelliousness and antagonism to authority are catalysts for conflict within the institution. Because of this, distinctions among his many functions as therapist, manager, and rehabilitator can become blurred and his allegiance confused.

Although the professional may quite accurately perceive his role as benefiting the individual, he may at the same time appear to have the institution, rather than the prisoner, as his primary client. The authors comment that often the goal of effective behaviour modification in penal institutions is the preservation of the institution's authoritarian control. Although some prison behaviour modification programmes are designed to educate the prisoners and benefit them in other ways, other programmes are directed towards making the prisoners less troublesome and easier to manage, thus adjusting the inmates to the needs of the institution.

A genuine and understandable concern is the one of bribery. Contingency contracting, for example, has been said to foster a manipulative, exchange orientation to social interaction, and token economies, an emphasis on materialistic evaluation of human efforts. The most comprehensive answers to these criticisms are provided by O'Leary, Poulos, and Devine (1972) and, as with other value issues which pervade these criticisms and counter-arguments, the reader must form his own conclusion.

It is perhaps fitting to conclude with words from the thoughful and compassionate statement of the moral issues in the review by Stolz, Wienckowski, and Brown (1975, p.1039):

> On the whole, the goal of behaviour modification, as generally practised, is not to force people to conform or behave in some mindless, automaton-like way. Rather, the goals generally include providing new skills and individualized options and developing creativity and spontaneity.

APPENDIXES

Appendix A

Assessment, Recording, and Evaluation

Without an objective assessment and record-keeping system, it is not possible to evaluate accurately and reliably the progress made by the child in the therapeutic situation. It is clear that many children's problems are transient and change can occur often as a function of time and non-specific placebo effects. For these reasons, a controlled evaluation of the therapeutic process is essential. Objective data make possible two important objectives: determining whether a child in treatment is changing, and the direction and extent of change. They also make possible an assessment of the relationship between different kinds of intervention within the overall therapeutic programme.

DIRECT OBSERVATION

Paper and pencils are much in evidence in busy day-to-day assessment. Other equipment includes stopwatches, counters to provide time samples and event recordings of behaviour, and tape-recorders, where appropriate. The available literature suggests that quite satisfactory measures can be obtained without having to resort to complex and expensive equipment. However, where video equipment is available, it can be very revealing to show parents and children what their behaviour looks like. To see yourself as others see you is often the beginning of a decision to change.

DATA COLLECTION

(1) Frequency

It is important to determine the frequency of a problem in quantifiable terms.

297

This should include not only the overall rate (i.e., how often it occurs — daily or weekly), but also any tendency of the problem to occur episodically (i.e. at particular times). Any evidence of clustering of behavioural events should lead to further investigation. A frequency recording procedure is the simplest type of data analysis. It is nothing more than a *tally* method. What the therapist does is to count the number of occurrences of the behaviour, as he has defined it. Recording the time at which the response occurred transforms the frequency data system into an even more useful instrument.

(a) Interval method

To use the interval method of recording, the observation period is broken down into small *equal* intervals and the behaviour is recorded as occurring or not occurring during each interval of time. The interval size will usually be from 5 seconds to 1 minute in duration, depending upon the rate of the response and the average duration of a single response.

(b) Time sampling

Many behaviours are not clearly discrete in nature. Some responses have no clear-cut beginning or ending. Time sampling provides the clearest analysis of such behaviours. For example, in the case of a student who makes many loud, disruptive noises, such as yelling out across the room, hitting his neighbour and pinching him, shuffling his chair around, it might be difficult either to make a tally of the number of times such responses occur or to measure their duration. After all, when does one instance of chair shifting end and another begin? However, it is feasible to record the presence or absence of such responses within a short time span at intervals during (say) a classroom lesson. In order to obtain a representative sample of observations one might record the presence or absence of the behaviour within short, uniform time intervals, such as the first 10 seconds in every minute of a half-hour classroom period.

(2) Intensity

It may be appropriate to measure the level of the problem in terms of its intensity rather than its frequency. Intensity can be assessed by asking two questions. (a) How long does the behaviour last? (b) How severe is it?

(a) Duration

Some problems are most usefully described in terms of how long the behaviour lasts or how long it has been since the behaviour occurred. A stopwatch is run continuously while the behaviour is occurring during an observation period of a specified length.

(b) Severity

This can be measured by constructing *ad hoc* severity rating scales of a graphical, numerical, or some other kind.

SYSTEMATIC VARIATION OF TREATMENT

The precise manipulation of therapeutic procedures is essential to the understanding of causation where behaviour modification is applied to individual cases. The way in which systematic treatment variation is arranged depends upon the type of 'experimental' design chosen. Many involve some form of own-control (single-subject) design (Greenwald, 1976). A particular advantage of the single-subject design is that it maximizes opportunity for innovation and flexibility in treatment, while laying the basis for the formulation of hypotheses. It also avoids one of the most powerful confounding factors in behavioural research: *individual differences* in child patients. The single-subject design allows comparisons to be made between a child under one condition and the same youngster under different conditions. The manner in which the therapeutic interventions are systematically varied directly affects the conclusion that can be drawn from the manipulation.

In the following discussion of the kind of own-control design to be used, symbol A represents a baseline during which the aggressive behaviour is monitored under uncontrolled conditions and the symbols, B, C, D, etc., represent different treatment programmes.

The AB design involves a comparison of the occurrence of the aggressive behaviour under a pre-treatment baseline condition and the application of a treatment programme.

The ABC design comprises comparisons of the occurrence of (say) aggressive behaviour under a pre-treatment baseline condition and two treatment programmes. It entails the problem of uncontrolled order effects across treatments, but it is of value when the B treatment in an AB design proves to be inadequate and a second treatment C is to be tried out to see if it is an improvement on treatment B.

The principal limitation of both the AB and the ABC designs is that one cannot be sure that any reduction in aggressive behaviour is due to treatment rather than to possible alternative factors. As the present project is concerned primarily with the development of treatment rather than with investigating its efficacy, this is not a vital limitation. Moreover, since a series of case studies will be conducted, if treatment is regularly followed by a reduction in aggression in a number of children, this renders less plausible certain of the alternatives to treatment as the source of change.

Intrasubject replication designs of a reversal kind do constitute a more rigorous form of own-control but they also have some considerable disadvantages for use in this project. Taking the very popular ABAB design as an example, the aggressive behaviour is first assessed to establish a baseline for predicting what the occurrence of the behaviour would have been in future if treatment had not been instituted. The second stage consists of applying the treatment and of assessing aggression during it. In the third stage the treatment is discontinued, and if the aggression returns to the original baseline level, this supports the prediction of the continuance of the behaviour at that level if the treatment had not been introduced. The fourth stage consists of reinstituting the treatment and if this is followed by another reduction in aggression, it suggests that it is the treatment which is producing the change in behaviour. Thus, this kind of design does yield *correlational* evidence of an association between a treatment and a reduction in aggression. However, one still cannot be certain that fluctuations in aggression which accompany the application and withdrawal of the treatment are in fact a function of this treatment. The changes might still be due to the operation of other factors which happen to co-vary with the treatment and baseline conditions. As in the case of the AB and ABC designs, this possibility is weakened if similar results are obtained in respect of a number of children.

Perhaps a more important problem attaching to the use of reversal designs in this project is the ethical dilemma of deliberately attempting to reverse any beneficial therapeutic changes by successive replications of the baseline conditions. In particular, these replications might train the child to retrieve his aggressive behaviour more quickly, might make it more resistant to extinction because the replications constitute an intermittent reinforcement schedule, and might also breed distrust and suspicion in the child because of the apparent capriciousness of the adults operating the programme. Another problem is that the aim of treatment is to produce an irreversible reduction in aggression which persists after treatment ends. If this is done successfully, then it will not be possible to recover the original baseline level of behaviour by withdrawing treatment in the third stage. Similarly, staff or foster parents may find it difficult to replicate the original baseline conditions in the third stage. Having learned to reduce the aggressive behaviour they may be unable or unwilling to revert to their pre-treatment practices.

In the light of these disadvantages attaching to reversal designs, it may be more appropriate to use a multiple baseline type of intrasubject replication design. In this type, instead of applying one or more treatments to a single baseline for aggressive behaviour, the same treatment is applied sequentially to several baselines for different forms of this behaviour. After obtaining baselines for two or more kinds of aggressive behaviour, the treatment is applied to one of these. If this reduces while the untreated forms remain unchanged, it suggests that the treatment is responsible for the reduction. This proposition is further tested by then applying the treatment sequentially to the other kind(s) of aggressive behaviour, and if reduction follows, this strengthens the case for attributing it to the treatment. However, as discussed above in the context of the ABAB design, the multiple baseline type of intrasubject replication design still only yields correlational evidence of an association between the treatment and any reduction in aggressive behaviour.

See other design options in Barlow and Hayes, 1979; Watson et. al., 1985)

CONTROL GROUP DESIGN

The control group design is another way to demonstrate the effect of an experimental contingency. There *is* a variety of control group designs suitable for applied settings (e.g., Campbell and Stanley, 1963). The most efficient procedure to control for systematic differences between groups before a treatment programme is implemented is to *randomly assign* children to one of the two groups. One receives the experimental therapeutic programme (the experimental group) and the other does not (the control group). If subjects are not randomly assigned to groups, the likelihood is greater that the groups may be different in their performance of the target behaviour prior to the therapy being implemented. Differential change in the target behaviour over time may occur for reasons other than the effect of the therapeutic intervention.

Appendix B

The Centre for Behavioural Work with Families, University of Leicester

The Centre (formerly the Child Treatment Research Unit) has evolved the following approach to behavioural work with families. It is presented in the form in which students receive their training handouts at the Centre (see Herbert, 1987).

OVERVIEW

In all there are 12 assessment and treatment steps:

Preliminary screnning

Step 1	Explain yourself and how you work
Step 2	Identify the problems
Step 3	Construct a problem profile
	Define and refine specific target behaviours
Step 4	Discover the desired outcomes
Step 5	Identify the child's assets
Step 6	Establish problem priorities

Baseline phase

Step 7	Provide client with appropriate recording material
	Find out more about the behaviour
	Find out how intense the behaviour is
Step 8	Assess the extent and severity of the problem

Baseline phase (*contd.*)

Step 9	Assess the contingencies
	Identify reinforcers
	Assess organismic variables
	Arrive at a diagnostic decision
Step 10	Formulate objectives
	Draw up a verbal agreement or written contract
Step 11	Formulate clinical hypotheses

Intervention and termination

Step 12	Plan your treatment programme
	Take into account non-specific therapeutic factors
	Work out the practicalities of the treatment programme
	Evaluate the programme
	Initiate the programme

ASSESSMENT PHASE

The first task in the assessment of problems is to specify precisely *what* the allegedly maladaptive behaviours or feelings and interactions are, defining them in terms of their frequency, intensity, number, and duration and the meaning (or sense) they have for the client (FINDS) (see Figure 3).

Who, in particular, constitutes the 'client' (or clients) in an intervention is often a moot point; it *may not* necessarily be the nominated person. It is useful to draw up a *problem profile* when working with families, to take account of problems other than those ascribed to (say) the target child and of perceptions of *all* members of the family. Clients tend to express their concern about their adolescent offspring's shortcomings and statements about *problems*: 'He is so thoughtless'; and/or *desired outcomes*: 'I wish he could come home at a respectable hour'. Encouraging the client to provide initial information about desired outcomes provides the raw material for the formulation (later) of more specific goals and objectives.

The therapist makes a note about who is complaining about particular problems: who desires a given outcome; the level of agreement/disagreement between (say) husband and wife with regard to how they would like things to be different; and the implications of change in the direction of the desired outcome.

She also tries to find out about the client's skills and prosocial behaviours. Next comes the selection (after negotiation with perhaps the whole family) of the problems on which to concentrate — at least initially. This requires the establishment of a hierarchy of problems/outcomes in order of their importance to the client/s and significant others. The therapist will have her own conception of a hierarchy of problems in terms of their implications as she perceives them.

The following stage involves a figurative 'change of gear' from the more static collection of data (interview) to the more active form of information gathering — *the baseline*. The therapist provides the client (and perhaps others in his environment) with appropriate charts for recording target behaviours, and explains how to observe, to code behaviour, and to record. This is *not* some academic exercise in keeping records and measuring change (important enough in themselves!) but it is part of a learning or, if you like, insight-gaining experience for the client.

It is advantageous for the therapist to *observe for herself* what is happening currently — if at all possible — in order to understand the controlling factors in the client's problem, and to set realistic treatment goals and make plans for achieving them. It is important to confirm the client's observations, checking on their reliability — especially those based on hearsay.

Let us now translate these general comments into concrete terms, a series of steps.

Step 1: Explain who you are, how you work

Explain to your client/s who you are, and your role as a psychologist or social worker, especially the fact that you will be engaging in a therapeutic *partnership*, in the sense of requiring their help and expertise, and of sharing the planning (and your thinking) with them. Describe the 'homework' that will be required of your clients if and when you embark on a detailed assessment; and the active part they will play in defining goals, and implementing any 'treatment'.

Step 2: Identify (tentatively) the problem/s

Gather information about the problems and the circumstances in which they occur. Try to establish whether the identified problems lend themselves to behavioural change. The crucial question here is 'what'? What are the problems? What are their implications in terms of what the client *does* and *says* or the interactions he has with other persons. There are, broadly speaking, three classes of problem:

   (i) Behaviour *that is excessive* (e.g., screaming, nagging, rowing, drinking, criticizing, hitting).
   (ii) Behaviour that is '*normal*' or 'appropriate' of itself but occurs in restricted or inappropriate contexts (e.g., compliant behaviour to criminal values but not prosocial community norms).
   (iii) Behaviour that is absent from, or *poorly represented*, in the client's behavioural repertoire (e.g., reinforcing actions: incontinence, poor parenting or social skills, low self-esteem).

Be cautious about assessing as necessarily 'problematic' the nominated client — a change of whose behaviours will make life easier for others but will not benefit himself. For example, teaching an adolescent to be quiet and malleable may make life easier for a teacher or for residential staff, who have not given enough thought to the problem and weaknesses in *their* systems which contribute to what is essentially a mutual difficulty.

Sometimes a behaviour which has advantages for one person may be detrimental to others. For example, helping a teenager (and others) to be more assertive may mean that she starts upsetting her parents and her friends.

Now this result (and the consequences of consciousness raising) for an 'oppressed' youngster — as you see it — may be no bad thing, by the tenets of your values. Nevertheless you are dealing with a sometimes fragile system, a family and the lives of people who have their own values and mores.

You need to decide, as a first priority, whether the problems being presented to you lend themselves to a behavioural assessment.

(i) Can you *operationalize* the stated problems ('my child is out of control'; 'my life isn't worth living'; 'my marriage is falling apart'; 'I can't stand my husband touching me'), in other words specify them in terms of responses which are accessible to the observation of your client, yourself, and other people? Work with 'problem' children often moves on to work with 'problem' marriages. To this end encourage (say) the husband to give descriptive examples of the problem. Ask him to define what he means in specific and observable terms when he uses a particular label. If the informant says: 'My wife is always getting at me', ask: 'In what way does she get at you? Tell me what she says and does that make you describe her as "getting at you".' Also: 'Give me some examples (preferably recent ones) of what happens when she behaves like this.' (It is usual in working with married couples to interview the couple. Here you might inquire: 'How do you respond to these remarks by your husband?'

(ii) Of course, not all problems lend themselves to behavioural change. Problems may be temporary ones, e.g., making a decision. Should I change my job? Can I let my disabled child go into a home? Should I abandon my family because my husband is battering me?

Try not to focus prematurely on *specific problems* (e.g., a highly focused problem like a child's misbehaviour) at the expense of an initially open-ended and reasonably full exploration of the range of difficulties that may be waiting to be expressed. It is critical that the first interview is sensitive to what the full extent and ramifications of a family's difficulties might be.

In trying to learn about the behaviour of other persons, the two principal ways are through questioning and observation.

(i) *Behaviour interview* Make use of interviewing techniques (because of the opportunity they give you to question and observe clients); they are among the prime instruments of the behavioural assessment.

(ii) *Direct observation*   Go and see for yourself at home, school, etc., what and where problematic behaviours are occurring.

(iii) *Record keeping*   Ask the client/s to keep a diary and/or chart indicating when/with whom/under what circumstances X occurs.

A technique used in order to obtain a general orientation into family interactions and behaviours is the 'typical day' in the life of the child and family. It is worked through in minute (indeed, pedantic) behavioural detail, pinpointing those areas which cause confrontations and concern. It also provides the times and places at which, and the persons with whom, they occur. A 'blow-by-blow' account is sought of the events surrounding problematic interactions. The typical day (or days) makes for a reasonable sampling of the events being complained of.

An adequate analysis requires a convincing demonstration that particular (i.e., specified) psychosocial factors are responsible for changes in the client's activities. This demonstration is usually accomplished through what are called *replication* and *control* procedures.

It is during the initial interview with the client/s that an account is given (with down-to-earth examples) of the theoretical rationale and practice policies of the therapist. In suitable form it is made clear to the client that some of the issues to be discussed (indeed, debated) concern *who* the client turns out to be (entire family, couple, or an individual member); the question of *what* the actual problem is and is not; the matter of doing 'homework'; and, in general, the desirability of a full partnership in the assessment and intervention.

Step 3: Construct a problem profile

Ask questions such as: Who is complaining and why? Who else perceives the presence of a problem? Exactly what is being complained of? In effect, you draw up a problem profile to take account of the problem of the 'client', and in addition those ascribed to others in (say) the family. In this way you will have a record of perceptions of *all* members of the family. Whether you conduct this exercise within the context of a group consisting of all or some family members is a matter of style (yours) and/or ideological conviction.

In any event, ask who desires a given outcome. Ascertain the level of agreement/disagreement between (for example) parents and child, or between husband and wife, as to how they would like things to be different. What are the implications of change in the direction of the desired outcome? Ask if anyone benefits; does anyone lose? A critical question is this one: What implications are there for the client and others if *no* change is brought about.

Step 4: Discover desired outcomes

Initial comments about desired outcomes provide the raw material for the formulation (later) of more specific goals and objectives. *Goals* are the behavioural changes to be sought; they define how the target behaviours (the ones you decide to concentrate on for your assessment) are to be changed.

Step 5: List client's assets

Make every effort to list the client's 'strong points'. The client himself, or significant others in his life, may be surprised at how many 'virtues', strengths, and resources he possesses when encouraged to think about them. Ask the client (or other informants) to imagine a credit and debit balance sheet with two columns. Get them to make a list of pluses and minuses. You most probably will have to say: 'There's a long list of items on his debit side; what can you think of to his credit?'

Consider direct or informal solutions, before deciding whether to continue

Your client's problems may be related to very practical issues which by no stretch of the imagination demand the intricacies of a behavioural assessment and intervention. A child may be wetting the bed because the toilet facilities are outside, and a cold winter's night acts as a deterrent to a nighttime trip to the lavatory. The electricity has been cut off and is causing rows between members of the family. What the parents need is help with budgeting and a mediator to negotiate with the Electricity Board. A battered wife may need to talk over her conflicting views as to whether to leave her husband or not. An exhausted, depressed mother may need day-care or baby-minding support. An adolescent youth may require a job or introduction to potential friends in a youth club.

Step 6: Establish problem priorities

It is important to select (after negotiation with the client/s) the problems on which to concentrate — at least initially. After the collection of baseline data you may find it necessary to alter the list.

(i) If there are many problems, select one or two on which to concentrate; have criteria to help you to decide which behaviours to work on, e.g.,
— Annoyance value of the current situation to the client.
— Danger value of the current situation.
— Interference of the current situation in the client's life.

— Centrality of the problem in a complex of problems.
— Accessibility of the problem. (Can you get at it?)
— Potential for change. (Can you do something about it?)
— Probable cost of intervention (time, money, energy, and resources).
— Relative frequency, duration, or magnitude of the problem.
— Ethical acceptability of the outcome to the counsellor.
— Likelihood that new behaviours will be maintained in the post-intervention environment.

(ii) Do not select behaviours that are under the exclusive control of events, situations, or people that you cannot control — e.g., if the parents of the child who hits other children are unwilling to participate in a programme which involves changes in their behaviour, it will be impossible to carry out this programme.

(iii) Select goals which are relevant to the person and which are likely to be maintained and encouraged after the programme ceases, i.e., behaviours that are likely to be adaptive for the person in the future. They should have reward and survival value for him or her.

(iv) Select goals that have a high probability of success. Success in changing behaviour is highly motivating to the client and others involved in the programme, and increases their confidence in attempting to deal with more difficult problems.

(v) Consider whether it is appropriate to select behavioural targets other than the major problem that is presented. Sometimes it may be more appropriate to concentrate on related behaviours which, if changed, will lead to improvements in the presenting problem. For example, with a person who experiences anxiety in a social situation it may be best to concentrate on training him to be more assertive than on eliminating the anxiety.

(vi) Try and have goals that involve the acquisition or strengthening of positive behaviours rather than (just) decreasing behaviours. It is generally easier to develop new behaviours than to eliminate old behaviours.

The therapist should indicate to clients before further detailed work begins that there could be disagreements over treatment objectives (reservations on their part or her part about the so-called 'target behaviours' — the specific objectives of change). The baseline records sometimes present surprises! Because behavioural work can be somewhat directive and often quite powerful, it is employed as a specific intervention or management procedure only after full and careful consideration of the desirability of the proposed changes. The objectives are decided primarily on personal, social, and ethical grounds. The therapist has a special responsibility for acting, in a sense, as an 'advocate' for her client, especially where a youngster is the primary target for change.

The common goal of behavioural work in the natural environment is to develop in the clients an awareness of their own importance in producing (a phenomenon referred to as 'attribution') and maintaining desirable and undesirable behaviours in themselves and in each other. Treatment, in the sense of clients obtaining an 'insight' into the principles and application of social learning theory, begins (whether the therapist desires it or not) before the actual intervention phase. After all, the therapist is encouraging the clients to think about behaviour sequentially (in ABC interactional terms) as they monitor.

BEGIN TO PLAN YOUR BASELINE

Let us assume that further assessment is necessary. This means that on the basis of your preliminary assessment (or screening) you feel there is prima facie evidence of a real, that is to say, significant, problem — one requiring more than advice or practical help.

Plan the baseline as part of, and flowing from, your assessment interview/s. You will now be moving from the more static collection of data (interview) to the more active, dynamic form of information gathering.

Behaviour modification is essentially about changing behaviour: the frequency with which the clients manifests a problematic activity may have to decrease, or increase — depending upon its nature. On the other hand, it may not be a matter of doing something less or more often, but of manifesting an action with different intensity.

In order to change behaviour *from* some level *to* another level, you need to be clear about the definition of the problem and to know how much there is of that problem. In this way you will know:

 (i) whether the problem is as extensive as the client, or others (e.g., say parents), says it is;
 (ii) Whether your therapeutic programme (when it gets going) is producing real change.

The period of careful and controlled data collection stemming from the early interview/s is called the *baseline*.

Observations by the therapist and/or mediator (e.g., parent) and/or client should be carried out for a period prior to beginning the intervention — the period should be long enough to obtain an accurate picture of the 'normal' frequency or intensity or duration of the behaviour. The baseline will enable the therapist to compare the occurrence of the target behaviour before and during treatment, and will indicate what effect intervention has had on the target behaviour.

Step 7: Provide client with appropriate material (charts, notebooks) to record problem behaviours, feelings, interactions

This marks the beginning of the so-called *baseline period*. You train the client to observe behaviour so that, in a sense, you can observe things through his eyes during the time you cannot be 'on the spot'.

Until now the main source of information has been the behavioural interview — a systematic approach to obtaining information about the problem, its nature, frequency, antecedents, consequences, etc. It may have been conducted at the office or in the client's home. Next the baseline data collected by interview are checked, supplemented, and quantified by:

(i) direct observation of the client in natural settings, e.g., home, school, youth club;
(ii) direct observation in other settings, e.g., office, reception centre, etc.;
(iii) self-recordings by the client (diaries, activity charts, self-ratings) in his day-to-day life or special situations;
(iv) use of questionnaires, rating scales, etc., completed by client or others;
(v) use of audio or video cassette recordings.

Event recording

For many behaviours, the easiest and most practical method of assessment is to count the number of occurrences of the behaviour over a particular period of time. For example, the number of times a young child has tantrums in a week, etc. This is known as *event recording* or *frequency counting* and is most appropriate for behaviours that have clearly definable beginnings and ends.

Some people claim that behaviours which can be quantified and counted are easiest to change; indeed, that problem behaviours which cannot be observed and counted are not likely to be changed by the therapeutic agent.

Write down the behaviour to be recorded (with symbols and definitions) as a reminder to the client. You might simply ask the parents to keep a count in the first week and then a more detailed ABC diary the next week (see Herbert, 1987).

Interval recording

In another method of recording, known as interval recording, periods of time are divided up into intervals of equal length and it is recorded whether or not the behaviour occurred within that interval. For example, recording in half-hour intervals. This procedure will provide you with information on both the relative frequency and the duration of the behaviour observed.

Generally data are collected for a set period of time, say 3 hours per day, and at a fixed time (e.g., from after supper to bedtime). In selecting a method for obtaining data bear in mind that you want to get a typical and representative picture of the problem. To achieve this you need to ask yourself how often you need to record, where you need to record, when you need to record, for how long you need to record.

Duration recording

Sometimes it is the duration of the behaviour — how long it occurs — that is the most important feature. For example, how long a child sucks her thumb, the length of time it takes to do homework, length of time a child cries, etc. Discover:

(a) The frequency of the problem.
(b) The overall rate at which the behaviour occurs — i.e., how often. The usual means of expressing this is frequency/time, e.g., confrontations per day, tantrums per day.
(c) Whether there is a tendency for the problem to occur episodically.
(d) Whether there is any evidence of a clustering of behavioural events.

Find out how intense (extreme) the behaviour is. Expressions of emotion and behavioural acts have certain allowable intensity levels. Very 'high' intensities — behavioural responses of excessive magnitude — which have unpleasant consequences for other people (e.g., incessant screaming, over-activity, fidgety behaviour) are likely to be viewed as socially inappropriate. These problems are sometimes referred to as 'aversive behavioural repertoires'.

Anxiety, up to a point, can be adaptive: think of the athlete who is 'toned up' by the adrenalin of apprehension or the actress who is 'keyed up' for a good performance by a certain amount of stage-fright. Too much anxiety can be crippling.

In checking for problematic actions look for 'interfering' behaviours, that is to say, actions which preclude or compete with the performance of socially adaptive behaviours. These actions are sometimes manifested so often and intensely that they reduce dramatically the probability of alternative responses being made.

Step 8: Assess the extent and severity of the problem

You do this by exploring the parameters of the problem behaviour. The acronym *FIND* refers to the specification of the target problems in terms of their frequency, intensity, number, and duration, and the sense they make from the client's point of view (see Figure 3). After an initial report from the client you require careful and controlled observation of the behaviours you think are important, as they are presently occurring.

You need to select appropriate behaviour assessment techniques. Choose a method of measuring or assessing the behaviour that will reliably estimate the extent of the problem, one that can be used easily and conveniently, and which does not involve the collection of redundant information. Although there are various sophisticated procedures for assessing behaviour, for most programmes straightforward and simple methods are adequate, such as those described in Step 7.

The two main methods of assessing behaviour are counting how often the behaviour occurs (known as frequency counting or event recording) and measuring the duration of the behaviour (known as duration recording). A third method, interval recording, involves elements of both event and duration recording.

Step 9: Assess the contingencies

In other words, identify the antecedent, and consequent factors (contingencies). The foundation for the behavioural approach is the contingency analysis, also referred to as a functinal analysis; it specifies the relationship between a behavioural performance, its precursors, and its outcomes. A contingency refers to the extent to which the occurrence of one event is dependent upon the occurrence of another event. Behaviour is not usually manifested on a random basis; the probability of a specific action occurring varies according to the surrounding environmental cues. You need to find out about the client and his responses to a variety of situations and environmental settings, in other words what you need is to specify the *functional* relationships between As and Bs and Cs.

(a) What happens just before the behaviour occurs; what sets it off?
(b) What happens immediately following the behaviour; what happens as a result of the behaviour?

A = antecedent events (prior stimulation)

These are the antecedent stimulus events which reliably precede the (target) behaviour. They may be *functionally* related to the behaviour by

(i) setting the stage for it (discriminative stimuli), or
(ii) evoking it (eliciting stimuli).

What factors (situations, persons, etc.) can 'push' or 'pull' — make more or less severe — the level of the problematic behaviour? In other words, what sets off the behaviour; what moderates it?

B = Discover the situations in which the problematic interactions/feelings/ behaviours are most likely to occur

To take one example: a child referred for troublesome behaviour may display this kind of behaviour in his home, his school classroom, his playground, and perhaps on the streets of his neighbourhood. Furthermore, there may be refinements of such specific situations in which the problem behaviour occurs.

For example, the child with severe temper-tantrums solely at home may show them only at bedtime and at mealtimes. He may be quite cooperative and pleasant at other times of the day when he is at home.

What all this means is that if you are to understand, predict, and prescribe, you need to find out how behaviour co-varies with different environmental stimuli, i.e., how *antecedent* situations affect a particular action.

C = Consequent events (outcomes)

Consequent events refer to the new conditions which the target behaviour was instrumental in bringing about. The effects of this behaviour on the person's internal and external environment are crucial determinants of whether or not the behaviour will recur.

An example

Here is an example (see Herbert, 1987) of an ABC analysis (obviously a small illustrative fragment) for a child named John, aged 6, and his 'demanding' behaviour.

A: antecedent events Demanding occurs in and out of the house. More frequently and intensively in public places like shops, friends' houses. At home it can happen any time, but more often when mother has got company or is very busy, cooking, washing, telephoning. Teatimes and mornings are particularly difficult. Demanding occurs seldom with his father and is less frequent when father is present. It never occurs with people he does not know well and never at school. Demanding is triggered off if mother does not respond immediately to his request or if she says 'no'.

B: Behaviour John will demand that mother give or buy him something, ask her to let him do something or go somewhere, things of which she does not approve, or demands she cannot fulfil immediately. He will go on and on repeating his 'request', getting very angry so that the request becomes a querulous command. He follows the mother, pulls her, eventually screams and shouts at her or becomes destructive, throwing things about, etc. The frequency is seven times a day on average, each episode lasting up to 20 minutes, and is very intensive — depending on what he wants and where it happens.

C: Consequences Mother interacts a good deal with John during these episodes, she pleads with him, disputes with him, tries to distract him, getting angrier and more frustrated, threatens him (threats are seldom carried out), screams and shouts at him, and occasionally hits him. He obviously gains a lot of attention. Eventually she gets tired and just for peace and quite she gives in. In public places, e.g., shops, she gives in quickly to avoid embarrassment, criticisms from other people and scenes. She gets very upset and at times ends up in tears.

You may get a hunch that your client's moods are part of the stimulus configuration of antecedents leading up to his own problematic behaviour (outbursts of verbal abuse), or fraught interactions between husband and wife. Try to quantify your hunch by getting the client to keep a diary.

The environment, as it is represented in words like stimulus (or antecedent events), occurs not simply as a physical or chemical agent impinging on the body or sense organs, but in terms of its *meaning* for the individual. The way in which the child interprets or categorizes (labels) events is likely to colour his emotional response to them. The same stimulus may have many different meanings, and many different stimuli may have the same meaning. It is the meanings that are important and not the stimulus in its own nature as a physical or chemical process.

If a parent tries to coax her child every time tantrums occur, the meaning for the child (and, indeed, the unwritten contract on the part of the mother) is that tantrumming will be reliably followed by parental attention. This represents a probabilistic relationship and it is the worker's task to assess and determine the probabilistic contract. The mother may not give attention *every* time, but *most* times! There is a high probability that she will reward her child with attention. These probabilistic relationships are frequently referred to as schedules of reinforcement.

Assess organismic variables

(Or obtain information from other sources.) You are not dealing with an 'empty vessel'; there are all sorts of things going on within the organism. The client's behaviour does not occur in a vacuum. He is responding to an external *and* internal environment. The way in which a client labels or categorizes events can influence his emotional reactions in such situations.

Although a person's beliefs, attitudes, and expectations may often be modified by changes in overt behaviour, there are times when such organismic (inferred, mediating) variables should themselves be the target for direct modification.

For example, there may be certain physiological and cognitive states of the client which might constitute the objective of a behavioural intervention. To take but one specific instance, phobic anxiety may involve avoidance or escape strategies, physiological signs of arousal, cognitive factors like faulty attribution or attitudes of helplessness, or combinations and permutations of all of them. Here then is a mixture of overt and covert events playing aetiological, maintaining, or mediational roles in the manifestation of the problem. Any of them might become the goal of the behavioural programme.

Step 10: Formulate goals and objectives

Do this if and when you have made a decision based on your interview and baseline findings that the problem requires an intervention.

Behavioural targets for change in the behavioural model are selected because they are socially important to either the client, those who bear the brunt of the client's behaviour, and/or those who care for him. The goal of behaviour modification is to help a person eventually to control his or her own behaviour and to achieve self-selected goals. The same applies to a group of individuals — a family seeking a viable way of living together.

Prior to designing a programme a goal should be translated into a set of behavioural objectives. Select as goals those behaviours which will be most likely to be encouraged and maintained and continue after the programme finishes. They should be relevant and seen as relevant by the client and those around him.

A behavioural objective is a precisely specified goal stating:

  (i) what the required (wanted) behaviour is;
 (ii) the situation in which it should occur;
(iii) the criteria for deciding whether the behavioural goal has been reached;
(iv) the direction of change (is the aim to increase, decrease, maintain, develop, or expand the target behaviours?).

Thus the contract is that the mother feeds her baby without expressing anger at her, in the quiet of her room, on each and every occasion that the child has her feed. This will involve the elimination of shouting, scolding, nagging, and force feeding.

Once treatment goals have been identified, they are ranked according to the negotiated consensus as to what are priorities. Balanced against the proposition that treatment must begin with the most troublesome behaviours is the proposition that nothing succeeds like success, and 'easier' problems if successfully tackled will motivate the client to 'stay with' the more intractable difficulties when the going gets hard.

Step 11: Treatment formulation

The therapist is by now in possession of a large amount of assessment data, and is in a position to construct a clinical formulation.

The clinical formulation attempts to answer the question: why? It involves a set of hypotheses, based upon assessment data, that explain the problem behaviour. It is a theory about how and why the child behaves in a particular situation. In a sense, treatment procedure 'tests' (although in no way conclusively) the hypotheses made in the clinical formulation, which will need to be reconsidered if treatment proves ineffectual. It provides a record of the therapist's initial conclusions.

The baseline period has given the therapist many opportunities to foster a working relationship with family members. In this book reference is often made to 'the parents' of the child. Ideally, the therapist should aim to work with all family members. In practice, it is often the mother who acts as main care-giver, and the involvement of father in assessment and treatment may be limited. If contact with the father is limited, he should at least be made aware of the strategies involved and be encouraged to join his wife as part of a 'united front' in order to provide consistency and support.

Prior to treatment, a list of suitable reinforcers should be obtained. Parents, child, and siblings can all contribute to the list of the target child's 'favourite things', to be checked with the child himself.

THE INTERVENTION

Step 12: Final goal plans are agreed between parents and therapist and initiated

The therapeutic task will involve a decrease in undesired behaviours, increase in desired behaviours, and sometimes the introduction of new behaviours into the child's repertoire. The therapist is now in a position to suggest certain treatment techniques that could be used in the home. These are discussed briefly with the parents in order to obtain agreement in principle for their use. The treatment programme should not incorporate any techniques that the parents feel would go against their personal values or be beyond their resources to operate. This discussion is most important as it is the parents who will control the contingencies. If the therapist and both parents are not in agreement over the tactics involved in a programme, it will easily decay through inconsistent application, or may even be sabotaged.

Parents should be warned of the possibility of extinction bursts during early treatment. The importance of consistency, persistence, and the timely application of techniques must be stressed (see Herbert, 1987).

Therapy at the Centres is a multifaceted package depending for its final shape on the behavioural assessment. It might include: differential reinforcement (positive reinforcement — social and sometimes material — of prosocial actions and removal of reinforcement or application of punishment contingent on antisocial behaviours), time-out form positive reinforcement (periods of 5 min for children below 10), response-cost and overcorrection procedures. Incentive systems (token economies) are negotiated and contracted between parents and children, and some are linked to behaviour at school. With the older children, we tend to use more cognitively orientated methods including self-control training (assertion and relaxation training, desensitizion of anger, role play, behaviour rehearsal, problem-solving and social skill training.

At the Centre parents *and* other family members figure *significantly* in the therapeutic programmes, not least because of their major contribution to the evolution of such problems. Parents of deviant children tend to display a significantly greater proportion of commands and criticisms and high rates of threats, anger, nagging, and negative consequences than parents of non-referred children. It is thus important to moderate these aversive interactions.

There is frequently a lack of contingent consequences among the distressed family members. The probability of receiving a positive, neutral or aversive consequence for coercive behaviour seems to be independent of the behaviour — a gross inconsistency. Indeed, there may be positive consequences for deviant behaviour and punishment for those rare prosocial actions.

It is only too often the case that the disturbed social interactions among the members of the family induce powerful feelings of frustration, anger and helplessness, and low self-esteem.

Parent training programmes thus include methods designed to reduce confrontations and antagonistic interactions among the family members, to increase the effectiveness (and moderate the intensity) of parental punishment, and establish consistent and genuinely rewarding patterns of reinforcement. Attention is paid to boosting parents' confidence and self-esteem and bolstering their expectations of success and sense of self-efficacy in their management of their offspring. Depending on the age of the child, he may be taught self-monitoring, the evaluation of his actions, and self-control techniques.

Frequent use is made of *alternative response training*, a method that provides children with alternative modes of response to cope with provocative and disturbing situations, or activities that are incompatible with the undesired behaviours. Contingency contracts between parents and their children (particularly adolescents) have also proved of great value, not least because of their function in modelling skills in finding solutions to conflicts. These are also useful in adoption and fostering situations and in residential settings, in which conduct problems often lead to a breakdown in substitute care.

Parents and significant others are trained to use reinforcement effectively, and are shown how to negotiate compromises and to bring about positive changes in ways other than violence. This type of work can also involve communication training.

One of the most dramatic advantages of using a behavioural model of assessment and treatment has become apparent (Iwaniec, 1983); namely, the parents' relief at finally finding professional personnel who showed an interest in finding out precisely (while enlisting *their* help) what was going wrong here and now, and who then continued to make very detailed suggestions as to ways of modifying the problems manifested by their child.

Bibliography

Abikoff, H. (1979). Cognitive training intervention in children: Review of a new approach. *Learning Disabilities*, 12(2), 123–135.

Achenbach, T.M. (1966). 'The classification of children's psychiatric symptoms: a factor analytic study'. *Psychological Monographs*, **80**, 6, Whole No. 615.

Achenbach, T.M. (1982). *Developmental Psychopathology*, Ronald Press, New York.

Achenbach, T.M., & Edelbrock, C.S. (1978). The classification of child psychopathology: A review and analysis of empirical efforts. *Psychological Bulletin*, 85, 1275–1301.

Alabiso, F. (1975). 'Operant control of attention behaviour: a treatment for hyperactivity'. *Behaviour Therapy*, **6**, 39–42.

Alexander, J.F., and Parsons, N.V. (1973). 'Short-term behavioural intervention with delinquent families: impact on family process and recidivism', *J. Abnormal Psychology*, **81**, 219–225.

Alexander, R.N., Corbett, T.F., and Smigel, J. (1976). 'The effects of individual group consequences on school attendance and curfew violations with predelinquent adolescents'. *J. Applied Behaviour Analysis*, **9**, 221–226.

Allen, K.E., Hart, B.M., Buell, J.S., Harris, F.R., and Wolf, M.M. (1965). 'Effect of social reinforcement of isolate behavior of a nursery school child'. In L.P. Ullmann and L. Krasner (Eds.), *Case Studies in Behavior Modification*, Holt, Rinehart and Winston, New York.

Allen, K.E., Henke, L.B., Harris, F.R., Baer, D.M., and Reynolds, N.J. (1967). 'Control of hyperactivity by social reinforcement of attending behavior'. *J Educational Psychology*, **58**, 231–237.

Anderson, C.M., and Plymate, H.B. (1962). 'Management of the brain damaged adolescent'. *Am. J. Orthopsychiatry*, **32**, 492–500.

Andry, R.C. (1960). *Delinquency and Parental Pathology*, Methuen, London.

Anthony, E.J. (1970). In P.H. Mussen (Ed.), *Carmichael's Manual of Child Psychology*, vol. 2, John Wiley, London.

Aronfreed, J. (1964), 'The origin of self-criticism'. *Psychological Review*, **71**, 193–218.

Aronfreed, J. (1968). *Conduct and Conscience*, Academic Press, New York.

Aronfreed, J., and Reber, A. (1965). 'Internalized behavioral suppression and the timing of social punishment' *J. Personality and Social Psychology*, **1**, 3–16.

Asher, S.R., Oden, S. and Gottman, J.M. (1976) Children's friendships in school settings. In: L.G. Katz (Ed.). *Current Topics in Early Childhood Education* (Vol. 1). Lawtrence Erlbaum, Hillsdale, N.J.

Asher, S.R. and Renshaw, P.D. (1981) Children without friends: Social knowledge and social skill training. In: S.R. Asher and J.M. Gottman (Eds.). *The Development of Children's Friendships.* Cambridge University Press, New York.

Ausubel, D. (1950). 'Negativism as a phase of ego development'. *Am. J. of Orthopsychiatry*, 796–805.

Ausubel, D.P., and Sullivan, E.V. (1970). *Theory and Problem of Child Development*, 2nd. ed. Grune and Stratton, London.

Avis, H.H. (1974). 'The neuropharmacology of aggression', *Psychological Bulletin*, **81**, 47–63.

Ayala, H.E. Minkin, N., Phillips, E.L., Fixsen, D.L., and Wolf, M.M. (1973). *Achievement Place: The Training and Analysis of Vocational Behaviors.* Paper read at the American Psychological Association, Montreal, Canada.

Ayllon, T., and Azrin, N.H. (1968). *The Token Economy: A Motivational System for Therapy and Rehabilitation,* Appleton-Century-Crofts, New York.

Ayllon, T., Layman, D., and Kandel, H.J. (1975). 'A behavioral–educational alternative to drug control of hyperactive children'. *J. Applied Behavior Analysis,* **8** (2), 137–146.

Azrin, N.H., and Holz, W.C. (1966), 'Punishment'. In W.K. Honig (Ed.), *Operant Behavior: Areas of Research and Application,* Appleton-Century-Crofts, New York.

Azrin, N.H., and Powers, M.A. (1975). 'Eliminating classroom disturbances of emotionally disturbed children by positive practice procedures'. *Behavior Therapy* **6**, 525–534.

Backeland, F., and Lundwall, L. (1975). 'Dropping out of treatment: a critical review'. *Psychological Bulletin*, **82**(5), 738–783.

Baer, D.M., and Wolf, M.M. (1970). 'The entry into natural communities of reinforcement'. In R. Ulrich, T. Stachnik, and J. Mabry (Eds.), *Control of Human Behavior: From Care to Prevention,* Scott, Foresman, Glenview, Illinois.

Baer, D.M., Wolf, M.M., and Risley, T.R. (1968). 'Some current dimensions of applied behavior analysis'. *J. Applied Behavior Analysis,* **1**, 91–97.

Bailey, J.S., Wolf, M.M., and Phillips, E.L. (1970). 'Home-based reinforcement and the modification of predelinquents' classroom behavior'. *J Applied Behavior Analysis,* **3**, 223–233.

Baker, B.L. (1969). 'Symptom treatment and symptom substitution in enuresis'. *J. Abnormal Psychology*, **74** (1), 42–49.

Baker, B.L., Brightman, A.J., Heifetz, L.J., and Murphy, D.M. (1976). *Steps to Independence Series.* Research Press, Champaign, Ill.

Bandura, A. (1965). 'Behavioral modifications through modeling procedures'. In L. Krasner and L.P. Ullmann (Eds.), *Research in Behavior Modification,* Holt, New York.

Bandura, A. (1969). *Principles of Behavior Modification,* Holt, Rinehart and Winston, New York.

Bandura, A. (1971a). *Social Learning Theory*, General Learning Press, Morristown, N.J.

Bandura, A. (1971b). 'Vicarious and self-reinforcement processes'. In R. Glaser (Ed.), *The Nature of Reinforcement,* Academic Press, New York.

Bandura, A. (1973). *Aggression: A Social Learning Analysis,* Prentice-Hall, Englewood Cliffs, N.J.

Bandura, A. (1977). *Social Learning Theory.* Prentice-Hall, Englewood Cliffs, N.J.

Bandura, A., and Perloff, B. (1967). 'Relative efficacy of self-monitored and externally imposed reinforcement systems'. *J. Personality and Social Psychology,* **7**, 111–116.

Bandura, A., and Walters, R.H. (1959). *Adolescent Aggression*. Ronald, New York.

Bandura, A., and Walters, R.H. (1963). *Social Learning and Personality Development*, Holt, Rinehart and Winston, New York.

Bannister, D., and Fransella, F. (1971). *Inquiring Man*, Penguin Books.

Barcai, A., and Rabkin, L.Y. (1974). 'A precursor of delinquency: the hyperkinetic disorder of childhood'. *The Psychiatric Quarterly*, **48**(3), 387–399.

Barcroft, J. (1970). *Behaviour Modification in the School*. Unpublished Thesis. University of London.

Bardill, D. (1972). Behaviour contracting and group therapy with preadolescent males in a residential treatment setting. *International Journal of Group Psychotherapy*, **22**, 333–342.

Barkley, R.A. (1977). A review of stimulant drug research with hyperkinetic children. *Journal of Child Psychology and Psychiatry*, **18**, 137–165.

Barkley, R.A. (1982). *Hyperactive Children: A Handbook for Diagnosis and Assessment*. Wiley, Chichester.

Barlow, D.H., and Hayes, S.C. (1979). 'Alternating treatments design'. *J. Applied Behaviour Analysis*, **12** 199–210.

Baron, R.M. (1966). 'Social reinforcement effects as a function of social reinforcement'. *Psychological Review*, **73**, 527–539.

Barrish, H.H., Saunders, M., and Wolf, M.M. (1969). 'Good behavior game. Effects of individual contingencies for group consequences on disruptive behavior in a classroom'. *J. Applied Behavior Analysis*, **2**, 119–124.

Baumrind, D. (1971). Current patterns of parental authority. *Developmental Psychology Monograph*, **4**(1), Pt. 2, pp.1–103.

Beck, A.T. (1970). 'Cognitive therapy: nature and relation to behavior therapy'. *Behavior Therapy*, **1**, 184–200.

Becker, H.S. (1963). *Outsiders: Studies in the Sociology of Deviance*, The Free Press, New York.

Beck, S., and Forehand, R. (1984). 'Social skills training for children: a methodological and clinical review of behaviour modification studies' *Behavioural Psychotherapy*, **12**, 17–45.

Becker, W.C. (1964). 'Consequences of different kinds of parental discipline'. In M.L. Hoffman and L.W. Hoffman (Eds.), *Review of Child Development Research*, Vol. 1. Russell Sage Foundation, New York.

Becker, W.C. (1971). *Parents are Teachers: A Child Management Program*, Research Press, Champaign, Illinois.

Becker, W.C., and Krug, R.S. (1964). 'A circumplex model for social behaviour of children'. *Child Development*, **35**, 371–396.

Becker, W.C., Madsen, C.H. Arnold, C.R., and Thomas, D.R. (1967). 'The contingent use of teacher attention and praise in reducing classroom behavior problems'. *J. Special Education*, **1**, 287–307.

Bell, R., and Harper, L. (1977). *Child Effects on Adults*, Erlbaum, Hillsdale, N.J.

Bell, R.Q. (1971). 'Stimulus control of parent or caretaker behavior by offspring'. *Development Psychology*, **4**, 63–72.

Bell, R.Q., Waldrop, M.F., and Weller, G.M. (1972), 'Rating system for the assessment of hyperactive and withdrawn children in preschool samples' *American J. Orthopsychiatry*, **42**(1), 23–34.

Bell, S.M., and Ainsworth, M.D.S. (1972). 'Infant crying and maternal responsiveness'. *Child Development*, **43**, 1171–1198.

Belson, W.A. (1975). *Juvenile Theft: The Causal Factors*, Harper and Row, London.

Bergin, A.E. (1969). 'Self-regulation technique for impulse control disorders'. *Psychotherapy: Theory Research and Practice*, **6**, 113–118.

Berkowitz, B.P., and Graziano, A.M. (1972). 'Training parents as behavior therapists: a review'. *Behaviour Research and Therapy*, **10**, 297–318.

Berkowitz, L., Parke, R.D., Leyens, J.P., West, S., and Sebastian, R.J. (1978). 'Experiments on the reactions of juvenile delinquents to filmed violance'. In L.A. Hersov and M. Berger (Eds.), *Aggression and Anti-social Behavior in Childhood and Adolescence.* Pergamon Press, Oxford.

Bernal, M.E., and North, J.A. (1978). 'A survey of parent training manuals' *J. Applied Behaviour Analysis,* **11,** 533–544.

Bernal, M.E., Duryee, J.S. Pruett, H.L., and Burns, B.J. (1968). 'Behavior modification and the brat syndrome'. *J Consulting and Clinical Psychology,* **32,** 447–455.

Beyer, M., Holt, S.A., Reid, T.A., and Quinlan, D.M. (1973). 'Runaway youths: families in conflict'. Paper presented at the convention of the Eastern Psychological Association, Washington, D.C., May, 1973.

Bijou, S.W. (1973). 'Behaviour modification in teaching the retarded child'. In C.E. Thoreson (Ed.) *72nd Year Book of the National Society for the Study of Education,* Chicago.

Bijou, S.W., and Baer, D.M. (1961). *Child Development: A Systematic and Empirical Theory,* Vol. 1. Appleton-Century-Crofts, New York.

Bijou, S.W., and Baer, D.M. (1966). 'Operant methods in child behavior and development'. In W.K. Honig (Ed.), *Operant Behavior: Areas of Research and Application,* Appleton-Century-Crofts, New York.

Birnbrauer, J.S. (1985). 'When social reinforcement fails'. *Unpublished manuscript.*

Birnbrauer, J.S., Bijou, S.W., Wolf, M.M., and Kidder, J.D. (1965). 'Programmed instruction in the classroom'. In P.L. Ullmann and L. Krasner (Eds.), *Case Studies in Behavior Modification,* Holt, Rinehart and Winston, New York.

Blanchard, E., and Johnson, R. (1973). 'Generalization of operant classroom control procedures'. *Behavior Therapy,* **4,** 219–229.

Blasi, A. (1980). Bridging moral cognition and moral action: A critical review of the literature. *Psychological Bulletin,* **88,** 1–47.

Boies, K.G. (1972). 'Role playing as a behavior change technique: Review of the empirical literature'. *Psychotherapy: Theory, Research and Practice,* **9,** 2.

Bolstad, O.D., and Johnson, S.M. (1972). 'Self-regulation in the modification of disruptive behavior'. *J. Applied Behavior Analysis,* **5,** 443–454.

Bornstein, P.H., and Quevillon, R.P. (1976). 'The effects of a self-instructional package on overactive preschool boys'. *J. Applied Behavior Analysis,* **9,** 179, 188.

Bornstein, M.R., Bellack, A.S., and Hersen, M. (1980), 'Social skills training for highly aggressive children'. *Behaviour Modification,* **4,** 173–186.

Bowers, K.S. (1973), 'Situationism in psychology: an analysis and a critique'. *Psychological Review,* **80,** 307–336.

Braukmann, C.J., and Fixsen, D.L. (1975). 'Behavior modification with delinquents'. In M. Hersen, R.M. Easler, and P.M. Miller (Eds.), *Progress in Behavior Modification,* Vol. 1. Academic Press, New York.

Braukmann, C.J., Maloney, D.M., Fixsen, D.L., Phillips, E.L., and Wolf, M.M. (1974). 'Analysis of a selection interview training package'. *Criminal Justice and Behavior* **1,** 30–42.

Brehm, J.W., and Cohen A.R. (1962). *Exploration in Cognitive Dissonance,* John Wiley, New York.

Broden, M., Hall, R.V., Dunlap, A., and Clark, R. (1970). 'Effects of teacher attention and a token reinforcement system in a junior high school special education class'. *Exceptional Children,* **36,** 341–349.

Broden, M., Hall, R.V., and Mitts, B. (1971). 'The effect of self-recording on the classroom behavior of two eighth-grade students'. *J. Applied Behavior Analysis,* **4** (3), 191–199.

Bronfenbrenner, U. (1967). 'Some familial antecedents of responsibility and leadership in adolescents'. In L. Petrullo and B.M. Bass (Eds.), *Leadership and Interpersonal Behaviour,* Holt, Rinehart and Winston, New York.

Bronfenbrenner, U. (1970). *Two Worlds of Childhood*, Foundation.

Brooks, B.D. (1974). 'Contingency contracts with truants'. *The Personnel and Guidance Journal,* **52**(5), 316–319.

Brooks, R.B., and Snow, D.L. (1972). 'Two case illustrations of the use of behaviour modification techniques in the school setting'. *Behavior Therapy,* **3**, 100–103.

Brown, G.D., and Tyler, V.O. (1968). 'Time out from reinforcement: a technique for dethroning the "duke" of an institutionalized delinquent group'. *J. Child Psychology and Psychiatry,* **9**, 203–211.

Brown, P., and Elliott, R. (1965). 'Control of aggression in a nursery school class'. *J. Experimental Child Psychology,* **2**, 103–107.

Brown, J.H., Gamboa, A.M., Birkimer, J., and Brown, R. (1976). 'Some possible effects of parent-self-control training on parent-child interactions'. In E.J. Mash, L.C. Handy and L.A. Hamerlynck (Eds.), *Behaviour Modification Approaches to Parenting,* Brunner/Mazel, New York, pp. 180–192.

Brown, G.W., Harris, T.O., and Peto, J. 1973: Life events and pyschiatric disorder, 2: Nature of causal links. *Psychological Medicine,* 3, 158–76.

Buehler, R.E., Patterson, G.R., and Furniss, J.M. (1966). 'The reinforcement of behavior in institutional settings'. *Behaviour Research and Therapy,* **4**, 157–167.

Burchard, J.D., (1967). 'Systematic socialization: a programmed environment for the habilitation of antisocial retardates'. *Psychological Record,* **17**, 461–476.

Burchard, J.D., and Barrera, F. (1972). 'An analysis of time out and response cost in a programmed environment'. *J. Applied Behavior Analysis,* **5**, 271–282.

Burchard, J.D., and Tyler, V. (1965). 'The modification of a delinquent behavior through operant conditioning'. *Behaviour Research and Therapy,* **2**, 245–250.

Burchard, J.D., & Harig, P.T. (1976). Behavior modification with juvenile delinquency. In H. Leitenberg (Ed.), *Handbook of Behavior Modification and Behaviour Therapy.* Prentice-Hall, Englewood Cliffs, N.J.

Caldwell, B.M. (1964). The effects of infant care. In: M.L. Hoffman and L.W. Hoffman (Eds.), *Review of Child Development Research,* Vol. 1. Russell Sage Foundation, New York.

Calhoun, K.S., Matherne, P. (1974). *An Investigation of the Effects of Varying Schedules of Time-out on Aggressive Behavior.* Unpublished manuscript, University of Georgia.

Camp, B., Blom, G., Herbert, F., and Van Doornenck, W. (1977) "Think aloud"; a program for developing self-central in young aggressive boys'. *J. Abnormal Child Psychology,* **5**, 157–169.

Campbell, D.T., and Stanley, J.C. (1973). *Experimental and Quasi-experimental Designs for Research,* Rand McNally, Chicago.

Campbell, J.D. (1964). 'Peer relations in early childhood'. In M.L. Hoffman and L.W. Hoffman (Eds.), *Review of Child Development Research,* Vol. 1. Russell Sage Foundation, New York.

Cannon, D., Sloane, H., Agosto, R., De Risi, W., Donovan, J., Ralph, J., and Della-Piana, G. (1972). *The Fred C. Nelles School for Boys Rehabilitation System,* Bureau of Educational Research, University of Utah, Salt Lake City.

Cantwell, D.P. (1972). 'Psychiatric illness in the families of hyperactive children'. *Archives of General Psychiatry,* **27**, 414–417.

Carlson, C.S., Arnold, C.R., Becker, W.C., and Madsen, C.H. (1968). 'The elimination of tantrum behavior of a child in an elementary classroom'. *Behaviour Research and Therapy,* **6**, 117–119.

Carrera, F. III, and Adams, P.L. (1970). 'An ethical perspective on operant conditioning'. *J. Am. Academy of Child Psychiatry,* **9**, 607–623.

Carter, R.D., and Thomas, E.J. (1973). 'Modification of problematic marital communication using corrective feedback and instruction', *Behavior Therapy,* **4**, 100–109.

Catania, A.C. (1966). 'Concurrent Operants'. In W.K. Honig (Ed.), *Operant Behavior: Areas of Research and Application*, Appleton-Century-Crofts. New York. pp. 213–270.

Cautela, J.R. (1965). 'Desensitization and insight'. *Behaviour Research and Therapy*, **3**, 59–64.

Cautela, J.R. (1967). 'Covert sensitization'. *Psychological Record*, **20**, 459–468.

Cautela, J.R. (1973a). 'Covert processes and behaviour mobification'. *J. Nervous and Mental Disease*, **157**, 27–35.

Cautela, J.R. (1973b). 'Covert sensitization'. In J.S. Stumphauzer (Ed.) *Behaviour Therapy with Delinquents*. Charles C. Thomas, Springield, Ill.

Chazan, M. (1959). 'Maladjusted children in grammar schools'. *Brit J. Educational Psychology*, **29**, 98–206.

Christensen, A., Johnson, S.M., and Glasgow, R.E. (1980). 'Cost effectiveness in behavioural family therapy.' *Behaviour Therapy*, **11**, 208–226.

Christensen, D.E. (1975). 'Effects of combining methylphenidate and a classroom token system in modifying hyperactive behavior'. *Am. J. Mental Deficiency*, **80** (3), 266–276.

Christy, D. (1975). 'Does the use of tangible rewards to individual children affect peer observers?' *J. Applied Behavior Analysis*, **8**, 187–197.

Clark, H.B. (1972). 'A program of delayed consequences for the management of class attendance and disruptive classroom behavior of 124 special education children'. In Semb, G. (Ed.), *Behavior Analysis and Education*, University of Kansas.

Clark, H.B., Rowbury, T., Baer, A.M., and Baer, D.M. (1973). 'Timeout as a punishing stimulus in continuous and intermittent schedules'. *J. Applied Behavior Analysis*, **6**, 443–455.

Clarke, Ann, and Clarke, A.D.B., (Eds.) (1976). *Early Experience: Myth and Experience*, Open Books Ltd., London.

Clarke, R.V.G., and Cornish, D.B. (1978). 'The effectiveness of residential treatment for delinquents', In L.A. Hersov, M. Berger, and D. Shaffer (Eds.). *Aggression and Antisocial Behaviour in Childhood and Adolescence*. Pergamon, Oxford.

Clement, P.W. (1976). 'Tailor-made peer therapy groups for children'. In B. Lubin (chairman). *Parents and Psychologists: The New Team*. Symposium, A.P.A. Convention, Washington, D.C., September, 1976.

Cobb, D.E., and Medway, F.J. (1978). 'Determinants of effectiveness in parent consultation'. *J. Community Psychology*, **6**, 229–240.

Cohen, A.K. (1955). *Delinquent Boys: The Culture of the Gang*, The Free Press, Glencoe, Illinois.

Cohen, H.L., and Filipczak, J. (1971). *A New Learning Environment*. Jossey Bass, San Francisco.

Cohen, H.L., Filipczak, J., and Bis, J.S. (1967). *Case 1: An Initial Study of Contingencies Applicable to Special Education*, Educational Facility Press, IBR, Silver Spring, Md.

Conners, C.K. (1972). 'Pharmacotherapy of psychopathology in children'. In H.C. Quay and J.S. Werry (Eds.), *Psycopathological Disorders of Childhood*, Wiley, New York.

Conners, C.K. (Ed.) (1974). *Clinical Use of Stimulant Drugs in Children*, Excerpta Medica, Amsterdam.

Coopersmith, S. (1967). *The Antecedents of Self-Esteem*, W.H. Freeman, London.

Cornish, D.B., and Clarke, R.V.G. (1975). *Residential Treatment and its Effects on Delinquency*, HMSO, No. 32.

Cowan, E., Gardner, E., and Zax, M. (Eds.) (1967). *Emergent Approaches to Mental Health Problems*. Appleton-Century-Crofts, New York.

Cowen, E.L., Pederson, A., Babigian, H., Izzo, L.D., and Trost, M.A. (1973). 'Long term followup of early detected vulnerable children. *Journal of Consulting and Clinical Psychology*, **41**, 438–44.

Cowan, P.A., and Walters, R.H. (1963). 'Studies in reinforcement of aggression: I. Effects of scheduling. *Child Development*, **34**, 543–551.

Crandall, V.J., and Bellugi, U. (1954). 'Some relationships of interpersonal and intrapersonal conceptualization to personal-social adjustement'. *J. Personality*, **23**, 224–232.

Cruickshank, W. (1968). 'Educational implications of psychopathology in brain injured children'. In J. Loring (Ed.), *Assessment of the Cerebral Palsied Child for Education*, W. Heinemann, New York.

Danaher, B.G. (1974). 'Theoretical foundations and clinical applications of the Premack Principle: review and critique'. *Behavior Therapy*, **5**, 307–324.

Dannefer, E., Brown, R., and Epstein, N. (1975). 'Experience in developing a combined activity and verbal group therapy program with latency-age boys'. *International Journal of Group Psychotherapy*, **25**, 331–337.

Das, J.P., and Nanda, P.C. (1963). 'Mediated transfer of attitudes'. *J. Abnormal and Social Psychology*, **66**, 12–16.

Davids, A. (1972). 'Effects of aggressive and non-aggressive male and female models on the behaviour of emotionally disturbed boys'. *Child Development*, **43** (4), 1443–1448.

Davidson, W.S., and Seidman, E. (1974). 'Studies of behavior modification and juvenile delinquency. Review. Methodological critique and social perspective'. *Psychological Bulletin*, **81** (12), 998–1011.

Davies, M., and Sinclair I. (1971). 'Families, hostels and delinquents: an attempt to assess cause and effect'. *Brit. J. Criminology*, **11**(3), 213–220.

Davison, G.C. (1969). 'A procedural critique of "desensitization and the experimental reduction of threat" '. *J. Abnormal Psychology*, **74**, 86–87.

Davison, G.C., and Taffel, S.J. (1972). *Effects of Behavior Therapy*. Paper presented at the Symposium on 'Recent evidence on the effects of divergent therapeutic methods' at the meeting of the American Psychological Association, Honolulu, September 1972.

Davidson, W.S., & Seidman, E. (1974). Studies of behavior modification and juvenile delinquency: Review, methodological critique and social perspective. *Psychological Bulletin*, **81**. 998–1011.

Dawe, H.C. (1934). 'An analysis of two hundred quarrels of pre-school children'. *Child Development*, **5**, 139–157.

Dean, G. (1976) 'Teaching self care skills to the mentally handicapped in children's homes.' *Child Treatment Research Unit* Paper No.6, Leicester University.

Delfini, L.F., Bernal, M.E. and Rosen, P.M. (1976) 'Comparison of deviant and normal boys in home settings'. In. E.J. Mash, L.A. Mammerlynck and L.C. Handy (Eds). *Behaviour Modification and Families*. Brunner/Mazel, New York.

De Risi, W.J., and Butz, G. (1975). *Writing Behavioural Contracts*, Research Press, Champaigne, Illinois.

Dinsmoor, J.A. (1966). 'Comments on Wetzel's treatment of a case of compulsive stealing'. *J. Consulting Psychology*, **30**, 378–380.

Dong, Y.L., Hallberg, E.T., and Hassard, H.U. (1979) Effects of assertion training on aggressive behavior of adolescents. *Journal of Counseling Psychology*, **26**(5), 459–461.

Doubros, S.G., and Daniels, G.J. (1966). 'An experimental approach to the reduction of overactive behaviour'. *Behaviour Research and Therapy*, **4**, 251–258.

Douglas, J.W.B. (1964). *The Home and the School*, MacGibbon and Kee, London.

Douglas, J.W.B., Ross, J.M., and Simpson, H.R. (1968). *All Our Future*, Peter Davies, London.

Drabman, R.S., and Spitalnik, R.S. (1973). 'Social isolation as a punishment', **16** (2), 236–249.

Drillien, C.M. (1964). *The Growth and Development of the Prematurely Born Infant*, Williams and Wilkins, Baltimore.

Dunlop, A. (1975). *The Approved School Experience,* H. London.

D'Zurilla, T.J., and Goldfried, M.R. (1971). 'Problem solving and behaviour modification', *J. Abnormal Psychology,* **78,** 107–126.

Eitzen, D.S. (1975). 'The effects of behavior modification on the attitudes of delinquents'. *Behavior Research and Therapy,* **13,** 295–299.

Elder, J.P., Edelstein, B.A. and Narick, M.M. (1979) 'Adolescent psychiatric patients: modifying aggressive behaviour with social skills training'. *Behaviour Modification,* **3,** 161–178.

Elmhorn, K. (1965). 'Study in self-reported delinquency among school-children'. In *Scandinavian Studies in Criminology,* Tavistock Publications, London.

Erwin, E. (1978). *Behaviour Therapy: Scientific, Philosophical, and Moral Foundations.* Cambridge University Press, Cambridge.

Eyberg, S.M., and Johnson, S.M. (1974). 'Multiple assessment of behavior modification with families: effects of contingency contracting and order of treated problems'. *J. Consulting and Clinical Psychology,* **42,** 594–606.

Farrington, D.P. (1978) 'The family backgrounds of aggressive youths'. In L.A. Hersov and M. Berger, (eds.), *Aggression and Anti-social Behavior in Childhood and Adolescence.* Pergamon Press, Oxford.

Farrington, D.P. 1979 Delinquent behavior modification in the natural environment'. *British Journal of Crimology,* **19,** 353–372.

Feldman, M.P. (1977). *Criminal behaviour; A psychological analysis.* Wiley, London.

Felixbrod, J.J., and O'Leary, K.D. (1973) Effects of reinforcement on children's academic behavior as a function of self-determined and externally imposed contingencies. *Journal of Applied Behavior Analysis,* **6,** 241–250.

Feldman, M.P. (1977). *Criminal Behaviour: A Psychological Analysis,* John Wiley, London

Feshbach, S. (1970). 'Aggression'. In P.H. Mussen (Ed.), *Carmichael's Manual of Child Psychology,* John Wiley, London.

Fixsen, D.L., Phillips, E.L., Harper, T., Mesigh, C., Timbers, G., and Wolf, M.M. (1972). *The Teaching-Family Model of Group Home Treatment.* Paper read at the American Psychological Association, Honolulu, Hawaii.

Fixsen, D.L., Phillips, E.L., and Wolf, M.M. (1973). 'Achievement Place: experiments in self-government with pre-delinquents'. *J. Applied Behavior Analysis,* **6,** 31–47.

Fo, S.O., and O'Donnell, C.R. (1974). 'The buddy system: relationship and contingency conditions in a community intervention program for youth with professionals as behavior change agents'. *J. Consulting and Clinical Psychology,* **42,** 163–169.

Fogelman, K. (1976). 'Bored children'. *New Society,* 15th July, 117–118.

Fogelman, K., and Richardson, K. (1974). 'School attendance: some results from the National Child Development Study'. in B. Turner (Ed.), *Truancy,* Ward Lock Educational, London.

Forehand, R. 'Child noncompliance to parental requests'. (1977). In M. Hersen, R.M. Eisler and P.M. Miller (Eds). *Progress in Behaviour Modification* (Vol 5). Academic Press, New York.

Forehand, R., and Atkeson, B. (1977). Generality of treatment effects with parents as therapists: A review of assessment and implementation procedures. *Behaviour Therapy,* **8,** 575–593.

Forehand, R., Cheney, T., and Yoder, P. (1974). 'Parent behavior training: effects on the non-compliance of a deaf child'. *Behavior Therapy and Experimental Psychiatry,* **5,** 281–283.

Forehand, R.L., and McMahon, R.J. (1981). *Helping the Noncompliant Child: A Guide to Parent Training.* Guilford Press, New York.

Foxx, R.M., and Azrin, N.H. (1972). 'Restitution: a method of eliminating aggressive-disruptive behavior of retarded and brain damaged patients'. *Behaviour Research and Therapy,* **10,** 15–27.

326

Foxx, R.M., and Azrin, N.H. (1973). 'The elimination of autistic self-stimulatory behavior by overcorrection'. *J. Applied Behavior Analysis*, **6**, 1–14.

Furnham, C. (1986). 'Social skill training with adolescents'. In C.R. Hollin and P. Trower (Eds.). *Handbook of Social Skills Training*, Volume I. Pergamon Press, Oxford.

Furniss, J.M. (1964). *'Peer reinforcement of behaviour in an institution for delinquent girls'*. Unpublished M.A. thesis, Oregon State University, Corvallis, Oregon.

Gagne, R.M. (1962). 'The acquisition of knowledge', *Psychology Review*, **69**, 355–365.

Gagne, R.M. (1965). *The Conditions of Learning*, Holt, Rinehart and Winston, New York.

Galloway, D. (1976). 'Size of school, socio-economic hardship, suspension rates, and persistent unjustified absence, from school'. *British J. Educational Psychology*, **6**, 40–47.

Gambrill, E.D. (1983). 'Behavioural intervention with child abuse and neglect'. In M. Hersen, R.M. Eisler, and P.M. Miller, (Eds). *Progress in Behaviour Modification*, Vol. 15. Academic Press, New York.

Gardner, J.M. (1976). 'Training parents as behaviour modifiers'. In S. Yen and R. McIntire (Eds.) *Teching Behaviour Modification*. Behaviordelia, Kalamazoo, Michigan.

Gelfand, D.M., and Hartmann, D.P. (1968). 'Behaviour therapy and children: a review and evaluation of research methodology'. *Psychological Bulletin*, **69**, 204–215.

Gelfand, D.M., and Hartmann, D.P. (1975). *Child Behaviour: Analysis and Therapy*, Pergamon Press, Oxford.

Germain, C. (1968). 'Social study, past and future'. *Social Casework*, **49**, 7 July 1968.

Gibbens, T.C.N. (1963). *Psychiatric Studies of Borstal Lads*, Oxford University Press, Oxford.

Gil, D.G. (1970). *Violence Against Children*, Harvard University Press, Cambridge, Mass.

Glasgow, R.E., and Rosen, G.M. (1978), 'Behavioural bibliotherapy: a review of self-help therapy manuals'. *Psychological Bulletin*, **85**, 1–23.

Gluck, M.R., Tanner, M.M., Sullivan, D.F., and Erickson, P.A. (1964). 'Follow-up and evaluation of 55 child guidance cases'. *Behaviour Research and Therapy*, **2**, 131, 134.

Glueck, E.T. (1966). 'Identification of potential delinquents at 2–3 years of age'. *International J. of Social Psychiatry*, **12**, 5–16.

Glueck, S., and Glueck G. (1950). *Unraveling Juvenile Delinquency*. Commonwealth Fund, New York.

Glueck, S., and Glueck, E.Y. (1960). *Predicting Delinquency and Crime*, Havard University Press.

Glynn, E.L., Thomas, J.D., and Shee, S.M. (1973). 'Behavioral self-control of on-task behavior in an elementary classroom'. *J. Applied Behavior Analysis*, **6**, 105–113.

Goetz, E.M., Homberg, M.C., and Leblanc, J.M. (1975). 'Differential reinforcement of other behavior and non-contigent reinforcement as control procedures during the modification of a pre-schooler's compliance'. *J. Applied Behavior Analysis*, **8**, 77–82.

Goldstein, A.P. (1978). 'Training aggressive adolescents in prosocial behaviour'. *Journal of Youth and Adolescence*, **7**(1). 73–92.

Goldstein, A.P., Heller, K., and Sechrest, L.B. (1966). *Psychotherapy and the Psychology of Behavior Change*, Wiley, New York.

Goocher, B.E., and Ebner, M. (1968). *A Behaviour Modification Approach Utilizing Sequential Response Targets in Multiple Settings*. Unpublished paper presented at Midwestern Psychological Association, Chicago, May 1968.

Goodenough, F.L. (1931). *Anger in Young Children*, Institute Child Welfare Monograph Series, No.9, University of Minnesota Press, Minneapolis.

Goodlet, G.R., and Goodlet, M.M. (1969). *Efficiency of Self-monitored and Externally Imposed Schedules of Reinforcement in Controlling Disruptive Behavior.* Unpublished manuscript, University of Guelph.

Goodwin, S.E., and Mahoney, M.J. (1975). 'Modification of aggression through modelling: an experimental probe'. *J. Behavior Therapy Experimental Psychiatry,* **6,** 200–202.

Gorer, G. (1955). *Exploring English Character,* Cresset Press, London.

Gottman, J.M., and Leiblum, S.R. (1974). *How to Do Psychotherapy and How to Evaluate it. A Manual for Beginners,* Holt, Rinehart and Winston, New York.

Graham, P., Rutter, M., and George, S. (1973). 'Temperamental characteristics predictors of behaviour disorders in children'. *Am. J. Orthopsychiatry,* **43,** 328–339.

Graubard, P.S., Rosenberg, H., and Miller, M.B. (1971). 'Student applications of behaviour modification to teachers and environments or ecological approaches to social deviancy.' In E.A. Ramp and B.L. Hopkins (Eds.) *A New Direction for Education: Behaviour Analysis.* Support and Development Centre for Follow Through, Lawrence, Kansas.

Graziano, A.M. (Ed.) (1971). *Behavior Therapy with Children,* Aldine Atherton, New York. pp. 1–29.

Greene R.J., and Pratt, J.A. (1972). 'A group contingency for individual misbehaviours in the classroom'. *Mental Retardation,* June 1972, 33–35.

Greenwald, A.G. (1976). 'Within-subjects designs: to use or not to use? *Psychological Bulletin,* **83**(2), 314–320.

Griest, D.L., and Wells, K.C. (1983). 'Behavioural family therapy with conduct disorders in children'. *Behaviour Therapy,* **14,** 37–53.

Grindee, K.D. (1970). 'Operant conditioning of "attending behaviors" in the classroom for two hyperactive Nego children'. In G.R. Patterson, D.T. Shaw, and M.J. Ebner (Eds.), *Teachers, Peers, and Parents as Agents of Change in the Classroom,* Department of Special Education, College of Education, Monograph No. 1, Eugene, Oregon. pp. 85–97.

Gronlund, N.E. (1959) *Sociometry in the Classroom.* Harper, New York.

Guthrie, E.R. (1935). *The Psychology of Learning,* Harper, New York.

Hall, R.V., and Copland, R.E. (1972). 'The responsive teaching model: a first step in shaping school personnel as behavior modification specialists'. In F.W. Clark et al. (Eds.), *Implementing Behavioural Programmes for Schools and Clinics,* Research Press, Champaign, Illinois, pp. 125–150.

Hall, R.V., Fox, R., Willard, D., Goldsmith, L., Emerson, M., Owen, M., Davis, F., and Porcia, E. (1971). 'The teacher as observer and experimenter in the modification of disputing and talking-out behaviors'. *J. Applied Behavior Analysis,* **4,** 141–149.

Hall, R.V., Lund, D., and Jackson, D. (1968). 'Effects of teacher attention on study behavior'. *J. Applied Behavior Analysis,* **1,** 1–12.

Hall, R.V., Lund, D., and Jackson, D. (1968). 'Effects of teacher attention on study behavior'. *J. Applied Behavior Analysis,* **1,** 1–12.

Hall, R.V., Panyan, M., Rabon, D., and Broden, M. (1968). 'Teacher applied contingencies and appropriate classroom behavior'. *J. Applied Behavior Analysis,* **1,** 315–322.

Halverson, C.F., and Waldrop, M.F. (1970). 'Maternal behaviour toward own and other preschool children: the problem of ownness.' *Child Development,* **41**(3), 839–845.

Hamilton, J.W., Stephens, L., and Allen, P. (1967). 'Controlling aggressive and destructive behavior in severely retarded institutionalized residents'. *Am. J. of Mental Deficiency,* **71,** 852–856.

328

Hanf, C. (1968). *Modifying Problem Behaviors in Mother–Child Interaction: Standardized Laboratory Situations*. Paper presented at the meeting of the Association of Behavior Therapies, Olympia, Washington.

Hardiker, P. (1972). 'Deviancy'. In D. Jehu, P. Hardiker, M.A. Yelloly, and A.M. Shaw (Eds.), *Behaviour Modification in Social Work*, Wiley, London.

Harlow, E. (1970). 'Intensive intervention: an alternative to institutionalization'. *Crime and Delinquency Literature*, **2**, 3–46.

Hartshorne, H., and May, M.A. (1928–1930). *Studies in the Nature of Character*, The Macmillan Co., New York.

Hartup, W.W. (1974). 'Aggression in childhood: developmental perspectives'. *American Psychologist*, **29**, 336–341.

Hartup, W.W. (1979) Peer relations and the growth of social competence. In: M.W. Kent and J.E. Role (Eds.). *Primary prevention of psychopathology (Vol. 3): Social competence in children*. University Press of New England, Hanover.

Hawkins, R.P. (1972). 'Its time we taught the young how to be good parents'. *Psychology Today*, November **1972**, 28–32.

Hawkins, R.P., Peterson, R.F., Schweid, E., and Bijou, S.W. (1966). 'Behavior therapy in the home: amelioration of problem parent–child relations with the parent in a therapeutic role'. *J. Experimental Child Psychology*, **4**, 99–107.

Henderson, M., and Hollin, C. (1983) A critical review of social skills training with young offenders. *Criminal Justice and Behaviour*, **10**, 316–341.

Henderson, W., and Silber, L. (1976) 'The behavioural contracting group: *Unpublished manuscript*. W.H. Trentman Mental Health Centre, Raleigh, N.C.

Herbert, E.W., Pinkston, E.M., Hayden, M.L. Sajwaj, T.E., Pinkston, S., Cordua, G., and Jackson C. (1973). 'Adverse effects of differential parental attention'. *J. Applied Behavior Analysis*, **6**, 15–30.

Herbert, M. (1964). 'The concept and testing of brain-damage in children: a review'. *J. Child Psychology and Psychiatry*, **5**, 197–216.

Herbert, M. (1974). *Emotional Problems of Development in Children*, Academic Press, London and New York.

Herbert, M. (1980a) Socialization for problem resistance. In P. Feldman & J. Orford (Eds.), *Psychological Problems: The social context*. Chichester: Wiley, 1980(a).

Herbert, M. (1980b) Hyperactivity in the classroom. *Special Education: Forward Trends*. **7**, 8–11.

Herbert, M. (1985a). Triadic work with children. In F. Watts (ed.), *New Developments in Clinical Psychology*, Chichester: John Wiley and Sons.

Herbert, M. (1985b). *Caring for Your Children: A Practical Guide*. Basil Blackwell, Oxford.

Herbert, M. (1986) 'Social skills training with children. In C.R. Hollin and P. Trower. (Eds.). *Handbook of Social Skills Training. Volume I: Applications Across the Life-Span*. Pergamon Press, Oxford.

Herbert, M. (1987a) *Behavioural Treatment of Children with Problems: A Practice Manual*. Academic Press, London.

Herbert, M. (1987b). *Living with Teenagers*. Basil Blackwell, Oxford.

Herbert, M., and Iwaniec, D. (1976). *The Formation of a Parents Group for Training in, and Discussion of, Child Management Procedures*. Child Treatment Research Unit (Leicester Section), No. 4, pp. 1–10.

Herbert, M., and Iwaniec, D. (1977). 'Children who are difficult to love'. *New Society*, **40**, (759), 111–112.

Herbert, M., and Iwaniec, D. (1981) Behavioural psychotherapy in natural homesettings: an empirical study applied to conduct disorders and incontinent children. *Behavioural Psychotherapy*, **9**, 55–76.

Herbert, M., Sluckin, W., and Sluckin, A. 1982: Mother-to-infant 'bonding'. *Journal of*

Child Psychology & Psychiatry, **23**, 205–21.

Herman, S.H., and Tramontana, J. (1971). 'Instructions and group versus individual reinforcement in modifying disruptive group behaviour'. *J. Applied Behavior Analysis*, **4**, 143–149.

Hersov, L.A. (1960). 'Persistent non-attendance at school/refusal to go to school'. *J. Child Psychology and Psychiatry*, **1**, 130–136.

Heussey, H.L. (1967). 'Study of the prevalance and therapy of choreatiform syndrome or hyperkinesis in rural Vermont'. *Acta Paedopsychiatrica*, **34**, 130–135.

Heussey, H., Metoyer, M., and Townsend, M. (1973). *Eight-to-Ten-Year Follow-up of 84 Children Treated for Behavior Disorder in Rural Vermont*. Paper read at the 50th Anniversary Annual Meeting of the American Orthopsychiatric Association, 29 May–1 June 1973.

Hewitt, L.E., and Jenkins, R.L. (1946). *Fundamental Patterns of Maladjustment: The Dynamics of Their Origin*, Thomas, Springfield, Ill.

Hobbs, N. (1962) 'Sources of gain in psychotherapy'. *American Psychologist*, **17**, 741–747.

Hobbs, S.A., and Forehand, R. (1975). 'Effects of differential release from time-out on children's deviant behavior'. *J. Behavior Therapy and Experimental Psychiatry*, **6**, 256–257.

Hobbs, T.R., and Holt, M.M. (1976). 'The effects of token reinforcement on the behavior of delinquents in cottage settings'. *J. Applied Behavior Analysis*, **9**, 189–198.

Hobbs, S.A., Moquin, L.E., Tyroler, M., and Lahey, B.B. (1980). 'Cognitive behaviour therapy with children'. *Psychological Bulletin*, **87**, 147–165.

Hoefler, S.A., and Bornstein, P.H. (1975). 'Achievement Place: an evaluative review'. *Criminal Justice and Behaviour*, **2**, 146–168.

Hoffman, M.L. (1970). 'Moral development'. In P.H. Mussen (Ed.), *Carmichael's Manual of Child Psychology*, Wiley, London, pp. 261–359.

Hoffman, M.L., and Saltzstein, H.D. (1967). 'Parent discipline and the child's moral development'. *J. Personality and Social Psychology*, **5**, 45–57.

Holder, C.E. (1969). 'Temper tantrum extinction: a limited attempt at behaviour modification'. *Social Work (U.K.)*, **26**, 8–11.

Holland, C.J. (1969). 'Elimination by the parents of fire-setting behavior in a seven-year-old boy'. *Behaviour Research and Therapy*, **7**, 135–137.

Holmes, A. (1979). 'The development and evaluation of hyperactive and conduct disordered children'. *Unpublished. Ph.D. thesis*, University of Leicester.

Holmes, A., and Roscoe, N. (1976). *A case-analysis of the Treatment of a Hyperactive Child*. CTRU report (unpublished), School of Social Work, University of Leicester.

Horton, L. (1982) 'Comparison of instructional components in behavioural parent training: a review. BEHAVIOURAL COUNSELLING QUARTERLY **2**, 131–147.

Homme, L., C'de Baca, P., Devine, J.V., Steinhorst, R., and Rickert, E.J. (1963). 'Use of Premack Principle in controlling the behavior of nursery school children'. *J. Experimental Analysis of Behavior*, **6**, 544.

Hoad, R., and Sparks, R. (1970). *Key Issues in Criminology*. Weidenfeld and Nicolson, London.

Hotchkiss, I. (1976). 'A Case-analysis of a Hyperactive Child. Unpublished paper, School of Social Work, University of Leicester.

Hudson B.L., and Macdonald (1986). *Behavioural Social Work*. Macmillan, London.

Iwaniec, D. (1983). Social and psychological investigation of the aetiology and management of children who fail to thrive'. *Unpublished PhD thesis*, University of Leicester.

Iwaniec, D., and Herbert, M. (1982). The assessment and treatment of children who fail to thrive. *Social Work Today*, **13**, 8–12.

330

Iwaniec, D., Herbert, M., and McNeish, (1985) 'Social work with failure-to-thrive children and their families'. Part II: Behavioural social work intervention. *Br. J. Social Wk.*, **15,** 375–389.

Iwata, B.A., and Bailey, J.S. (1974). *Reward Versus Cost Token Systems: An Analysis of the Effects on Students and Teacher.* Unpublished manuscript, Florida State University.

Jacobson, E. (1938). *Progressive Relaxation,* University of Chicago Press, Chicago, Ill.

James, W.H., and Rotter, J.B. (1958). 'Partial and 100% reinforcement under chance and skill conditions'. *J. Experimental Psychology,* **55,** 397–403.

Jehu, D. (1974). *A Behavioural Approach in the Treatment of Childhood Aggression.* Unpublished paper, University of Leicester School of Social Work.

Jehu, D., Hardiker, P., Yellowly, M., and Shaw, Mf. (1972). *Behaviour Modification in Social Work,* Wiley, London.

Jenkins, R.L. (1966). 'Psychiatric syndromes in children and their relation to family background'. *Am. J. Orthopsychiatry,* **36,** 450–457.

Jessness, C.F. (1975). 'Comparative effectiveness of behaviour modification and transactional analysis programs for delinquents'. *Journal of Consulting and Clinical Psychology,* **43,** 758–779.

Jessness, C.F., and De Risi, W.J. (1973). 'Some variations in techniques of contingency management in a school for delinquents'. In J.S. Stumphauzer (Ed.), *Behavior Therapy with Delinquents,* Charles C. Thomas, Springfield, Ill. pp. 105–121.

Johansson, S., Johnson, S.M., Wahl, G., and Martin, S. (Undated). *Compliance and Non-Compliance in Young Children: A Behavioural Analysis,* University of Oregon, Eugene, Oregon.

Johnson, C.A., and Katz, C. (1973). 'Using parents as change agents for children: a review. *J. Child Psychology and Psychiatry,* **14,** 181–200.

Johnson, D.W. (1980) 'Attitude modification methods'. In F.H. Kanfer and A.P. Goldstein (Eds). *Helping People Change* (2nd edn.) Pergamon Press, Oxford.

Johnson, R.C., and Medinnus, G.R. 1968: *Child Psychology: Behaviour and Development.* New York: John Wiley and Sons.

Johnson, S.M. (1970). 'Self reinforcement versus external reinforcement in behaviour modification with children'. *Development Psychology,* **3,** 147–148.

Johnson, S.M., and Brown, R.A. (1969). 'Producing behavior change in parents of disturbed children'. *J. Child Psychology and Psychiatry,* **10,** 107–121.

Johnson, S.M., and Lobitz, G.K. (1974). 'Parental manipulation of child behavior in home observations'. *J. Applied Behavior Analysis,* **7,** 23–31.

Johnson, S.M., Wahl, G., Martin, S., and Johansson, S. (1973). 'How deviant is the normal child: a behavioral analysis of the preschool child and his family'. In R.D. Rubin, J.P. Brady, and J.D. Henderson (Eds.), *Advances in Behavior Therapy,* Vol. 4. Academic Press, New York. pp. 37–54.

Johnston, J.M. (1972). 'Punishment of human behavior'. *American Psychologist,* **27,** 1033–1054.

Jurkovic, G.J. (1980). The juvenile delinquent as a moral philosopher: A structural-developmental perspective. *Psychological Bulletin,* **88,** 709–727.

Jones, R., and Kazdin, A.E. (1981) 'Childhood behaviour problems in the school'. In S.M. Turner, K.S. Calhoun, and H.E. Adams (Eds). *Handbook of Clinical Behaviour Therapy.* Wiley, New York.

Kagan, J., and Moss, H.A. (1962). *Birth to Maturity: A Study in Psychological Development,* Wiley, New York.

Kahn, J.H., and Nursten, J.P. (1964). *Unwillingly to School.* Pergamon Press, Oxford.

Kallarackal, A.M., and Herbert, M. (1976). 'The adjustment of Indian Immigrant Children'. In *Growing Up: A New Society Social Studies Reader,* IPC, London. pp. 6–9.

Kanfer, F.H., and Karoly, P. (1972). 'Self-control: a behavioristic excursion into the lion's den'. *Behavior Therapy*, **3**, 398–416.

Kanfer, F.H., and Saslow, G. (1969). 'Behavioral diagnosis'. In C.M. Franks (Eds.), *Behavior Therapy: Appraisal and Status*, McGraw-Hill, New York. pp. 417–444.

Kaspar, J.C., Millichap, J.G., Backus, R., Child, D., and Schulman, J.L. (1971). 'A study of the relationship between neurological evidence of brain damage in children and activity and distractibility'. *J. Consulting and Clinical Psychology*, **36**, 329–337.

Kaufman, K.F., and O'Leary, K.D. (1972). 'Reward, cost, and self-evaluation procedures for disruptive adolescents in a psychiatric hospital school'. *J. Applied Behavior Analysis*, **5**, 293–309.

Kazdin, A.E. (1972). 'Response cost: the removal of conditioned reinforcers for therapeutic change'. *Behaviour Therapy*, **3**, 533–546.

Kazdin, A.E. (1973). 'Methodological and assessment considerations in evaluating reinforcement programs in applied settings'. *J. Applied Behavior Analysis*, **6**, 517–531.

Kazdin, A.E., and Bootzin, R.R. (1972). 'The token economy: an evaluative review'. *J. Applied Behavior Analysis*, **5**, 343–372.

Kazdin, A.E. (1978). *History of Behaviour Modification*. University Park Press, Baltimore.

Kazdin, A.E. (1979a) 'Advances in child behaviour therapy: applications and implications. *American Psychologist*, **34**, 981–987.

Kazdin, A.E. (1979b) *Behaviour Modification in Applied Settings*. Dorsey Press, Homewood, Ill.

Kazdin, A.E. (1982), *Single-Case Research Designs: Methods for Clinical and Applied Settings*, Oxford University Press, New York.

Kelly, G.A. (1955). *The Psychology of Personal Constructs*, Vols. 1 and 2. Van Nostrand Reinhold, New York.

Kendall, P.C. (1977). 'On the efficacious use of verbal self-instructional procedures with children'. *Cognitive Therapy and Research*, **1**, (4), 331–341.

Kendall, P.C. (1981). 'Cognitive-behavioural interventions with children'. In B. Lahey and A.E. Kazolin (Eds). *Advances in Clinical Child Psychology*, Vol. 4., Plenum, New York.

Kendall, P.C., and Braswell, L. (1982) 'On cognitive-behavioural assessment: model, method and madness'. In C.D. Spielberger and J.N. Butcher. (Eds.). *Handbook of Research Methods in Clinical Psychology*. Wiley, New York.

Kent, R.N., and O'Leary, K.D. (1976). 'A controlled evaluation of behavior modification with conduct problem children'. *J. Consulting and Clinical Psychology*, **44**, (6), 586–596.

Kifer, R.E., Lewis, M.A., Green, D.R., and Phillips, E.L. (1974). 'Training predelinquent youths and their parents to negotiate conflict situations'. *J. Applied Behavior Analysis*, **7**, 357–364.

Kirigin, K.A., Timbers, G.D., Ayala, H.E., Fixsen, D.L., Phillips, E.L., and Wolf, M.M. (1973). *The Negative Effects of 'Positive' Tutoring on the Independent Reading Behavior of Delinquent Adolescents*. Unpublished manuscript, University of Kansas.

Knight, B.J., and West, D.J. (1975). 'Temporary and continuing delinquency'. *British J. Criminology*, **15**, 43–50.

Kohlberg, L. (1970). *Moral Development*, Holt, Rinehart and Winston, New York.

Kohlberg, L. (1976). Moral stages and moralization. In T. Lickona (Ed.), *Moral Development and Behavior: Theory Research and Social Issues*. Holt, Rinehart & Winston, New York.

Kohn, M. (1969). *Congruent Competence and Symptom Factors in the Preschool Child*.

Paper presented at the meeting of the American Psychological Association, Washington, D.C., September 1969.

Kraft, T. (1970). 'Treatment of drinamyl addiction'. *J. Nervous Mental Disease*, **150**, 138–144.

Koller, K.M., and Castanos, J.N. (1970). Family background in prison groups: A comparative study of parental deprivation. *British Journal of Psychiatry*, **117**, 371–380.

Kovitz, K.E. (1976). 'Comparing group and individual methods for training parents in child management techniques'. In E.J. Mash, L.C. Handy and L.A. Hammerlynk (Eds) *Behaviour Modification Approaches to Parenting*. Brunner/Mazel, New York.

Krebs, K. (1976). 'Children and their pecking order'. In *Growing Up: A New Society Social Studies Reader*, IPC, London. pp. 14–16.

Kubany, E.S., Weiss, L.E., and Sloggett, B. (1971). 'The good behaviour clock: reinforcement/timeout procedure for reducing disruptive classroom behavior'. *J. Behavior Therapy and Experimental Psychiatry*, **2**, 173–174.

Kuypers, D.S., Becker, W.C., and O'Leary K.D. (1968). 'How to make a token system fail'. *Exceptional Children*, **35**, 101–109.

Lahaderne, H.E. (1968). 'Attitudinal and intellectual correlates of attention: a study of four sixth grade classrooms'. *J. Educational Psychology*, **59**, 320–324.

Lahey, B.B., Delamater, A., and Kupfer, D. (1981) 'Intervention strategies with hyperactive and learning disabled children'. In S.M. Turner, R.S. Calhoun and H.E. Adams (Eds.) *Handbook of Clinical Behaviour Therapy*. Wiley, New York.

Lahe, D.B., McNees, M. P. and Brown, C.C. (1973) Modification of deficits in reading for comprehension. *Journal of Applied Behaviour Analysis*, **6**, 475–480.

Lapouse, R., and Monk, M.A. (1958). 'An epidemiological study of behaviour characteristics in children'. *Am. J. Public Health*, **48**, 1134–1144.

Lazarus, A.A. (1966). 'Behavioral rehearsal versus non-directive therapy versus advice in effecting behavior change'. *Behaviour Research and Therapy*, **4**, 209–212.

Lazarus, A.A., and Abramovitz, A. (1962). 'The use of "emotive imagery" in the treatment of children's phobias'. *J. Mental Science*, **108**, 191–195.

Lefkowitz, M.M., Eron, L.D., Walder, L.O., and Huessmann, L.R. (1977). *Growing up to be Violent: A Longitudinal Study of Aggression*. Pergamon Press, Oxford.

Lee, S.G.M., and Herbert, M. (Eds) (1970). *Freud and Psychology*, Penguin Books, Harmondsworth.

Leitenberg, H. (1965). 'Is time-out from positive reinforcement an aversive event? A review of the experimental evidence'. *Psychological Bulletin*, **64**, 428–441.

Leung, F.L. (1975). 'The ethics and scope of behaviour modification'. *Bulletin Br. Psychological Soc.*, **28**, 376–379.

Levitt, E.E. (1963). 'Psychotherapy with children: a further evaluation'. *Behaviour Research and Therapy*, **1** (1), 45–51.

Levitt, E.E. (1971). 'Research on psychotherapy with children'. In A.E. Bergin and S.L. Garfield (Eds.), *Handbook of Psychotherapy and Behaviour Change*, John Wiley, London.

Levy, D.M. (1955). 'Oppositional syndromes and oppositional behavior'. In P.H. Hoch and J. Zubin (Eds.), *Psychotherapy in Childhood*, Greene and Stratton, New York.

Lewis, C. (1986) 'Paternal behaviour', In W. Sluckin and M. Herbert (Eds.) *Parental Behaviour*, Basil Blackwell, Oxford.

Lobitz, G.K., and Johnson, S.M. (1973). *Normal Versus Deviant Children. A Multimethod Comparison*. Unpublished manuscript, University of Oregon. Cited in Johnson, S.M., and Lobitz, G. (1974). 'Parental manipulation of child behavior in home observations'. *J. Applied Behavior Analysis*, **7**, 23, 31.

Lobitz, W.C., and Johnson, S.M. (1975). 'Parental manipulation of the behavior of normal and deviant children'. *Child Development*, **46**, 719–726.

Loevinger, J. (1966). 'The meaning and measurement of ego development'. *American Psychologist*, **21**, 195–206.

Logan, C.H. (1972). 'Evaluation research in crime and delinquency: a reappraisal'. *J. Criminal Law, Criminology and Police Science*, **63**, 378.

Luria, A.R. (1961). *The Role of Speech in the Regulation of Normal and Abnormal Behaviour,*. Pergamon Press, Oxford.

McCandless, B. (1969). *Children: Behaviour and Development.* Holt, Rinehart and Winston, London.

McAllister, L.W., Stachowiak, J.G., Baer, D.M., and Conderman, L. (1969). 'The application of operant conditioning techniques in a secondary school classroom'. *J. Applied Behaviour Analysis*, **2**, 277–285.

McAuley, R. (1982); 'Training parents to modify conduct problems in their children'. *Journal of Child Psychology and Psychiatry*, **23**, 335–342.

McCord, W., and McCord, J. (1959). *The Origins of Crime: A New Evaluation of the Cambridge–Somerville Youth Study*, Columbia University Press, Columbia.

McCord, W., and McCord, J. (1964). *The Psychopath*, Van Nostrand, London.

MacFarlane, J.W., Allen, L., and Honzik, M.P. (1954). *A Developmental Study of the Behavior Problems of Normal Children between Twenty-one Months and Fourteen Years*, University of California Press, Berkeley and Los Angeles.

McIntyre, R.W., Jensen, J., and Davis, G. (1968). *Control of Disruptive Behaviour with a Token Economy*. Paper presented to Eastern Psychological Association, Philadelphia.

McKenzie, H.S., Clark, M., Wolf, M.M., Kothera, R., and Benson, C. (1968). 'Behavior modification of children with learning disabilities using grades as tokens and allowances as back up reinforcers'. *Exceptional Children*, **35** (Summer), 745–752.

McMillan, D.E. (1967). 'A comparison of the punishing effects of response-produced shock and response-produced time-out'. *J. Experimental Analysis of Behavior*, **10**, 430–449.

Madsen, C.H. Jr., Becker, W.C., and Thomas, D.R. (1968). 'Rules, praise and ignoring: elements of elementary classroom control'. *J. Applied Behavior Analysis*, **1**, 139–150.

Madsen, C.H. Jr., Becker, W.C., Thomas, D.R. Koser, L., and Plager, E. (1968). 'An analysis of the reinforcing function of 'Sit-down' commands'. In R.K. Parker (Ed.), *Readings in Educational Psychology*, Allyn and Bacon, Boston, pp. 265–278.

Mahoney, M.J. (1972). 'Research issues in self-management'. *Behavior Therapy*, **3**, 45–63.

Mahoney, M.J., and Thoresen, C.E. (1974). *Self-control: Power to the Person*, Brooks, Cole, Monterey, Cal.

Malewska, H.E., and Muszynski, H. (1970). 'Children's attitudes to theft'. In K. Danziger (Ed.), *Readings in Child Socialization*, Pergamon Press, Oxford.

Marlatt, G.A., and Perry, M.A. (1975) 'Modeling methods'. In F.H. Kanfer and A.P. Goldstein (Eds.), *Helping People Change*, Pergamon Press, Oxford.

Marshall, M.H. (1965). 'The effects of punishment on children: a review of the literature and a suggested hypothesis'. *J. Genetic Psychology*, **106**, 23–33.

Marshall, T.M. (1976). 'Vandalism: the seeds of destruction', *New Society*, 17 June, 625–627.

Martin, M., Burkholder, R., Rosenthal, T., Tharp, R., and Thorne, G. (1968). 'Programming behavior change and reintegration into school milieux of extreme adolescent deviates'. *Behaviour Research and Therapy*, **6**, 371–384.

Martinson, R. (1974). 'What works? — questions and answers about prison reform'. *The Public Interest*, **Spring**, 22–34.

Masters, J.C. (1970). 'Treatment of adolescent rebellion by the reconstrual of stimuli', *Journal of Consulting and Clinical Psychology*, **35**, 213–216.

Meehl, P.E. (1960). 'The cognitive activity of the clinician'. *American Psychologist*, **15**, 19–27.

Meichenbaum, D.H. (1973). 'Cognitive factors in behavior modification: modifying what clients say to themselves'. In R.D. Rubin, J.P. Brady, and J.D. Henderson (Eds.), *Advances in Behavior Therapy*, Vol. 4, Academic Press, New York, pp. 21–36.

Meichenbaum, D.H., & Burland, S. (1979). Cognitive behavior modification with children. *School Psychology Digest*, **8**(4), 426–433.

Meichenbaum, D.H., and Cameron, R. (1974). 'The clinical potential of modifying what clients say to themselves'. In M.J. Mahoney and C.E. Thoresen (Eds.), *Self-control: Power to the Person*, Wadsworth, Belmont, California, pp. 263–290.

Meichenbaum, D., and Goodman, J. (1971). 'Training impulsive children to talk to themselves: a means for developing self-control'. *J. Abnormal Psychology*, **77**, 155–126.

Mendelson, W., Johnson, N., and Stewart, M.A. (1971). 'Hyperactive children as teenagers: a follow-up study'. *J. Nervous Mental Disease*, **153**, 273–279.

Menkes, M.M., Rowe, J.S., and Menkes, J.H. (1967). 'A 25-year follow-up study on the hyperkinetic child with minimal brain dysfunction'. *Pediatrics*, **39**, 393–399.

Mickelson, D.J., and Stevic, R.R. (1971). 'Differential effects of facilitative and non-facilitative behavioural counsellors'. *J. Counselling Psychology*, **18**, 314–319.

Mira, M. (1970). 'Results of a behaviour modification training program for parents and teachers'. *Behaviour Research and Therapy*, **8**(3), 309–311.

Mischel, W. (1968). *Personality and Assessment*, Wiley, New York.

Moore, T.W. (1966). 'Difficulties of the ordinary child in adjusting to primary school'. *J. Child Psychology and Psychiatry*, **7**, 299.

Morgn, R.T.T. (1984). *Behavioural Treatments with Children*. William Heinemann Medical Books, London.

Morrison, J.R., and Stewart, M.A. (1971). 'A family study of the hyperactive child syndrome'. *Biol. Psychiatry*, **3**, 189–195.

Mowrer, O.H. (1960). *Learning Theory and Symbolic Processes*. Wiley, New York.

Nawas, M.M. (1970). 'Wherefore cognitive therapy? A critical scrutiny of three papers by Beck, Bergin, and Ullmann'. *Behavior Therapy*, **1**, 359–370.

O'Dell, S., Flynn, J., and Benlolo, L. (1977). A comparison of parent training techniques in child behavior modification. *Journal of Behavior Therapy and Experimental Psychiatry*, **8**, 261–268.

O'Dell, S. (1974). 'Training parents in behavior modification: a review'. *Psychological Bulletin*, **81** (7), 418–433.

O'Donnell, C.R., and Worell, L. (1973). 'Motor and cognitive relaxation in the desensitization of anger'. *Behaviour Research and Therapy*, **11**, 473–481.

O'Leary, K.D. (1972). 'The entree of the paraprofessional in the classroom'. In S.W. Bijou and E. Ribes-Inesta (Eds.), *Behavior Modification: Issues and Extensions*, Academic Press, New York, pp. 93–108.

O'Leary, K.D., and Becker, W.C. (1967). 'Behavior modification of an adjustment class: a token reinforcement program'. *Exceptional Children*, **33**, 637–642.

O'Leary, K.D., Becker, W.C., Evans, M.B., and Saudargas, R.A. (1969). 'A token reinforcement program in a public school: a republication and systematic analysis'. *J. Applied Behavior Analysis*, **2**, 3–13.

O'Leary, K.D., and Drabman, R.S. (1971). 'Token reinforcement program in the classroom: a review'. *Psychological Bulletin*, **75**, 379–398.

O'Leary, K.D., Kaufman, K.F., Kass, R.E., and Drabman, R.S. (1970). 'The effects of loud and soft reprimands on the behaviour of disruptive students'. *Exceptional Children*, **37**, 145–155.

O'Leary, K.D., and Kent, R. (1973). 'Behaviour modification for social action:

research tactics and problems'. In L.A. Hamerlynck, L.A. Handy, and E.J. Mash, (Eds.), *Behaviour Change: Methodology, Concepts and Practice*, Research Press, Ill. pp. 69–96.

O'Leary, K.D., and O'Leary, S.G. (1972). *Classroom Management: The Successful Use of Behavior Modification*, Pergamon Press, New York.

O'Leary, S.G., and O'Leary, K.D. (1976). 'Behavior modification in the school'. In H. Leitenberg (Ed.), *Handbook of Behavior Modification and Therapy*, Prentice-hall, Englewood Cliffs, N.J.

O'Leary, K.D., O'Leary, S.G., and Becker, W.C. (1967). 'Modification of a deviant sibling interaction pattern in the home'. *Behaviour Research and Therapy*, **5**, 113–120.

O'Leary, K.D., Pelham, W.E., Rosenbaum, A., and Price, G.H. (1976). 'Behavioral treatment of hyperkinetic children: an experimental evaluation of its usefulness'. *Clinical Pediatrics*, **15**, 510–515.

O'Leary, K.D., Poulos, R.W., and Devine, V.T. (1972). 'Tangible reinforcers: bonuses or brides?' *J. Consulting and Clinical Psychology*, **38**, 1–8.

O'Leary, K.D., Turkewitz, H., and Taffel, S.J. (1973). 'Parent and therapist evaluation of behavior therapy in a child psychological clinic'. *J. Consulting and Clinical Psychology*, **41**, 279–283.

O'Leary, K.D., and Wilson, G.T. (1975). *Behavior Therapy: Application and Outcome*, Prentice-Hall, London.

Ollendick, T.H., and Cerny, J.A. (1981). *Clinical Behaviour Therapy with Children*. Plenum, New York.

O'Malley, J.E., and Eisenberg, L. (1973). 'The hyperkinetic syndrome'. *Seminars Psychiatr.*, **5**, 95.

O'Neal, P., and Robins, L.N. (1958). 'The relation of childhood behaviour problems to adult psychiatric status: a 30-year follow-up study of 150 subjects'. *Am. J. Psychiatry*, **114**, 961–969.

Paine, R., Werry, J., and Quay, H. (1968). 'A study of "Minimal Cerebral Dysfunction" '. *Developmental Medicine and Child Neurology*, **10**, 505–520.

Pasamanick, B., and Knobloch, A.M. (1961). 'Epidermiologic studies on the complication of pregnancy and the birth process'. In G. Caplan (Ed.), *Prevention of Mental Disorders in Childhood*, Basic Books, New York.

Patterson, G.R. (1965). 'An application of conditioning techniques to the control of a hyperactive child'. In L.P. Ullmann L. Krasner (Eds.), *Case Studies in Behavior Modification*, Holt, Rinehart and Winston, New York. pp. 370–375.

Patterson, G.R. (1974). 'Interventions for boys with conduct problems: multiple settings, treatments, and criteria'. *J. Consulting and Clinical Psychology*, **42**(4), 471–481.

Patterson, G.R. (1975). 'The coercive child: architect or victim of a coercive system?' In L. Hamerlynck, L.C. Handy, and E.J. Mash (Eds.), *Behavior Modification and Families. I. Theory and Research. II. Applications and Developments*, Brunner and Mazell, New York.

Patterson, G.R. (1982). *Coercive Family Process*. Castalia, Eugene, Oregon.

Patterson, G.R., and Brodsky, G. (1966). 'A behavior modification programme for a child with multiple problem behaviors'. *J. Child Psychology and Psychiatry*, **7**, 277–295.

Patterson, G.R., and Cobb, J.A. (1971). 'A dyadic analysis of "aggressive" behaviors'. In J.P. Hill (Ed.), *Minnesota Symposia on Child Psychology*, Vol. V. University of Minnesota Press, Minneapolis. pp. 73–129.

Patterson, G.R., Cobb, J.A., and Ray, R.S. (1972). 'Direct intervention in the classroom: a set of procedures for the aggressive child'. In F. Clark, D. Evans, and L. Hamerlynck (Eds.), Research Press, Champaign, Ill. pp. 151–210.

Patterson, G.R., Cobb, J.A., and Ray, R.S. (1973). 'A social engineering technology for retraining the families of aggressive boys'. In H.E. Adams and I.P. Unikel (Eds.), *Issues and Trends in Behavior Therapy*, C.C. Thomas, Springfield, Ill. pp. 139–224.

Patterson, G.R., and Fleischman, M.J. (1979). 'Maintenance of treatment effects: some consideration concerning family systems and follow-up data.' *Behaviour Therapy*, **10**, 168–185.

Patterson, G.R., and Gullion, M.E. (1968). *Living with Children: New Methods for Parents and Teachers*, Research Press, Champaign, Ill.

Patterson, G.R., Jones, R., Whittier, J., and Wright, M.A. (1965). 'A behaviour modification technique for the hyperactive child'. *Behaviour Research and Therapy*, **2**, 217–226.

Patterson, G.R., Littman, R.A., and Bricker, W. (1967). 'Assertive behaviour in children: a step toward a theory of aggression'. *Monographs of the Society for Research in Child Development*, **32**, 5 (Whole No. 113). 1–38.

Patterson, G.R. Ray, R.S., and Shaw, D.A. (1968). 'Direct intervention in families of deviant children'. *Oregon Research Institute Research Bulletin*, **8** (9).

Patterson, G.R., Ray, R.S., Shaw, D.A., and Cobb, J.A. (1969). *Manual for Coding Family Interactions, 6th rev.*, Available from ASIS National Auxiliary Publications Service, in care of CCM Information Service, Inc., 909 Third Avenue, New York, N.Y. 10022, Document 01234.

Patterson, G.R., and Reid, J.B. (1970). 'Reciprocity and coercion: two facets of social systems'. In C. Neuringer and J. Michael (Eds.), *Behaviour Modification in Clinical Psychology*, Appleton-Century-Crofts, New York, pp. 133–177.

Patterson, G.R., and Reid, J.B. (1973). 'Intervention for families of aggressive boys: a replication study', *Behavior Research and Therapy*, **11**, 383, 394.

Patterson, G.R., Reid, J.B. Jones, J.J., and Conger, R.E. (1975). *A Social Learning Approach to Family Intervention:* Vol. 1, *Families with aggressive children*, Castalix Publishing Co., Eugene.

Patterson, G.R., Shaw, D.A., and Ebner, M.J. (1969). 'Teachers, peers, and parents as agents of change in the classroom'. In F.A.M. Benson (Ed.), *Modifying Deviant Social Behaviors in Various Classroom Settings*, No.1. University of Oregon, Eugene, Oregon, pp.13–47.

Pavlov, I.P. (1927). *Conditioned Reflexes and Psychiatry* (Trans. W.H. Gantt). International Publications, New York.

Persons, R.W. (1966). 'Psychological and behavioural change in delinquents following psychotherapy'. *J. Clinical Psychology*, **22**, 337–340.

Peterson, D.R. (1961). 'Behaviour problems of middle childhood'. *J. Consulting Psychology*, **25**, 205–209.

Phillips, E.L., Phillips, E.A., Fixsen, D.L., and Wolf, M.M. (1971). 'Achievement Place: modification of the behaviors of pre-delinquent boys within a token economy'. *J. Applied Behavior Analysis*, **4**, 45–59.

Phillips, E.L., Wolf, M.M., and Fixsen, D.L. (1973). Achievement Place: development of the elected manager system'. *J. Applied Behavior Analysis*, **6**, 541–561.

Piaget, J. (1932). *The Moral Judgement of the Child*, Harcourt, Brace, New York.

Pinkston, E.M., Reese, N.M., LeBlanc, J.M., and Baer, D.M. (1973). 'Independent control of a preschool child's aggression and peer interaction by contingent teacher attention'. *J. Applied Behavior Analysis*, **6**, 115–124.

Power, M.J., Ash, P., Shoenberg, E., and Sircy, C. (1974). 'Delinquency and the family'. *Brit. J. Social Work*, **4**, 13–38.

Power, M.J., Benn, R.T., and Morris, J.N. (1972). 'Neighbourhood, school and juveniles before the courts'. *Brit. J. Criminology*, **12**, 111–132.

Premack, D. (1965). 'Reinforcement theory'. In D. Levine (Ed.), *Nebraska Symposium on Motivation*, University of Nebraska Press, Lincoln, pp. 123–180.

Quay, H.C., Morse, W.C., and Cutler, R.L. (1966). 'Personality patterns of pupils in special classes for the emotionally disturbed'. *Exceptional Children*, **32**, 297–301.

Ray, R.S., Shaw, D.A., and Cobb, J.A. (1970). 'The work-box: an innovation in teaching attentional behavior'. *The School Counselor*, **18**, 15–35.

Repp, A.C., and Dietz, S.M. (1974). 'Reducing aggressive and self-injurious behavior of institutionalized retarded children through reinforcement of other behaviors'. *J. Applied Behavior Analysis*, **7**, 313–325.

Repucci, N.D., and Saunders, J.T. (1974). 'Social psychology of behavior modification: problems of implementation in natural settings'. *American Psychologist*, **29**, 649–660.

Reynolds, M.M. (1928). 'Negativism of preschool children: an observational and experimental study'. *Contributions to Education*, No.228, Bureau of Publications. Teachers College, Columbia University, New York.

Rich, J. (1956). 'Types of stealing'. *Lancet*, **1956**, 496.

Riemer, M.D. (1940). Runaway children'. *American Journal of Orthopsychiatry*, **10**, 522–526.

Riddle, K.D., and Rapoport, J.L. (1976). 'A 2-year follow-up of 72 hyperactive boys. Classroom behavior and peer acceptance'. *J. Nervous and Mental Disease*, **162**(2), 126–134.

Rimm, D.C., De Groot, J.C., Boord, P., Heiman, J., and Dillow, P.V. (1971). 'Systematic desensitization of an anger response'. *Behaviour Research and Therapy*, **9**, 273–280.

Rimm, D.C., and Masters, J.C. (1974). *Behavior Therapy: Techniques and Empirical Findings*, Academic Press, New York and London.

Robins, L.N. (1966). *Deviant Children Grown Up*, Williams and Wilkins, Baltimore.

Robins, L.N. (1970). 'Antecedents of character disorder'. In M. Roff and D.F. Ricks (Eds.), *Life History Research in Psychopathology*, University of Minnesota Press, Minneapolis.

Robins, L.N. (1972). 'Follow-up studies of behavior disorders in children'. In H.C. Quay and J.S. Werry (Eds.), *Psychopathological Disorders of Childhood*, Wiley, New York, pp. 414–450.

Roscoe, N. (1976). *A Behavioural Case Analysis of a Non-compliant Child*. Unpublished paper, School of Social Work, University of Leicester.

Rose, S.D., (1974). *Treating Children in Groups*, Jossey-Bass, San Francisco.

Rosenbaum, A., O'Leary, K.D., and Jacob, R.G. (1975). 'Behavioral intervention with hyperactive children: group consequences as a supplement to individual contingencies'. In C.M. Franks (Ed.), *Behavior Therapy*, Vol. 6, No. 3, Academic Press, New York and London, pp. 315–323.

Rosenkrans, M.A., and Hartup, W.W. (1967). 'Imitative influences of consistent and inconsistent response consequences to a model on aggressive behavior in children'. *J. Personality and Social Psychology*, **7**, 429–434.

Ross, A.O. (1968). 'Conceptual issues in the evaluation of brain damage'. In J.L. Khanna (Ed.), *Brain Damage and Mental Retardation: A Psychological Evaluation*.

Rotter, J.B. (1966). 'Generalized expectations for internal versus external control of reinforcement'. *Psychological Monographs: General and Applied*, **80** (Whole No. 609).

Rotter, J.B. (1971). 'External control and internal control'. *Psychology Today*, **5**, 37–42, 58–59.

Russo, S. (1964). 'Adaptations in behavioral therapy with children'. *Behaviour Research and Therapy*, **2**, 43–47.

Rutter, M. (1966). *Children of Sick Parents*, Oxford University Press, London.

Rutter, M. (1972). 'Parent–child separation: psychological effects on the children'. *J. Child Psychology and Psychiatry*, **12**, 233–260.

Rutter, M.L. Prospective studies to investigate behavioral change. In J.S. Strauss,

338

H.M. Babigian, and M. Roff (Eds.), *The origins and course of psychopathology*. New York: Plenum Press, 1977. (a).

Rutter, M.L. Individual differences. In M.L. Rutter and L.A. Hersov (Eds.), *Child psychiatry: Modern approaches*. Oxford: Blackwell Scientific, 1977 (b).

Rutter, M.L. Family, area and school influences in the genesis of conduct disorders. In L. A. Hersov and M. Berger (Eds)., *Aggression and anti-social behavior in childhood and adolescence*, Oxford: Pergamon Press, 1978.

Rutter, M., and Brown, G.W. (1966). 'The reliability and validity of measures of family life and relationships in families containing a psychiatric patient'. *Social Psychiatry*, **1**, 38–53.

Rutter, M. and Giller, H., (1983) *Juvenile Delinquency: Trends and Perspectives* Penguin, Harmondworth.

Rutter, M., Maughan, B., Mortimore, P. and Ouston, J. (1979). *Fifteen Thousand Hours*. Open Books, London.

Rutter, M., Tizard, J., and Whitmore, K. (Eds.) (1970). *Education, Health and Behaviour*, Longman, London.

Ryall, R. (1974). 'Delinquency: the problem for treatment'. *Social Work Today*, **5** (4), 98–104.

Sachs, D.A. (1973). 'The efficacy of time-out procedures in a variety of behavior problems'. *J. Behavior Therapy and Experimental Psychiatry*, **4**, 237–242.

Safer, D.J., and Allen, R.P. (1975). 'Stimulant drug treatment of hyperactive adolescents', *Diseases of the Nervous System* **36**, 454–460.

Sajwaj, T., Culver, P., Hall, C., and Lehr, L. (1972). 'Simple punishment techniques for the control of classroom disruptions'. In G. Semb *et al.* (Eds.), *Behaviour Analysis and Education*, University of Kansas.

Sajwaj, T., Twardosz, S., and Burke, M. (1972). 'Side effects of extinction procedures in a remedial preschool'. *J. Applied Behavior Analysis*, **5**, 163–175.

Sameroff, A.J. (1975). 'Early influences on development: fact or fancy?' *Merrill-Palmer Quarterly*, **21**, 275–301.

Sandberg, S.T., Rutter, M.L., and Taylor, E. (1978) Hyperkinetic disorder in psychiatric clinic attenders. *Developmental Medicine and Child Neurology*, 1978, **20**, 278–299.

Santogrossi, D.A., O'Leary, K.D., Romanczyk, R.G., and Kaufman, K.F. (1973). 'Self-evaluation by adolescents in a psychiatric hospital school token program'. *J. Applied Behavior Analysis*, **6**, 277–287.

Sarason, I.G. (1968). 'Verbal learning, modeling and juvenile delinquency'. *American Psychologist*, **23**, 254–266.

Sarason, I.G.., and Ganzer, V.J. (1973). 'Modeling and group discussion in the rehabilitation of juvenile delinquents'. *J. Counseling Psychology*, **20**, 442–449.

Schaefer, E.S. (1959). 'A circumplex model of maternal behaviour'. *Journal of Abnormal Social Psychology*, **59**, 226–235.

Scarboro, M.E., and Forehand, R. (1975). 'Effects of two types of response, — contingent time-out on compliance and oppositional behaviour of children. *Journal of Experimental Child Psychology*, **19**, 252–264.

Schmidt, F.W., and Ulrich, R.E. (1969). 'Effects of group contingent events upon classroom noise'. *J. Applied Behavior Analysis*, **2**, 171–179.

Schmidt, K. (1975). 'The effect of continuous stimulation on the behavioural sleep of infants'. *Merrill-Palmer Quarterly*, **21**, 77–88.

Schneider, M. (1973). 'Turtle technique in the classroom'. *In Exceptional Children*, **42**, 201.

Schrag, P., and Divoky, D. (1975). *The Myth of the Hyperactive Child*, Pantheon, New York.

Schreibman, L., and Koegel, R.L. (1981). 'A guideline for planning behaviour modification programmes for autistic children'. In S.M. Turner, K.S. Calhoun and H.E. Adams. *Handbook of Clinical Behaviour Therapy*. Wiley, New York.

Schulman, J.L., Kaspar, J.C., and Thorne, F.M. (1965). *Brain Damage and Behaviour. A Clinical Experiment Study,* C. Thomas, Springfield, Ill.

Schwartz, M.L., and Hawkins, R.P. (1970). 'Application of delayed reinforcement procedures to the behavior of an elementary school child'. *J. Applied Behavior Analysis,* **3,** 85–96.

Schwitzgebel, R.L. (1964). *Streetcorner Research,* Harvard Press, Cambridge.

Schwitzgebel, R.L., and Kolb, D.A. (1964). 'Inducing behavior change in adolescent delinquents'. *Behavior Research and Therapy,* **1,** 297–304.

Scott, P.D. (1966). 'The child, the family and the young offender'. *Brit. J. Criminology,* **6** (2), 105–111.

Sears, R.R., Rau, L., and Alpert, R. (1965). *Identification and Child Rearing,* Stanford University Press, Stanford.

Seligman, M.E.P. (1975) *Helplessness,* Freeman, San Francisco.

Senn, M.J.E. (1959). 'Conduct disorders'. In W.E. Nelson (Ed.), *Textbook of Pediatrics.* W.B. Saunders, Philadelphia.

Shah, S.A. (1971). 'A behavioral approach to outpatient treatment of offenders.' In H.C. Rickard (Ed.), *Behavioral Intervention in Human Problems,* Pergamon. New York. pp. 223–265.

Shapiro, D.A. (1975). 'Some implications of psychotherapy research for clinical psychology'. *Br. J. Medical Psychology,* **48,** 199–206.

Sheldon, B. (1982). *Behaviour Modification* Tavistock, London.

Shepherd, M., Oppenheim, B., and Mitchell, S. (1971). *Childhood Behaviour and Mental Health,* University of London Press.

Shirley, M. (1939). 'A behavior syndrome characterizing prematurely-born children'. *Child Development,* **10,** 115–128.

Simpson, D.D., and Nelson, A.E. (1974). 'Attention training through breathing control to modify hyperactivity'. *J. Learning Disabilities,* **7** (5), 274–283.

Skinner, B.F. (1953). *Science and Human Behavior,* Macmillan, New York.

Slater, E. (1939). 'Types, levels and irregularities of response to a nursery school situation'. *Monograph of the Society for Research in Child Development,* **4**(2), 207.

Sluckin, W., and Herbert, M. (Eds.) (1986) *Parental Behaviour,* Basil Blackwell, Oxford.

Sluckin, W., Herbert, M., and Sluckin, A. (1983). *Maternal Bonding,* Oxford: Blackwell.

Sloane, H.N., Johnston, M.K., and Bijou, S.W. (1967). 'Successive modification of aggressive behaviour and aggressive fantasy play by management of contingencies'. *J. Child Psychology and Psychiatry and Allied Disciplines,* **8,** 217–226.

Smith, M.B., and Hobbs, H. (1966). 'The community and the community mental health center'. *American Psychologist,* **21,** 499–509.

Snyder, J.J. and White, J.J. (1979). The use of cognitive self-instruction in the treatment of behaviorally disturbed adolescents. *Behavior Therapy,* **10,** 227–235.

Snyder, J.J. (1977). 'Reinforcement analysis of interaction in problem and non-problem families'. *Journal of Abnormal Psychology,* **86,** 528–535.

Solomon, R.W., and Wahler, R.G. (1973). 'Peer reinforcement control of classroom problem behavior'. *J. Applied Behavior Analysis,* **6,** 49–56.

Spence, S.H. and Marzillier, J.S. (1979). 'Social skills training with adolescent male offenders: 1. Short-term effects'. *Behaviour Research and Therapy,* **17,** 7–16.

Spivack, G., Platt, J.J., and Shure, M.B. (1976). *The Problem-Solving Approach to Adjustment.* Jossey-Bass, San Francisco.

Spivack, G., and Shure, M.B. (1973). *Social Adjustment of Young Children: Cognitive Approach to Solving Real Life Problems,* Jossey-Bass, San Francisco.

Sprague, R.L., and Sleator, E.E. (1973). 'Effects of pharmacological agents on learning disabilities'. *Pediatrics Clinic of North America,* **20,** 719–735.

340

Staub, E. (1975). *The Development of Prosocial Behaviour in Children*, General Learning Press, Morrison, N.J.

Stayton, D.J., Hogan, R., and Ainsworth, M. (1971). 'Infant obedience and maternal behaviour: the origin of socialization reconsidered'. *Child Development*, **42**, 1057–1069.

Stern, D. (1977). *The First Relationship: Infant and Mother*. Fontana/Open Books, London.

Stewart, M.A., de Blois, C.S., and Cummings, C. (1980). Psychiatric disorder in the parents of hyperactive boys and those with conduct disorder. *Journal of Child Psychology and Psychiatry*, **21**, 283–292.

Stewart, M.A., Pitts, F.N., Craig, A.G., et al. (1966). 'The hyperactive child syndrome'. *Am. J. Orthopsychiatry*, **36**, 861–867.

Stolz, S.B. (1976). 'Evaluation of therapeutic efficacy of behavior modification in a community setting'. *Behaviour Research and Therapy*, **14**, 479–481.

Stolz, S.B., Wienckowski, L.A., and Brown, B.S. (1975). 'Behavior modification: a perspective on critical issues'. *American Psychologist*, November **1975**, 1027.

Stuart, R.B. (1967). Behavioral control of overeating'. *Behaviour Research and Therapy*, **5**, 357–365.

Stuart, R.B. (1971a). 'Behavioral contracting within the families of delinquents'. *J. Behavior Therapy and Experimental Psychiatry*, **2**, 1–11.

Stuart, R.B. (1971b). 'Behavioral control of delinquency: critique of existing programs and recommendations for innovative programming'. In L.A. Hamerlynck and F.C. Clark (Eds.), *Behavior Modification for Exceptional Children and Youth*, University of Calgary Press, Calgary, Alberta, pp. 97–128.

Stuart, R.B. (1974). 'Behavior modification for the educational technologist'. In R. Ulrich, T.E. Stachnik and J. Mabry (Eds.), *Control of Human Behavior*, Vol. 3. Scott, Foresman, New York.

Stuart, R.B., Jayaratne, S., and Tripodi, T. (1976). 'Changing adolescent deviant behaviour through reprogramming the behaviour of parents and teachers: an experimental evaluation'. *Canadian J. Behavioural Science*, **8** (2), 132–144.

Stumphauzer, J.S. (1970). 'Behaviour modification with juvenile delinquents: a critical review'. *FCI Technical and Treatment Notes*, **1** (2), Federal Correctional Institution, Tallahassee, Florida.

Stumphauzer, J.S. (Ed.) (1973). *Behaviour Therapy with Delinquents*, Charles C. Thomas, Springfield, Ill.

Sulzbacher, S.I. (1975). 'The learning-disabled or hyperactive child: diagnosis and treatment', *J.A.M.A.*, **234**, 938–941.

Tavormina, J.B., (1974). 'Basic models of parent counselling: a critical review'. *Psychological Bulletin*, **81** (11), 827–835.

Tedeschi, J.T., Smith, R.B., and Brown, R.C. (1970). 'A reinterpretation of research on aggression'. *Psychological Bulletin*, **77**, 301.

Terrace, H.S. (1966). 'Stimulus control'. In W.K. Honig (Ed.), *Operant Behavior: Areas of Research and Application*, Appleton-Century-Crofts, New York. pp. 299–302,317–323.

Tharp, R.G., and Wetzel, R.J. (1969). *Behavior Modification in the Natural Environment*, Academic Press, New York.

Tharp, R.G., Wetzel, R.J., and Thorne, G. (1968). *Behavioural Research Report: Final Report*, Office of Juvenile Delinquency and Youth Development, Health, Education, and Welfare Grants, 65023 and 66020.

Thomas, D.R., Becker, W.C., and Armstrong, M. (1968). 'Production and elimination of disruptive classroom behavior by systematically varying teacher's behavior'. *J. Applied Behavior Analysis*, **1**, 35–45.

Thomas, A., and Chess, S. (1977). *Temperament and Development*, Brunner/Mazel, New York.

Thomas, A., Chess, S., and Birch, H.G. (1968). *Temperament and Behaviour Disorders in Children*, University of London Press, London.

Thoresen, C.E., and Mahoney, M.J. (1974). *Behavioral Self-control*, Holt, Rinehart and Winston, New York.

Thorne, G.L., Tharp, R.G., and Wetzel, R.J. (1967). 'Behavior modification techniques: new tools for probation officers'. *Federal Probation*, **31**, 21–27.

Tolman, C.W., and Mueller, M.R. (1964). 'Laboratory control of toe-sucking in a young rhesus monkey by two kinds of punishment'. *J. Experimental Analysis of Behaviour*, **1**, 323–325.

Truax, C.B. (1966). 'Reinforcement and non-reinforcement in Rogerian psychotherapy'. *J. Abnormal Psychology*, **71**, 1–9.

Truax, C.B., and Carkhuff, R.R. (1967). *Toward Effective Counselling and Psychotherapy*, Aldine, Chicago.

Tsoi, M. (1974). *Behaviour Modification in the Classroom Using Group Reinforcement Contingencies*. Unpublished M. Phil. Thesis. University of London.

Tutt, N. (1976). 'You and research'. *Social Work Today*, **7**(7), 198–199.

Tyerman, M.J. (1968). *Truancy*, University of London Press, London.

Turney, A. (1985). 'Treatment manuals'. In F. Watts (Ed.) *New Developments in Clinical Psychology*. British Psychological Society, Leicester (in association with Wiley, Chichester).

Ullmann, L.P. (1970). 'On cognitions and behavior therapy'. *Behavior Therapy*, **1970**, 201–204.

Ulrich, R.E. (1966). 'Pain as a cause of aggression'. *American Zoologist*, **6**, 643–662.

Ulrich, R.E., and Azrin, N.H. (1962). 'Reflexive fighting in response to aversive stimulation'. *J. Experimental Analysis of Behaviour*, **5**, 511–521.

Urbain, E.S., and Kendall, P.C. (1980). Review of social-cognitive problem-solving interventions with children. *Psychological Bulletin*, 1980, **88**(1), 109–143.

Varlaam, A. (1974). Educational attainment and behavior at school. *Greater London Intelligence Quarterly*, December 1974, pp.29–37.

Vitalo, R.L. (1970). 'Effects of facilitative interpersonal functioning in a conditioning paradigm'. *J. Counseling Psychology*, **17**, 141–144.

Wadsworth, M. (1979). *Roots of delinquency: Infancy, adolescence and crime*. Martin Robertson, Oxford.

Wahler, R.G. (1969a). 'Oppositional children: a quest for parental reinforcement control'. *J. Applied Behaviour Analysis*, **2**, 159–170.

Wahler, R.G. (1969b). 'Setting generality: some specific and general effects of child behavior'. *J. Applied Behavior Analysis*, **2**, 239–246.

Wahler, R.G. (1976). 'Deviant child behavior within the family'. In H. Leitenberg (Ed.), *Handbook of Behavior Modification and Therapy*, Prentice-Hall, Englewood Cliffs, NJ.

Wahler, R.G., and Erickson, M. (1969). 'Child behaviour therapy: a community programme in Appalachia'. *Behaviour Research and Therapy*, **7**(1), 71–78.

Wahler, R.G., and Fox, J.J. (1980). Solitary toy play and time out: A family treatment package for; children with aggressive and oppositional behavior'. *Journal of Applied Behavior Analysis*, **13**, 23–39.

Walder, L.O., Cohen, S.I., Breiter, D.E., Darton, P., Hirsch, I., and Liebowitz, J. (1969). 'Teaching behavioral principles to parents of disturbed children'. In B. Gurney, Jr. (Ed.), *Psychotherapeutic Agents: New Roles for Non-professionals, Parents and Teachers*, Holt, Rinehart and Winston, New York.

Walker, H.M., and Buckley, N.K. (1973). 'Teacher attention to appropriate and inappropriate classroom behavior: an individual case study'. *Focus on Exceptional Children*, **5**(3), 5–11.

Walker, H.M. and Buckley, N.K. (1974). *Token Reinforcement Techniques*. Engelmann-Becker, Eugene, Oregon.

Walker, H.M., Hops, H., and Fiegenbaum, E. (1976). 'Deviant classroom behavior as a function of combinations of social and token reinforcement and cost contingency'. *Behavior Therapy*, **7**, 76–88.

Walker, H.M., Mattson, R.H., and Buckley, N.K. (1971). 'The functional analysis of behavior within an experimental class setting'. In W.C. Becker (Ed.), *An Empirical Basis for Change in Education*. Science Research Associates, Chicago. pp. 236–263.

Walker, N.D. (1972). *Sentencing in a Rational Society*. Penguin Books, Harmondsworth.

Walker, R.N. (1962). 'Body build and behaviour in young children'. *Monographs of the Society for Research in Child Development*, **27**, No. 3 (Serial No. 84).

Walter, H.I., and Gilmore, S.K. (1973). 'Placebo versus social learning effects in parent training procedures designed to alter the behavior of aggressive boys'. *Behavior Therapy*, **4**, 361–377.

Walters, R.H., and Brown, M. (1963). 'Studies of reinforcement of aggression'. *Child Development*, **34**, 563–571.

Walters, R.H., Cheyne, J.A., and Banks, R.D. (Eds.) (1972). *Punishment*. Penguin Books, Harmondsworth.

Ward, J. (1971). 'Modification of deviant classroom behaviour'. *Brit. J. Educational Psychol.*, **41**, 304–313.

Watson, J.E., Singh, N., and Winton, A.S.W. (1985). 'Comparing interventions using the alternating treatment design' *Behaviour Change*, **2**, 13–20.

Weatherby, B., and Baumeister, A.A. (1981). 'Mental retardation' In S.M. Turner, K.S. Calhoun, and H.E. Adams (Eds.). *Handbook of Clinical Behaviour Therapy*. Wiley, New York.

Weathers, L., and Liberman, R. (1975). 'Contingency contracting with families of delinquent adolescents'. *Behaviour Therapy*, **6**, 212.

Weiss, G., Minde, K., Werry, J.S. Douglas, V., and Nemeth, E. (1971b). 'Studies on the hyperactive child: VIII. Five-year follow-up'. *Archives of General Psychiatry*, **24**, 409–414.

Weithorn, C.J. (1973). 'Hyperactivity and the cns: an etiological and diagnostic dilemma'. *J. Learning Disability*, **6**, 41–45.

Wells, K.C., Griest, D.L., and Forehand, R. (1980). 'The use of self-control package to enhance temporal generality of a parent training program.' *Behavior Research and Therapy*, **18**, 347–353

Welsh, R.S. (1968). 'The use of stimulus satiation in the elimination of juvenile fire-setting behaviour'. Paper read at Eastern Psychological Association, Washington, D.C. April.

Wender, P.H. (1971). *Minimal Brain Dysfunction in Children*, Wiley Interscience, New York.

Wender, P.H. (1973). *The Hyperactive Child: A Handbook for Parents*. Crown, New York.

Werry, J.S. (1968). 'Studies of the hyperactive child: IV. An empirical analysis of the minimal brain dysfunction syndrome'. *Archives of General Psychiatry*, **19**, 9–16.

Werry, J., Minde, K., Guzman, A., Weiss, G., Dogan, K. and Hoy, E. (1972) 'Studies on the hyperactive child: VII. Neurological status compared with neurotic and normal children'. *Am. J. Orthopsychiatry*, **42**, 441–451.

Werry, J.S., and Sprague, R.L. (1970). 'Hyperactivity'. In C.G. Costello (Ed.), *Symptoms of Psychopathology Handbook*, John Wiley, London.

Werry, J., Weiss, G., Douglas, V., and Martin, J. (1966). 'Studies on the hyperactive child: III. Effect of chlorpromazine on behavior and learning'. *J. of the American Academy of Child Psychiatry*, **5**, 292–312.

West, D.J. (1967). *The Young Offender*, Penguin, Harmondsworth.

West, D.J., and Farrington D.P. (1973). *Who Becomes Delinquent?*, Heinemann, London.

Wetzel, R. (1966). 'Use of behavioral techniques in a case of compulsive stealing'. *J. Consulting Psychology*, **30**, 367–374.

White, G.D., Nielsen, G., and Johnson, S.M. (1972). 'Timeout duration and the suppression of deviant behavior in children'. *J. Applied Behavior Analysis*, **5**, 111–120.

Wildman, R.W. II., and Wildman, R.W. (1975). 'The generalization of behavior modification procedures: a review — with special emphasis on classroom applications'. *Psychology in the Schools*, **12**, 432–448.

Williams, C.D. (1959). 'The elimination of tantrum behavior by extinction procedures'. *J. Abnormal and Social Psychology*, **59**, 269.

Wiltz, N.A. (1969). *Modification of Behaviour of Deviant Boys Through Parent Participation in a Group Technique*. Unpublished Ph.D. dissertation. College of Education, University of Oregon.

Wolf, M.M., Hanley, E.L., King, L.A., Lachowicz, J., and Giles, D.K. (1970). 'The timer-game: a variable interval contingency for the management of out-of-seat behavior'. *Exceptional Children*, **37**, 113–117.

Wolf, M.M., Phillips, E.L., and Fixsen, D.L. (1972). 'The teaching family: a new model for the treatment of child behaviour in the community'. In S.W. Bigod and E.L. Ribes-Inesta (Eds.), *Behaviour Modification*. Academic Press, New York.

Wolf, M.M., Phillips, E.L., & Fixsen, D.L. (1975). *Achievement Place Phase II: Final reort*. Lawrence: Department of Human Development, University of Kansas,

Wolf, M.M., Risley, T.R., and Mees, H. (1964). 'Application of operant conditioning procedures to the behavior problems of an autistic child'. *Behaviour Research and Therapy*, **1**, 305–312.

Wolff, S. (1971). Dimensions and clusters of symptoms in disturbed children. *British Journal of Psychiatry*, **118**, 421–427.

Wolff, S. (1977). Nondelinquent disturbances of conduct. In M.L. Rutter & L.A. Hersov (Eds.), *Child psychiatry: Modern approaches*. Blackwell Scientific, Oxford

Wolkind, S., and Rutter, M.L. (1973). Children who have been 'in care': An epidemiological study. *Journal of Child Psychology and Psychiatry*, **14**, 95–105.

Woolfolk, A.E., and Woolfolk, R.L. (1974). 'A contingency management technique for increasing student attention in a small group setting'. *J. School Psychology*, **12**, 3.

Wright, D.S. (1971). *The Psychology of Moral Behaviour*, Penguin Books. Harmondsworth.

Yarrow, L.J. (1968). 'The crucial nature of early experience'. In D.C. Glass (Ed.), *Environmental Influences*, Rockefeller University Press, New York.

Yarrow, M.R., Campbell, J.D., and Burton, R.V. (1968). *Child Rearing: An Inquiry into Research and Methods*, Jossey, Bass, San Francisco.

Yelloly, M. (1972). 'Chapter 5: The concept of insight'. In D. Jehu, P. Hardiker, M. Yelloly, and M. Shaw (Eds.), *Behaviour Modification in Social Work*, Wiley, London.

Yerkes, R.M., and Dodson, J.D. (1908). 'The relation of strength of stimulus to rapidity of habit formation'. *J. Comparative Neurology and Psychology*, **18**, 459–482.

Yule, W. (1979). 'Behavioural approaches to the treatment and prevention of school refusal' *Behavioural Analysis and Modification*, **3**, 55–68.

Zeilberger, J., Sampen, S.E., and Sloane, H.N. (1968). 'Modification of a child's problem behaviors in the home with the mother as therapist'. *J. Applied Behavior Analysis*, **1**, 47–53.

Zigler, E., and Child, I.L. (1969). 'Socialization'. In G. Lindzey and E. Aronson (Eds.), *Handbook of Social Psychology*, Vol. 3, Addison-Wesley, New York.

344

Zimmerman, E.H., and Zimmerman, J. (1962). 'The alteration of behavior in a special classroom situation'. *J. Experimented Analysis of Behavior,* **5,** 59, 60.

Zubin, J. (1967). 'Classification and the behaviour disorders'. In P.R. Farnsworth. O McNemar, and Q. McNemar (Eds.), *Annual Review of Psychology,* California Annual Reviews Inc., Palo Alto.

Subject Index

345